Towards a Public Health Wellness:
Psychosocial & Physical Health in
Community

# Towards a Public Health Wellness: Psychosocial & Physical Health in Community

Editors

**Won Ju Hwang**
**Mi Jeong Kim**

MDPI • Basel • Beijing • Wuhan • Barcelona • Belgrade • Manchester • Tokyo • Cluj • Tianjin

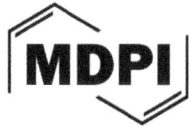

*Editors*
Won Ju Hwang
Kyung Hee University
Seoul
Korea

Mi Jeong Kim
Hanyang University
Seoul
Korea

*Editorial Office*
MDPI
St. Alban-Anlage 66
4052 Basel, Switzerland

This is a reprint of articles from the Special Issue published online in the open access journal *International Journal of Environmental Research and Public Health* (ISSN 1660-4601) (available at: https://www.mdpi.com/journal/ijerph/special_issues/Psychosocial_Physical).

For citation purposes, cite each article independently as indicated on the article page online and as indicated below:

LastName, A.A.; LastName, B.B.; LastName, C.C. Article Title. *Journal Name* **Year**, *Volume Number*, Page Range.

**ISBN 978-3-0365-5043-5 (Hbk)**
**ISBN 978-3-0365-5044-2 (PDF)**

© 2022 by the authors. Articles in this book are Open Access and distributed under the Creative Commons Attribution (CC BY) license, which allows users to download, copy and build upon published articles, as long as the author and publisher are properly credited, which ensures maximum dissemination and a wider impact of our publications.

The book as a whole is distributed by MDPI under the terms and conditions of the Creative Commons license CC BY-NC-ND.

# Contents

**About the Editors** . . . . . . . . . . . . . . . . . . . . . . . . . . . . . . . . . . . . . . . . . . . . . . . vii

**Won Ju Hwang, Ji Sun Ha and Mi Jeong Kim**
Research Trends on Mobile Mental Health Application for General Population: A Scoping Review
Reprinted from: *Int. J. Environ. Res. Public Health* **2021**, *18*, 2459, doi:10.3390/ijerph18052459 . . . 1

**Kees Blase, Eric Vermetten, Paul Lehrer and Richard Gevirtz**
Neurophysiological Approach by Self-Control of Your Stress-Related Autonomic Nervous System with Depression, Stress and Anxiety Patients
Reprinted from: *Int. J. Environ. Res. Public Health* **2021**, *18*, 3329, doi:10.3390/ijerph18073329 . . . 19

**Won Ju Hwang and Minjeong Kim**
Work-Related Stress, Health Status, and Status of Health Apps Use in Korean Adult Workers
Reprinted from: *Int. J. Environ. Res. Public Health* **2022**, *19*, 3197, doi:10.3390/ijerph19063197 . . . 33

**Mei-Chun Lu, Wei-Ching Fang, Wen-Cheng Li, Wei-Chung Yeh, Ying-Hua Shieh and Jau-Yuan Chen**
The Association between Insulin Resistance and Cardiovascular Disease Risk: A Community-Based Cross-Sectional Study among Taiwanese People Aged over 50 Years
Reprinted from: *Int. J. Environ. Res. Public Health* **2020**, *17*, 7195, doi:10.3390/ma17197195 . . . . 41

**Yu-Chung Tsao, Wen-Cheng Li, Wei-Chung Yeh, Steve Wen-Neng Ueng, Sherry Yueh-Hsia Chiu and Jau-Yuan Chen**
The Association between Metabolic Syndrome and Related Factors among the Community-Dwelling Indigenous Population in Taiwan
Reprinted from: *Int. J. Environ. Res. Public Health* **2020**, *17*, 8958, doi:10.3390/ma17238958 . . . . 53

**Hai-Hua Chuang, Rong-Ho Lin, Wen-Cheng Li, Wei-Chung Yeh, Yen-An Lin and Jau-Yuan Chen**
High-Sensitivity C-Reactive Protein Elevation Is Independently Associated with Subclinical Renal Impairment in the Middle-Aged and Elderly Population—A Community-Based Study in Northern Taiwan
Reprinted from: *Int. J. Environ. Res. Public Health* **2020**, *17*, 5878, doi:10.3390/ma17165878 . . . . 67

**Ivory H. Loh, Vanessa M. Oddo and Jennifer Otten**
Food Insecurity Is Associated with Depression among a Vulnerable Workforce: Early Care and Education Workers
Reprinted from: *Int. J. Environ. Res. Public Health* **2021**, *18*, 170, doi:10.3390/ijerph18010170 . . . 77

**Gun Ja Jang, Ginam Jang and Sangjin Ko**
Factors Influencing the Preventive Practice of International Students in South Korea against COVID-19 during the Pandemic
Reprinted from: *Int. J. Environ. Res. Public Health* **2021**, *18*, 2259, doi:10.3390/ijerph18052259 . . . 91

**Eun Jung Kim, Won Ju Hwang and Mi Jeong Kim**
Determinants of Perceived Accessibility of Maternity Leave and Childcare Leave in South Korea
Reprinted from: *Int. J. Environ. Res. Public Health* **2021**, *18*, 10286, doi:10.3390/ijerph181910286 . 101

**Lina Lee and Mary Lou Maher**
Factors Affecting the Initial Engagement of Older Adults in the Use of Interactive Technology
Reprinted from: *Int. J. Environ. Res. Public Health* **2021**, *18*, 2847, doi:10.3390/ijerph18062847 . . . 117

**Seonju Kam and Youngsun Yoo**
Patient Clothing as a Healing Environment: A Qualitative Interview Study
Reprinted from: *Int. J. Environ. Res. Public Health* **2021**, *18*, 5357, doi:10.3390/ijerph18105357 . . . **139**

**Mikyung Kim, Kyeonghee Kim and Eunjeong Kim**
Problems and Implications of Shelter Planning Focusing on Habitability: A Case Study of a Temporary Disaster Shelter after the Pohang Earthquake in South Korea
Reprinted from: *Int. J. Environ. Res. Public Health* **2021**, *18*, 2868, doi:10.3390/ijerph18062868 . . . **155**

**Eun Ji Lee and Sung Jun Park**
Toward the Biophilic Residential Regeneration for the Green New Deal
Reprinted from: *Int. J. Environ. Res. Public Health* **2021**, *18*, 2523, doi:10.3390/ijerph18052523 . . . **171**

**Matheus Oliveira de Jesus, Thatiane Lopes Valentim Di Paschoale Ostolin, Neli Leite Proença, Rodrigo Pereira da Silva and Victor Zuniga Dourado**
Self-Administered Six-Minute Walk Test Using a Free Smartphone App in Asymptomatic Adults: Reliability and Reproducibility
Reprinted from: *Int. J. Environ. Res. Public Health* **2022**, *19*, 1118, doi:10.3390/ijerph19031118 . . . **193**

# About the Editors

**Won Ju Hwang**

Dr. Won Ju Hwang is a professor of community health nursing at Kyung Hee University College of Nursing Science. She received her bachelor's degree and master's degree from Yonsei University and her Ph.D. in the Community Health Systems at University of California San Fancisco (UCSF), USA. Her primary scientific area is the development and evaluation of community health promotion and wellness on a basis of an ecological perspective for individuals, families, and populations who are at risk for vulnerable environments such as workers in small workplace. Her research features a series of cardiovascular epidemiological studies to identify socioeconomic, behavioral, and environmental factors associated with cardiovascular health outcomes. Furthermore, a series of randomized controlled trials to improve health behaviors, cardiovascular outcomes, and mental health in vulnerable population groups. Dr. Hwang has published numerous articles in professional journals and some books. She also edited special issues in international journals as a guest editor and has been on editorial boards in international journals.

**Mi Jeong Kim**

Mi Jeong Kim is a professor of the School of Architecture at Hanyang University in Korea. She received her bachelor's degree and master's degree from Yonsei University and her Ph.D. in the Key Centre of Design Computing and Cognition at the University of Sydney. She worked as a postdoc fellowship in the Department of Engineering Research Support Organization at UC Berkeley before joining Kyung Hee University. She was previously a visiting fellow at NYU, MIT, and Curtin University. She is an Editor-in-Chief of the Journal of the Korean Institute of Interior Design. Her current research interest includes convergence issues such as sensing architecture, human-computer interaction (HCI) for spatial design, virtual reality (VR) & augmented reality (AR), design education & strategies for creativity, health smart homes & smart communities, and cognitive studies related to design & environment. She has published over 100 journal papers and chapters of six international architectural books in the field. She edited special issues in international journals as a guest editor and has been on editorial boards in international journals.

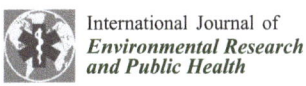 

*Review*

# Research Trends on Mobile Mental Health Application for General Population: A Scoping Review

**Won Ju Hwang [1,*], Ji Sun Ha [1,*] and Mi Jeong Kim [2]**

1. College of Nursing Science, Kyung Hee University, 26 Kyungheedae-ro, Dongdaemun-gu, Seoul 02447, Korea
2. School of Architecture, Hanyang University, 222 Wangsimni-ro, Seongdong-gu, Seoul 04763, Korea; mijeongkim@hanyang.ac.kr
* Correspondence: hwangwj@khu.ac.kr (W.J.H.); hajs@khu.ac.kr (J.S.H.)

**Abstract:** Background: Scoping reviews of the literature on the development and application of mental health apps based on theoretical suggestions are lacking. This study systematically examines studies on the effects and results of mental health mobile apps for the general adult population. Methods: Following PICOs (population, intervention, comparison, outcome, study design), a general form of scoping review was adopted. From January 2010 to December 2019, we selected the effects of mental health-related apps and intervention programs provided by mobile to the general adult population over the age of 18. Additionally, evaluation of methodological quality was assessed using the Scottish Intercollegiate Guidelines Network (SIGN) checklist. Results: Fourteen studies were analyzed of 1205 that were identified; duplicate and matching studies were excluded. One was a descriptive study and 13 were experimental, of which randomized control trials (RCTs) accounted for 71.4%. Four of the mobile apps were developed based on cognitive behavior theory, one based on stress theory, and one on ecological instant intervention theory. These apps included breathing training, meditation, and music therapy. Stress, depression, and anxiety decreased using these apps, and some were effective for well-being. Conclusion: With the rapid development of technology related to mental health, many mobile apps are developed, but apps based on theoretical knowledge and well-designed research are lacking. Further research and practices should be conducted to develop, test, and disseminate evidence-based mHealth for mental health promotion. RCT studies are needed to expand the application to mental health services to various populations.

**Keywords:** mobile mental health; mobile app; m-health; stress management; mental health app

## 1. Introduction

The demand to improve mental quality of life has increased along with the recent increase in interest in and awareness of mental health [1]. Consequently, the concept of mental health services emerged, along with an increased demand to manage mental health using information and communication technology (ICT) such as mobile communication and social network services (SNS) [2]. Mobile social media is a rapidly growing internet sector, in which, according to the Ministry of Science and ICT and the Ministry of the Interior and Safety, the number of smartphone users accounted for 94.0% of the total Korean population in 2017, with 86.8% of smartphone users using applications (apps). As such, the use of smartphones and apps have become a part of daily life. Recently, clinical use of mental health-related apps and intervention programs based on mobile apps have been implemented as an approach to managing mental health [3,4].

Mobile health (m-Health) is not yet well known in South Korea. The World Health Organization (WHO) defined mobile health (m-Health, mHealth) or mobile healthcare as medical and public health services provided through mobile devices including smartphones. In other words, mobile healthcare is the exchange of medical services between physicians and patients using IT and mobile devices, free from restrictions of time and space [5]. In that sense, the use of mobile apps for mental health management is expected to have various advantages [6]. In South Korea specifically, smartphone usage is approximately 90% and thus, interventions using readily available smartphones may grant excellent accessibility. It also offers economic advantages of reducing medical costs and can help overcome limitations of accessibility compared to the in-person cognitive behavioral therapy previously used for mental health management [7]. Furthermore, mobile apps enable user-friendly access through their various functions. According to FLURRY, a mobile app information analysis company, the use of health and fitness apps increased by more than 330% from 2014 to 2016 as smartphone usage became diversified—needless to say, apps have become an important tool in for pursuing a healthy lifestyle [8,9]. Mental health-related mobile apps are referred to as "Mental Health apps (MHapps)," and their types and numbers are diverse [10]. Nevertheless, mental health apps that have insufficient medical evidence or are for commercial use are common, and it is to be expected that such apps will continue to be developed and distributed in the future. Therefore, in order to efficiently manage the mental health of citizens, the development and distribution of apps with proven effectiveness and reliability are needed. Mental health specialists, in particular, should demonstrate leadership in studying, evaluating, and integrating such apps [3]. Nonetheless, there is a lack of scoping review identifying trends in research and evidence-based app development and application on topics such as the effects of mental health apps. Thus, this study aimed to perform a scoping review of previous research on the application of mental health apps on the general adult population and systematically analyze the content, methods, and effectiveness of the proposed intervention programs.

In this study, a scoping literature review was conducted on studies that examined the effectiveness of interventions that used mental health-related apps, using mobile devices such as smartphones or tablets, within the general adult population aged over 18 years, to outline the necessary implications for mental health practitioners and health promotion.

## 2. Methods

A scoping review of various databases was conducted, as outlined below, to identify intervention studies that used mental health apps for the general adult population over the age of 18, with the purpose of presenting directions and possible research questions for future research. It consists of six steps of identifying the research question, identifying relevant studies, study selection, charting the data, collecting, summarizing, and reporting results and recommendations [11,12].

### 2.1. Identifying the Research Question

The focus of this study is reflected in the following research questions: "What trends have intervention studies followed when using mental health-related apps for the general adult population?" and "What is the effectiveness of interventions that use mental-health related apps?"

### 2.2. Identifying Relevant Studies

A literature search was conducted by 2 independent researchers from 1 October 2019 to 30 December 2019 on mental health app-related intervention articles published in a journal between January 2010 to 2019. For data collection, Korean search engines (RISS (Research Information Sharing Service) and DBpia) and international search engines (MEDLINE, CINAHL, EMBASE, PsycINFO, Cochrane Library) were used. Google Scholar was used to manually search and verify the references of selected articles for inclusion of grey literature. Language was limited to English and Korean.

The keywords used for searches using international search engines were: m-health or "mobile health;" "mobile app*"/or mms*/or smartphone*/or "ipad" or "ipod" or "iphone*"/or "ipod*"; mental health* or "mental health treatment" and "program*" stress* depress* or depression or exp "depressive disorder, general * anxi*" or "social anxi*"/exp anxiety disorders, well-being or wellbeing, emotional labor or emotional labor, resilience or resiliency or resilient. The keywords used for searches using Korean search engines were: mobile app, mobile application mobile*, smartphone, mental health, mobile health. The search strategy combined keywords using the Boolean operators "AND" and "OR," and limited results to articles published in English or Korean. Furthermore, studies in which the subjects were not adults, studies in which subjects received psychiatric medication or treatment, studies without interventions using apps, studies without intervention outcomes, studies that did not provide original text, qualitative studies, review papers, and studies with irrelevant topics were excluded.

*2.3. Study Selection*
2.3.1. Study Population

This study selected articles that targeted the general adult population aged over 18 years, thus excluding nonadult subjects, neuropsychiatric drug users or those undergoing treatment, studies without app interventions, and studies without research outcomes. Studies that did not involve original research, qualitative studies, review articles, and studies not related to the research area were also excluded.

2.3.2. Interventions

The selected interventions were mental health apps that showed improvements through mobile use. This study was general in that all sorts of intervention methods that involved mobile use for the purpose of mental health promotion were selected.

2.3.3. Comparisons

Comparative interventions included all intervention studies in which a comparison was made to nonintervention groups, waiting lists, and groups that received conventional treatment.

2.3.4. Outcomes

The selected outcome was the effectiveness of the mental health app intervention, where studies that presented results of measurements using tools such as stress, depression, anxiety, and well-being were selected.

2.3.5. Study Design

The selected study designs were randomized controlled trials (RCTs), nonrandomized controlled trials (NRCT), and research studies; 28 articles were selected based on the data selection criteria. The initial search by inputted keywords in respective databases yielded the following results: in the Korean literature, 37 articles in RISS and 59 articles in DBpia; in the international literature, 85 articles in MEDLINE, 344 articles in CINAHL, 493 articles in EMBASE, 116 articles in PsycINFO, and 54 articles in Cochrane Library; a total of 1205 articles.

There were 258 articles that overlapped in the initial search, leaving 930 articles for review. Upon review of the titles and abstracts of the 930 articles, 28 articles met the selection criteria; 11 articles were selected upon further exclusion of studies based on app accessibility, studies that only presented preliminary research, study design, and case reports. Three articles were then added for inclusion of grey literature, based on a review of references used in major journals, consequently leading to a final selection of 14 articles for analysis (Figure 1). The literature search and selection process were independently reviewed by two researchers, and, in case of a disagreement, sufficient discussion on the reasons for article selection and exclusion was conducted.

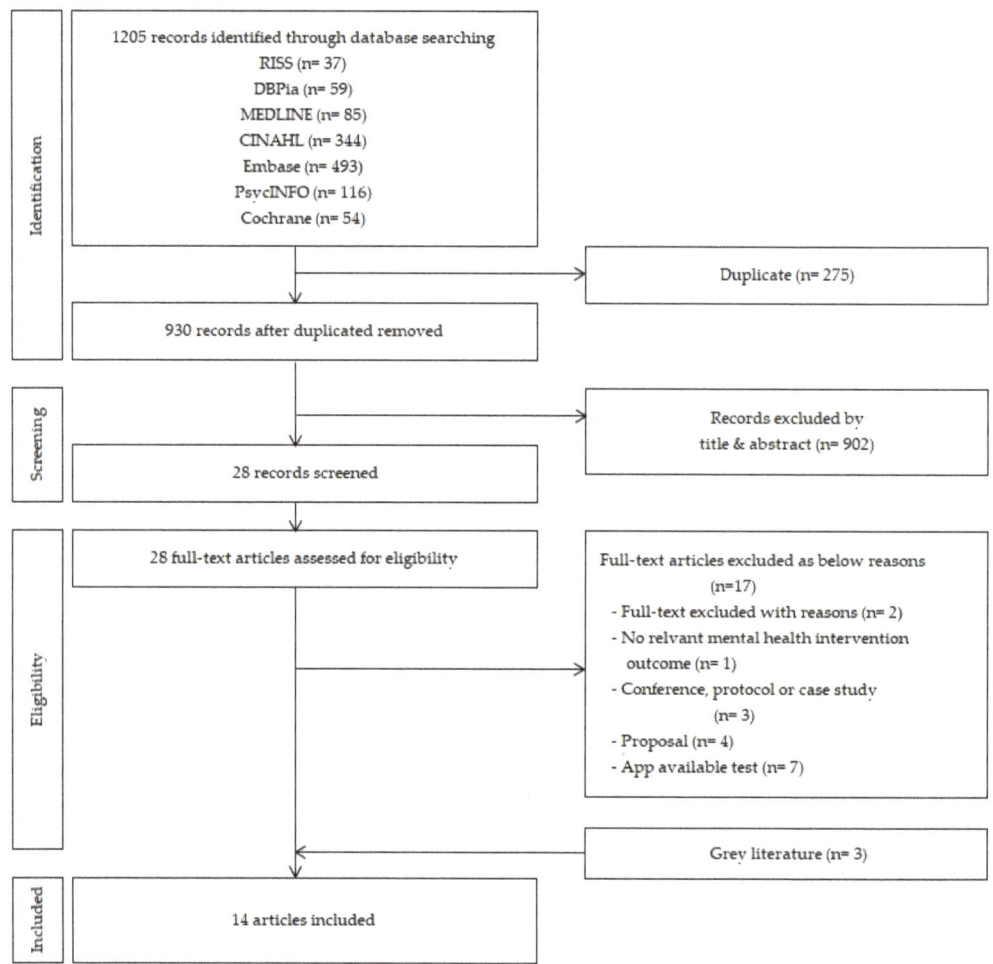

**Figure 1.** Flow diagram of the study selection processes for scoping review.

*2.4. Quality Evaluation of Selected Literature*

To evaluate the quality of the selected literature, a critical review was conducted using the Scottish Intercollegiate Guidelines Network (SIGN) Checklist, a methodological quality assessment tool [13]. The SIGN Checklist involves a comprehensive evaluation of methodological quality of a study, a general evaluation of quality based on potential bias, and combined approach evaluating the type of study design and its execution [14]. The SIGN Checklists are comprised of the following 10 sections: appropriate and clear questions; randomization; adequate concealment; blinding; similarity of treatment and control group; treatment differentiation; standard, validity, and reliability of measurement devices; dropout rate; intention to treat analysis (ITT); and confidence between results at all sites. The primary evaluation consisted of "Yes" or "No," "Cannot say," and "Not applicable" as according to the checklist, while the overall quality of the studies were ranked based on the number of sections that received a "Yes," for a final evaluation based on the following guidelines: studies with more than seven sections rated "Yes" were considered ++(high quality); studies with 5~6 'Yes's were +acceptable; studies with

2~4 'Yes's were –(low quality); and studies with less than one 'Yes' were unacceptable and therefore deleted. The quality evaluation process was independently conducted by two researchers; in case of a disagreement, the final decision was reached after consultation and sufficient discussion with a third researcher.

## 2.5. Charting the Data

Two researchers analyzed and encoded the 14 selected articles. The encoded data were analyzed by serial number, researcher(year), name of the app, application program and theoretical evidence, study design, variables, number of samples, intervention subject, intervention period, and results.

Two researchers independently analyzed the 14 studies selected before December 2019, followed by a cross-analysis to ensure the appropriateness and accuracy of the content of the primary analysis. If discussions on omissions, errors, or inconsistencies were deemed necessary, the analysis was conducted after an agreement was reached following enough discussion. If there was any conflict, it was consulted to another author.

## 3. Results

### 3.1. General Characteristics of the Literature

As there were articles analyzed up until 2013 [15], articles from studies conducted after 2010 were included in the search. The general characteristics of the final 14 articles selected to analyze the effectiveness of mental health apps in adults, are as shown in Table 1. There was one article published between 2010 and 2015 (7.1%) [16] and 13 articles published after 2016 (92.9%) [17–29], which made up most of the selected papers. The study designs of the selected articles were one research study (7.1%) [17], 10 RCTs (Randomized Controlled Trial) (71.4%) [16,19,20,22,24–29], and three NRCTs (Nonrandomized Controlled Trial) (21.4%) [17,20,22]. In terms of the intervention subjects, there were various types, with three studies on normal adults (21.4%) [17,24,25], three studies on symptomatic cases (21.4%) [18,19,21], two workers (14.3%) [16,22], two nurses (14.3%) [23,29], one soldier (7.1%) [26], and three students (21.4%) [20,27,28]. The duration of intervention varied from 2 to 24 weeks, with nine studies less than four weeks long (64.3%), three 8-week studies (21.4%) [20,21,26], one 12-week study (7.1%) [25], and one 24-week study (7.1%) [22]. Over 60% of the selected studies lasted for less than four weeks [16–19,23,24,27–29].

Table 1. General characteristics of selected 14 studies.

| Variables | Categories | N (%) |
|---|---|---|
| Publication Year | 2013~2015 | 1 (7.1) |
| | 2016~2019 | 13(92.9) |
| Research Designs | Randomized controlled trials | 10(71.4) |
| | Nonrandomized controlled trials | 3(21.4) |
| | Survey | 1 (7.1) |
| Intervention Group | The general adult population | 3(21.4) |
| | Psychological clients | 3(21.4) |
| | Employees | 2(14.3) |
| | Students | 3(21.4) |
| | Nurses | 2(14.3) |
| | Soldiers | 1 (7.1) |
| Intervention Duration | below 4 weeks | 9 (64.3) |
| | 8 weeks | 3 (21.4) |
| | 12 weeks | 1 (7.1) |
| | 24 weeks | 1 (7.1) |

### 3.2. Quality Evaluation of the Literature

Overall, the quality assessment of 13 of the selected articles, excluding one research study, yielded the following results: two studies [18,21] received a (-); one study [16] received a (+); and 10 studies [19,20,22–29] received a (++) (Table 2). The evaluation of the methodological quality of each of the selected studies indicated that all studies had adequately and clearly stated research questions [16–29]. Additionally, limitations in the quality assessment included issues regarding blinding and adequate concealment [19,26]), as well as cases in which a clear description of the survey procedure on app usage was not provided [16,29]. The dropout rate of study participants varied, from 0% [16,19,23,26] to 69.7% [25].

*3.3. Summary of the Literature*

One study [17] analyzed the effects of a mobile app (MoodPrism) through hierarchical regression analysis. MoodPrism is a self-monitoring app that examines the impact of subjects' emotional self-awareness on their mental health. A program involving 234 participants demonstrated an impact of 18%, 20%, and 37% on depression, anxiety, and mental well-being, respectively (Table 3).

*3.4. Experimental Research Using Mobile Apps*

In total, there were 13 intervention studies using mobile apps [16,18–29]. The purposes of such mobile app interventions varied, including stress management, reduction of anxiety, reduction in depression, increase in well-being, and provision of feedback on mental health apps. The intervention period also varied, ranging from 2 to 24 weeks in duration. More specifically, there was one 2-week study [18], one 3-week study [16], three 30-day studies [17,20,24,28], two 4-week studies [19,23,27,29], two 8-week studies [21,26], one 12-week study [25], and one 24-week study [22].

For studies in which the purpose of the intervention was to provide feedback on the application of mental health apps, the results were measured in several ways. The result variables from the measurements of the effectiveness of the mobile app are as follows— 13 articles on stress [16–18,20–29], nine articles on depression [17,18,21,24–29], 10 articles on anxiety [17–19,21,24–29], and five articles on well-being [17,20,24,27,29]. Furthermore, quality of life [19,20], self-efficacy [17,24,29], alcohol dependency [25], hyperventilation [19], sleep quality [27], work productivity [27], resilience [28], fatigue [23], mental health literacy [17,24], and emotional labor [29] were examined, and five articles [17,18,23,26,29] explored the accessibility and functional characteristics of the mobile applications (Table 3).

Table 2. Quality evaluation of the selected studies.

| Controlled Trial | Carissoli (2015) [16] | David (2018) [17] | Levin (2017) [18] | Pham (2016) [19] | Yang (2018) [20] | Mohr (2017) [21] | Ebert (2016) [22] | Wylde (2017) [23] | Bakker (2018) [24] | Arean (2016) [25] | Winslow (2016) [26] | Lee (2018) [27] | Flett (2019) [28] | Hwang (2019) [29] |
|---|---|---|---|---|---|---|---|---|---|---|---|---|---|---|
| 1.1 The study addresses an appropriate and clearly focused question. | Y | | Y | Y | Y | Y | Y | Y | Y | Y | Y | Y | Y | Y |
| 1.2 The assignment of subjects to treatment groups is randomized. | Y | | NA | Y | Y | Y | Y | Y | Y | Y | Y | Y | Y | Y |
| 1.3 An adequate concealment method is used. | CS | | NA | Y | Y | NA | Y | NA | Y | Y | N | Y | Y | CS |
| 1.4 The design keeps subjects and investigators 'blind' about treatment allocation. | CS | | NA | N | Y | NA | Y | NA | Y | Y | N | Y | Y | CS |
| 1.5 The treatment and control groups are similar at the start of the trial | Y | | * | Y | Y | NA | Y | Y | Y | Y | Y | Y | Y | Y |
| 1.6 The only difference between groups is the treatment under investigation. | Y | | NA | Y | Y | NA | Y | Y | Y | Y | Y | Y | Y | Y |
| 1.7 All relevant outcomes are measured in a standard, valid, and reliable way. | N | | Y | Y | Y | Y | Y | Y | Y | CS | Y | Y | Y | Y |
| 1.8 What percentage of the individuals or clusters recruited into each treatment arm of the study dropped out before the study was completed? | 0.0% | | 7.1% | 0.0% | 6.8% | 5.7% | 0.4% | 0.0% | 35.8% | 55.4% (4 weeks) 64.3% (8 weeks) 69.7% (12 weeks) | 0.0% | 20.9% | 1.0% | 6.7% |
| 1.9 All the subjects are analyzed in the groups to which they were randomly allocated (often referred to as intention to treat analysis). | Y | | Y | Y | Y | Y | Y | Y | Y | Y | Y | Y | Y | Y |

Table 2. Cont.

| | Carissoli (2015) [16] | David (2018) [17] | Levin (2017) [18] | Pham (2016) [19] | Yang (2018) [20] | Mohr (2017) [21] | Ebert (2016) [22] | Wylde (2017) [23] | Bakker (2018) [24] | Arean (2016) [25] | Winslow (2016) [26] | Lee (2018) [27] | Flett (2019) [28] | Hwang (2019) [29] |
|---|---|---|---|---|---|---|---|---|---|---|---|---|---|---|
| Controlled Trial | | | | | | | | | | | | | | |
| 1.10 Where the study is carried out at more than one site, results are comparable for all sites. | CS | | Y | | Y | Y | Y | Y | Y | Y | Y | Y | Y | Y |
| Overall assessment of the study. | + | | ++ | ++ | ++ | ++ | ++ | ++ | ++ | ++ | ++ | ++ | ++ | ++ |

Y = YES; N = No; CS = cannot say; NA = Not applied; * = intervention group.

Table 3. Characteristics and outcomes of selected 14 studies.

| | Author (Year) | Name | Program/Evidence | Research Design | Intervention Group (N) | Period | Measure Tools | Results (Significant *) |
|---|---|---|---|---|---|---|---|---|
| 1 | Carissoli et al. (2015) [16] | "it's time to relax!" | Mindful apps, MindApps, both released from iTunes | Randomized Controlled Trial | Italian workers (56) | 3 weeks | MSP, HR | Meditation group: improvement in coping with stress, reduction in hyperactivity and accelerated behaviors and heartbeats * Listened to music: improvement in coping with stress. Reduction in pain and physical problems and heartbeats * |
| 2 | Bakker and Rickard (2018) [17] | MoodPrism | MoodPrism | Survey | General adults (234) | 30 days | PHQ-9, GAD-7, WEMWBS ESAS-R, MHLQ CSES, SDS | Reduction in depression * Reduction in anxiety * Increase in mental well-being * |
| 3 | Levin et al. (2017) [18] | ACT Daily | ecological momentary intervention, acceptance and commitment therapy(ACT) | Nonrandomized Controlled Trial | Depressed/ anxious clients (14) | 2 weeks | DASS, AAQ-II CFQ, VQ PHLMS, SUS | Reduction in depression * Reduction in anxiety * Reduction in overall psychological inflexibility * Reduction in cognitive fusion * Reduction in obstacles * Reduction in acceptance * |

Table 3. Cont.

| | Author (Year) | Name | Program/Evidence | Research Design | Intervention Group (N) | Period | Measure Tools | Results (Significant *) |
|---|---|---|---|---|---|---|---|---|
| 4 | Pham, Khatib, Stansfeld, Fox, and Green (2016) [19] | Flowy | breathing exercises Diaphragmatic breathing | Randomized Controlled Pilot Trial | Adults with Common Mental Health Disorders (63) | 4 weeks | eHEALS, GAD-7, OASIS, ASI-3, PDSS-SR, QLES-Q-SF Nijmegen Questionnaire | Reduction in anxiety, panic, hyperventilation * Increase in quality of life * |
| 5 | Yang, Schamber, Meyer, and Gold (2018) [20] | Headspace | mindfulness | Randomized controlled trial | Medical students (88) | 60 days | PSS, FFMQ GWBS | Reduction in perceived stress * Increase in well-being and sustainment * |
| 6 | Mohr et al. (2017) [21] | IntelliCare | acceptance commitment therapy, cognitive-behavioral therapy, positive psychology Lazarus' transactional model | Nonrandomized Controlled Trial | Adults With depressive/anxiety symptoms (96) | 8 weeks | PHQ-9 GAD-7 | Reduction in depression * Reduction in anxiety * |
| 7 | Ebert et al. (2016) [22] | iSMI (internet-based stress management intervention) | problem-solving therapy, emotion regulation | Randomized controlled trial | Employees with stress symptoms (264) | 6 months | PSS-10 | Reduction (7 weeks) in stress and sustainment * |
| 8 | Morrison Wylde, Mahrer, Meyer, and Gold (2017) [23] | SDM (smartphone delivered mindfulness) | Cognitive Behavior Therapy | Nonrandomized Controlled Trial | Novice pediatric Nurse (95) | 4 weeks | CFST LEC PCL-C FFMQ | Reduction in burnout Increase in compassion satisfaction Increase in "acting with awareness" and "nonreactivity to inner experienc" * |

Table 3. Cont.

| | Author (Year) | Name | Program/Evidence | Research Design | Intervention Group (N) | Period | Measure Tools | Results (Significant *) |
|---|---|---|---|---|---|---|---|---|
| 9 | Bakker, Kazantzis, Rickwood, and Rickard (2018) [24] | MHapp - MoodKit, - MoodPrism, - MoodMission | Cognitive Behavior Therapy | Randomized controlled trial | General adults (226) | 30 days | PHQ-9, GAD-7 WEMWBS, ESAS-R, CSES MHLQ | Increase in mental well-being Increase in coping self-efficacy Reduction in depression (MoodKit and MoodMission group) * Improvement in anxiety * |
| 10 | Arean et al. (2016) [25] | EVO iPST Health Tips | EVO: Cognitive Control Therapy iPST: Problem-Solving Therapy Health Tips: Information Control | Randomized controlled trial | General adults with depressive symptoms (626) | 12 weeks | PHQ-9, SDS GAD-7, IMPACT AUDIT-C | No difference at weeks 4 and 8 for the project EVO yielded higher rates of recovery at 4 weeks compared with the Health Tips group * Similar recovery between the iPST and Health Tips arms |
| 11 | Winslow et al. (2016) [26] | mHealth | Cognitive behavioral therapy | Randomized Controlled Trial | US military veterans (16) | 8 weeks | SUDS, DASS PROMIS, TSST | Reduction in stress * Reduction in anxiety * Reduction in stress and depression (between time points) * |
| 12 | Lee and Jung (2018) [27] | DeStressify | Mindfulness | Randomized controlled trial | University students (163) | 4 Weeks | PSS, STAI QIDS-SR, MDD PSQI, RAND WPAI | Reduction in trait anxiety * Improvement in general health, energy, emotional well-being * |
| 13 | Flett, Hayne, Riordan, Thompson, and Conner (2019) [28] | Headspace Smile Mind | Mindfulness | Randomized controlled trial | University students (208) | 30 Days | CES-D HADS-A PSS, BRS FS, CAT CAMS-R | Improvement in depressive symptoms and resilience * |

**Table 3.** *Cont.*

| | Author (Year) | Name | Program/Evidence | Research Design | Intervention Group (N) | Period | Measure Tools | Results (Significant *) |
|---|---|---|---|---|---|---|---|---|
| 14 | Hwang and Jo (2019) [29] | Mind Healer | Meditation, sound, yoga, health information | Randomized controlled trial | nurses (56) | 4 Weeks | PSS-10, KOSS PHQ-9, GAD-10 | Reduction in perceived stress and occupational stress * Reduction in emotional labor * Increase in self-efficacy, well-being * |

* MSP: Measure du Stress Psychologique; HR: Heart Rate; PHQ-9: Patient Health Questionnaire-9; GAD-7: Generalized Anxiety Disorder 7-item scale; WEMWBS: Warwick-Edinburgh Mental Well-Being Scale; ESAS-R: Emotional Self-Awareness Scale- Revised; MHLQ: Mental Health Literacy Questionnaire; CSES: Coping Self-Efficacy Scale; SDS: Social Desirability Scale; DASS: Depression, Anxiety, and Stress Scale. AAQ-II: Acceptance and Action Questionnaire; CFQ: Cognitive Fusion Questionnaire; VQ: Valuing Questionnaire; PHLMS: Philadelphia Mindfulness; SUS: System Usability Scale; eHEALS.: eHealth Literacy Scale; OASIS: Overall Anxiety Severity and Impairment Scale; ASI-3: Anxiety Sensitivity Index-3; PDSS-SR: Panic Disorder Severity Scale-Self Report; QLES-Q-SF: Quality of Life Enjoyment and Satisfaction Questionnaire-Short Form; PSS: Perceived Stress Scale: FFMQ: Five-Facet Mindfulness Questionnaire; GWBS: General Well-Being Schedule.* CFST: Compassion Fatigue Self-Test; LEC: Life Events Checklist; PCL-C: Posttraumatic stress disorder Checklist-Civilian; FFMQ: Five Facet Mindfulness Questionnaire; WEMWBS: Warwick-Edinburgh Mental Well-Being Scale; ESAS-R: Emotional Self-Awareness Scale- Revised; CSES: Coping Self-Efficacy Scale; MHLQ: Mental Health Literacy Questionnaire; SUDS: Subjective Units of Distress Scale; DASS: Depression, Anxiety, and Stress Scale; PROMIS: Patient-Reported Outcomes Measurement Information Scale; TSST: Trier Social Stress Test; PHQ-9: Patient Health Questionnaire 9-Item; SDS: Sheehan Disability Scale; GAD-7: Generalized Anxiety Disorder 7-item scale; IMPACT: Improving Mood-Promoting Access to Collaborative Treatment; AUDIT-C: Alcohol Use Disorders Identification Test.* PSS: Perceived Stress Scale; QIDS-SR: Quick Inventory of Depressive Symptomatology Self-Report; MDD: Major depressive disorder; PSQI: Pittsburg Sleep Quality Index; WPAI: Work Productivity and Activity Impairment; CES-D: Ceter for Epidemiological Studies Depression Scale; HADS-A: Hospital Anxiety and Depression Scale-Anxiety Subscale; BRS: Brief Resilience Scale; FS: Flourishing Scale; CAT: College Adjustment Test: CAMS-R: Cognitive Affective Mindfulness Scale-Revised; KOSS: Korean Occupational Stress Scale.

*3.5. Mobile App Programs and Theoretical Evidence*

The mobile apps used in the studies were, "It's time to relax!" [16], "MoodPrism" [17], "ACT Daily" [18], "Flowy" [19], "Headspace" [20], "IntelliCare" [21], "internet-based stress management intervention (iSMI)" [22], "smartphone delivered mindfulness (SDM)" [23], "Mhapp (MoodKit, MoodPrism, MoodMission)" [24], "Cognitive Control App" [25], "mHealth" [26], "DeStressify" [27], "Headspace & Smiling Mind" [28], and "Mind Healer" [28]. Of the 14 articles, the most used apps were based on mindful meditation, used in five studies [16,20,23,27,28] (35.7%). Four studies used [23–26] cognitive behavioral therapy apps; one study [22] used a complex program involving problem-solving, relaxation, and acceptance tolerance therapy based on stress theory; one study [18] used an acceptance tolerance therapy app based on ecological momentary intervention (EMI); and another study [29] used a complex program involving meditation, yoga, and sound. There were two studies in which theoretical evidence was not provided, each using a breathing exercise app [19] and a mood-monitoring app [17].

- "It's time to relax!" [16] is a stress management program developed by an Android smartphone app. Based on a mindfulness protocol, the app was designed so that users could follow instructions and practice meditation for free.
- "MoodPrism" [17] is an app developed to monitor and provide feedback on the user's emotional state by converting the daily mood report to incorporate health aspects. The app also provides links on mental health information and resources.
- "ACT Daily" [18] is an EMI app designed to support the improvement and generalization of ACT (Acceptance and Commitment Therapy) technology, on which the users self-report emotions such as depression, anger, violent thoughts, and feelings of being trapped, and rate them on a Likert scale. Information is then provided on ways to alleviate such emotions.
- "Flowy" [19] is an app developed as a set of breathing-retraining exercises to manage anxiety, and uses simulations such as games to enable the user to subconsciously utilize breathing techniques.
- "Headspace" [20] and "smartphone delivered mindfulness (SDM)" [23] are based on mindful meditation techniques designed to encourage users to meditate for a few minutes each day to reduce stress, and provides information for a good night's sleep.
- "IntelliCare" [21] is an app developed with the purpose of reducing depression or anxiety caused by sleep disorders, social isolation, or lack of physical activity, based on acceptance and commitment, conscious behavior, optimism, and problem-solving techniques.
- "iSMI (Internet-based stress management intervention)" [22] is an internet-based stress management program aimed to reduce stress, comprised of eight modules using problem-solving, relaxation, and acceptance tolerance therapy. Through adherence monitoring by an E-coach and presenting feedback pertaining to the user's needs, an opportunity for the user to develop self-guided health promotion and behavioral change is provided.
- "Mhapp (MoodKit, MoodPrism, MoodMission)" [24] is a study involving the use of 3 apps—"MoodKit" and "MoodMission" are apps designed to manage depression, anxiety, and stress based on cognitive behavioral therapy. Upon analyzing mood, activity, values, and sentiment, it provides individualized goals that the user can choose and work towards.
- "Cognitive Control App" [25] is an app designed for the user to actively self-regulate behavior through choosing appropriate activities and refusing activities deemed inappropriate. It uses Cognitive Control Therapy (EVO), Problem-Solving Therapy App (iPST), Information Control (Health Tips) apps to facilitate both problem-solving abilities and provision of health information.
- "mHhealth" [26] is a mobile app with a combination approach involving wearables and cognitive behavioral therapy to reduce stress, depression, anxiety, and rage, developed to compensate for limitations observed in traditional approaches involving

only cognitive behavioral therapy, such as dropout and loss, as well as the shortage of objective data between user experience and cognitive behavioral therapy sessions. Additionally, it provides objective data for the users and providers by identifying the user's condition through cardiovascular and electrodermal input from wearable devices, enabling the detection of psychological stress.

- "DeStressify" [27] is a commercially available meditation app that provides guided meditation through audio, video, and text files. There are free and pro versions of the app, both of which are organized into visualization, gratitude, imagining one's ideal life, and finding purpose. In the pro version, additional functions including the options "my friends," "nutrition," and "shop" are offered. Such functions are intended to manage symptoms of stress, anxiety, and depression.
- "Headspace & Smiling Mind" [28] is a preregistered meditation app with over 100,000 downloads on the Google play app with high-quality mobile ratings. 'Headspace' is designed for users to download the app and complete a basic 10-day training session on mindful breathing, body scan (systematically focusing on certain parts of the body), practice of nonjudgement of thoughts and emotions, and sitting meditation, then access other meditation tracks for the following 30 days using a prepaid voucher. "Smiling Mind" is a smartphone app developed by a psychologist and an educator that provides a variety of meditation programs for a diverse audience in different age groups. The adult program is designed for everyday use for 10 days, followed by continuous use for another 30 days to manage mental health using "Smiling Mind." If the content is deemed insufficient, the user can select contents of their choice.
- "Mind Healer" [29] is an app developed for workers and the general adult population to manage stress and involves a psychological test and a PPG sensor that measures heart rate, enabling users to measure their mental health status, thus increasing workers' self-awareness. Additionally, if stress, anxiety, or depression is detected, a short-term healing program is offered, providing breathing, meditation, music, and yoga practices for healing and management of mental health. By also providing materials for mental health education, the app enables users to promote mental health by themselves.

### 3.6. Effectiveness of Mental Health Interventions using Mobile Apps

The analysis of the 14 articles demonstrated that mobile mental health promotion apps were indeed effective in improving mental health. More specifically, mindful meditation apps [16,20] commonly demonstrated a significant reduction in stress, and when 56 Italian workers were subject to performing meditation for three weeks, significant reductions were observed in hyperactivity and accelerated behaviors in addition to stress [16]. Meanwhile, a 30-day trial of mindful meditation in 88 medical students also demonstrated a significant reduction in stress and increased well-being, displaying lasting effects of mindful meditation [20]. In a study involving a 4-week trial of mindful meditation in university students, a significant reduction in trait-anxiety and significant improvements in general health, energy, and emotional wellbeing were observed [27]. The use of an intervention app based on the stress model by 264 workers demonstrated a significant reduction in stress after seven weeks of use, which was maintained in follow-up observations from seven weeks to six months of use [22]. Furthermore, in a study involving the distribution of 626 normal adults into three groups, each using a Cognitive Control Therapy app, a Problem-solving Therapy app, and an Information Control app, no significant differences were observed between weeks 4 and 8, but a higher recovery rate was observed in the group using the Cognitive Control Therapy app at four weeks compared to the group using a health information app [25]. When adults with mental health disorders were subject to using apps that provided a 4-week training program on breathing, a significant improvement in quality of life was reported, along with reductions in anxiety, panic, and hyperventilation, though the observed differences were not significant [19]. In the case of the study on the IntelliCare app [21], in which interventions on commitment to acceptance, cognitive behavioral therapy, and positive psychology were provided to 96 adults, significant reductions were observed in both depression and anxiety. A 2-week intervention using an app providing EMI-based Acceptance and Commitment Therapy in 14 depressed and anxious patients demonstrated significant reductions in anxiety, psychological inflexibility, cognitive fusion, obstacle, and acceptance [18]. A study involving an 8-week provision of cognitive behavioral therapy through an app to 35 American soldiers demonstrated significant reductions in stress, anxiety, and depression [26], and when cognitive behavioral therapy was provided to 226 normal adults through an app, improvements in emotional well-being and self-efficacy in coping were observed, along with reduced anxiety. In the Moodkit and Moodmission groups, especially, significant reductions in depression were reported [24]. When cognitive control therapy was provided to normal adults with depressive symptoms for 12 weeks, significantly higher rates of recovery were observed after four weeks, compared to the control group [25]. When cognitive behavioral therapy was provided to 95 newly appointed pediatric nurses for 4 weeks, significant increases were observed in acting with awareness and nonreactivity to inner experience, along with reduced in burnout and increased compassion satisfaction. Additionally, in a 4-week trial of the Mind Healer app in workers, significant reductions were observed in stress and emotional labor, while significant improvements were observed in well-being and self-efficacy following app use [29].

## 4. Discussion

Given the recent emergence of mobile apps as a tool for mental health intervention, this study presents a scoping review of intervention studies that used mental health-related apps for the general adult population over 18 years, to present directions for future research.

The study identified intervention methods and their effectiveness, as well as implications for the further development and application of intervention programs for improving mental health in the general adult population, by analyzing intervention studies using mobile apps.

Mobile mental health application research has accelerated since 2016, which appears to be related to the rapid growth in the number of smartphone users [3,4]. Subsequently, the number of studies has increased as more people have access to mobile applications, and as the interest in and demand for mental health services has increased [1].

Experimental studies (92.8%) were the most used research design, of which well-designed RCTs accounted for 71.4%. On the contrary, in another systematic review of smartphone apps for treatment of mental disorders, it was found that RCTs are still a minority, at 15.8% [30]. In the future, a well-designed RCT study is needed to expand the application of mental health services to various populations and to present evidence for the effectiveness of these apps.

The participants in the reviewed studies were the general adult population, psychological clients, employees, students, nurses, and soldiers. Particularly, mobile mental health applications were applied as a primary preventive method for mental health management, not for patients diagnosed with mental illness but for the general population. In the future, studies that compare and analyze the trends of mobile application use and the primary preventive effects for general populations should be conducted.

Intervention studies on mobile apps involved the development of new apps as well as existing apps, depending on the purposes of the study. Approaches using wearables were also included to promote mental health. Nonetheless, real-life applications of such apps on the general adult population are currently limited, with most of the developed apps designed to target subjects who already have mental health problems or to support clinical treatments [29]. Additionally, screening apps designed to classify high-risk adult subjects in relation to stress, depression, and anxiety were being developed and operated [31]. It was demonstrated that various attempts on assessments and interventions using mobile apps were being made in a variety of aspects, with the majority targeting the general adult population [32]. As the stigma around psychological treatment is the biggest factor that hinders the mental health promotion, there is an urgent need for the use of mobile apps for the provision of intervention, education, and consultation services for mental health promotion in Korea [31]. Addressing mental health using mobile apps has the advantages of providing researchers with a database to make up-to-date observations and develop future interventions from, and providing users with a way to become self-aware of their current status and changes, considering most users must download and sign into the apps [33].

Although the duration of app use varied from two weeks to six months and the effectiveness of the apps were evaluated following the intervention in existing studies, there was a lack of research on the lasting effects of mobile app interventions. The analysis of the existing studies indicated a shortage of research on the prolonged use of the apps. Furthermore, Donker et al. [15] indicated that the rates of prolonged use of mHealth apps were low. Therefore, considering the sustainability aspect of the mental health promotion apps and the fact that rates of continuous use decrease with longer intervention periods, there is a need to identify ways that support the continuous use of the apps. As a response, there have been studies that have applied the information–motivation–behavioral skills model to mental health apps [31,34], which indicate that because motivation strengthens behavior [35], subjects who acquire both health information and motivation gain the capacity needed to continue to perform healthy behaviors, which brings about actual behavioral skills [36]. Therefore, it can be presumed that strategies involving active efforts to increase the effectiveness of interventions and sustainability will need to be inserted into the context of the app during development, provided through immediate motivation, or provided through continuous relevant feedback for emotional support in future mobile app applications [29]. On the other hand, it was difficult to compare the effectiveness of mobile apps as there were variables other than stress, depression, anxiety, and mental well-being measured to evaluate the effectiveness of the mobile app use and interventions, not to mention inconsistent results.

Recently, there has been a lot of meta-analysis of the effectiveness of mobile interventions in specific mental disorders and in health psychology [37–39]. Although meta-analysis was performed on the general population, the effects of mobile app intervention itself could not be confirmed because the effects of the interventions, mixed by mobile app and web-based interventions, were identified [40,41]. Meta-analysis of the effectiveness of mobile app intervention in the general population is still not enough. In the future, a meta-analysis on the effectiveness of mobile app interventions for the general population may be needed.

Upon analysis of the programs and theoretical evidence involved in mental health apps, it was evident that most mental health apps were developed based on therapy rather than a theoretical framework. There are more than 3000 mental health apps available for Android, Apple, and Microsoft [15,42]. In a recent review of the existing commercial mHealth apps for the most prevalent health conditions on the Global Burden of Disease list provided by the World Health Organization, it was concluded that the development of mHealth apps was driven by commercial and economic motives, rather than scientific motives, as observed by previous studies [43]. Therefore, there is a need for the development and distribution of mobile apps with evidence-based content [32], along with consumer education, to enable users to select reliable, effective high-quality apps [44].

Additionally, despite the large amount of mobile app development due to the rapid growth and development of mental health technology, there remain important issues and risks involving insufficient quality control [45]. As such, more research and processes for the development, testing, and distribution of evidence-based mHealth are needed to promote mental health effectively. Furthermore, there is a need for nationwide support in developing and distributing high-quality content for mental health management apps. Additional efforts are required to identify the best ways a mobile app can be used to address components [46] such as the development and application of methods to evaluate interactive mechanisms from physical measurements [47,48]. Mental health problems arise not only from congenital factors, but through a complex mechanism of various factors [49]. Thus, there is a need not only for customized apps that take the demands of the users into account, but also for mobile apps that enable the simultaneous management of physical and mental health alongside stress prevention [29,50].

Recently, there have not been many mental health intervention studies using mobile apps on the general adult population. Therefore, caution is required when generalizing and interpreting the results of this study. In the meantime, as the mobile app approaches and usage are increasing, mental health workers must continue to evaluate whether various apps are developed upon sound, scientific evidence [42,44,51] and whether the effectiveness of the interventions was examined using appropriate and reliable tools [32], and enforce reliability through further research [52]. Continuous management and attention may also be needed from the government to enable the use of efficient and effective mobile apps [53]. Additionally, efforts should be made to prevent health inequalities related to age, socioeconomic status, and health literacy by identifying and encouraging a wide range of smartphone and health app users [54]. The development and use of mobile apps taking such points into consideration will enable the effective and systematic management of adult mental health, and ultimately prevent and alleviate mental health problems.

This paper analyzed studies on apps used for mental health promotion in the general population to present a scoping review, which is a research methodology used to present future research directions to clinical practitioners and guide further studies. In addition, since the scoping review study does not perform quality assessments, there is a potential risk of methodological bias. To overcome methodological limitations, a quality assessment for practical studies was performed after selecting the literature.

This study included RCT, non-RCT, and descriptive studies for the literature review on the subject scope, and excluded theses and academic conference presentations, among other possible variants of presentational forms, because the analysis was focused on journal articles. Moreover, unpublished studies were not included in the analysis.

## 5. Conclusions

According to the results obtained in the study, there were a total of 14 studies pertaining to mobile healthcare service research done using mobile health promotion apps developed by mobile app providers on healthy adults to examine its effectiveness. The analysis of the literature demonstrated that mindful meditation was most applied in mental health intervention programs using mobile apps. Other intervention programs included cognitive behavioral therapy apps, complex programs made up of a variety of different components, and apps based on the stress model and breathing exercises. Mental health apps encouraged awareness of self and provided information pertaining to the user's current status, and were comprised of components such as music, meditation, breathwork, quotes, videos, nature sounds, and health information. Such apps reduced stress, anxiety, and depression and improved well-being, but faced challenges in that there were only a small number of intervention studies, making the generalization of the study findings difficult. They may be helpful in the development and application of mobile apps for adults in the future.

Based on the results, the following suggestions can be made. A meta-analysis should be conducted on the research studies on mobile apps to confirm the effectiveness of apps. Moreover, the validity of mobile apps for mental health promotion for the general population can be improved by the development and application of mobile apps that satisfy the needs of users through further research on user demand.

**Funding:** This research was supported by the Basic Science Research Program through the National Research Foundation of Korea (NRF) funded by the Ministry of Science ICT and Future Planning (No. 2017R1A2B4008496) and Korea Health Industry Development Institute (HI18C1317). The funding agencies had no role in the study design, the collection, analysis, or interpretation of data, the writing of the report, or the decision to submit the article for publication.

**Conflicts of Interest:** The authors declare that the research was conducted in the absence of any commercial or financial relationships that could be construed as a potential conflict of interest.

## References

1. Pricewaterhouse Coopers. Emerging mHealth: Paths for Growth. 2014. Available online: pwc.com/gx/en/healthcare/mhealth/assets/pwc-emerging-mhealth-full.pdf (accessed on 1 March 2021).
2. Commission, E. Green Paper on Mobile Health ('m-Health'). 2014. Available online: ec.europa.eu/digital-single-market/en/node/69759 (accessed on 2 March 2020).
3. East, M.L.; Havard, B.C. Mental Health Mobile Apps: From Infusion to Diffusion in the Mental Health Social System. *JMIR Ment. Health* **2015**, *2*, e10. [CrossRef] [PubMed]
4. Marley, J.; Farooq, S. Mobile telephone apps in mental health practice: Uses, opportunities and challenges. *BJPsych Bull.* **2015**, *39*, 288–290. [CrossRef]
5. Kay, M.; Santos, J.; Takane, M. mHealth: New horizons for health through mobile technologies. *World Health Organ.* **2011**, *64*, 66–71.
6. Chandrashekar, P. Do mental health mobile apps work: Evidence and recommendations for designing high-efficacy mental health mobile apps. *mHealth* **2018**, *4*, 6. [CrossRef]
7. Newman, M.G.; Szkodny, L.E.; Llera, S.J.; Przeworski, A. A review of technology-assisted self-help and minimal contact therapies for anxiety and depression: Is human contact necessary for therapeutic efficacy? *Clin. Psychol. Rev.* **2011**, *31*, 89–103. [CrossRef]
8. Khalaf, S. Health and Fitness Apps Finally Take Off, Fueled by Fitness Fanatics. 2014. Available online: http://www.flurry.com/blog/health-and-fitness-apps-finally-take-off-fueled/ (accessed on 1 January 2021).
9. Jang, J.S.; Cho, S.H. Mobile health (m-health) on mental health. *Korean J. Stress Res.* **2016**, *24*, 231–236. [CrossRef]
10. Bakker, D.; Kazantzis, N.; Rickwood, D.; Rickard, N. Mental Health Smartphone Apps: Review and Evidence-Based Recommendations for Future Developments. *JMIR Ment. Health* **2016**, *3*, e7. [CrossRef] [PubMed]
11. Seo, H.J.; Kim, S.Y. What is scoping review? The Korean association for health technology assessment. *J. Health Technol. Assess.* **2018**, *6*, 16–21.
12. Arksey, H.; O'Malley, L. Scoping studies: Towards a methodological framework. *Int. J. Soc. Res. Methodol.* **2005**, *8*, 19–32. [CrossRef]
13. Scottish Intercollegiate Guidelines Network, S. SIGN 50: A Guideline Developer's Handbook (Vol. SIGN Publication No. 50). Edinburgh: SIGN. Available online: http://www.sign.ac.uk (accessed on 1 December 2019).
14. Kim, K.; Kim, J.H.; Lim, K.-C.; Lee, K.-S.; Jeong, J.-S.; Choe, M.; Chae, Y.R. Quality assessment tools and reporting standards in nursing research. *J. Korean Biol. Nurs. Sci.* **2012**, *14*, 221–230. [CrossRef]
15. Donker, T.; Petrie, K.; Proudfoot, J.; Clarke, J.; Birch, M.R.; Christensen, H. Smartphones for Smarter Delivery of Mental Health Programs: A Systematic Review. *J. Med. Internet Res.* **2013**, *15*, e247. [CrossRef] [PubMed]
16. Carissoli, C.; Villani, D.; Riva, G. Does a meditation protocol supported by a mobile application help people reduce stress? Suggestions from a controlled pragmatic trial. *Cyberpsychol. Behav. Soc. Netw.* **2015**, *18*, 46–53. [CrossRef] [PubMed]
17. Bakker, D.; Rickard, N. Engagement in mobile phone app for self-monitoring of emotional wellbeing predicts changes in mental health: MoodPrism. *J. Affect. Disord.* **2018**, *227*, 432–442. [CrossRef] [PubMed]
18. Levin, M.E.; Haeger, J.; Pierce, B.; Cruz, R.A. Evaluating an Adjunctive Mobile App to Enhance Psychological Flexibility in Acceptance and Commitment Therapy. *Behav. Modif.* **2017**, *41*, 846–867. [CrossRef] [PubMed]
19. Pham, Q.; Khatib, Y.; Stansfeld, S.; Fox, S.; Green, T. Feasibility and Efficacy of an mHealth Game for Managing Anxiety: "Flowy" Randomized Controlled Pilot Trial and Design Evaluation. *Games Health J.* **2016**, *5*, 50–67. [CrossRef] [PubMed]
20. Yang, E.; Schamber, E.; Meyer, R.M.L.; Gold, J.I. Happier Healers: Randomized Controlled Trial of Mobile Mindfulness for Stress Management. *J. Altern. Complement. Med.* **2018**, *24*, 505–513. [CrossRef] [PubMed]
21. Mohr, D.C.; Tomasino, K.N.; Lattie, E.G.; Palac, H.L.; Kwasny, M.J.; Weingardt, K.; Schueller, S.M. IntelliCare: An Eclectic, Skills-Based App Suite for the Treatment of Depression and Anxiety. *J. Med Internet Res.* **2017**, *19*, e10. [CrossRef]
22. Ebert, D.D.; Lehr, D.; Heber, E.; Riper, H.; Cuijpers, P.; Berking, M. Internet- and mobile-based stress management for employees with adherence-focused guidance: Efficacy and mechanism of change. *Scand. J. Work Environ. Health* **2016**, *42*, 382–394. [CrossRef]
23. Morrison Wylde, C.; Mahrer, N.E.; Meyer, R.M.L.; Gold, J.I. Mindfulness for Novice Pediatric Nurses: Smartphone Application Versus Traditional Intervention. *J Pediatr. Nurs.* **2017**, *36*, 205–212. [CrossRef] [PubMed]
24. Bakker, D.; Kazantzis, N.; Rickwood, D.; Rickard, N. A randomized controlled trial of three smartphone apps for enhancing public mental health. *Behav. Res. Ther.* **2018**, *109*, 75–83. [CrossRef] [PubMed]
25. Arean, P.A.; Hallgren, K.A.; Jordan, J.T.; Gazzaley, A.; Atkins, D.C.; Heagerty, P.J.; Anguera, J.A. The use and effectiveness of mobile apps for depression: Results from a fully remote clinical trial. *J. Med. Internet Res.* **2016**, *18*, e330. [CrossRef]
26. Winslow, B.D.; Chadderdon, G.L.; Dechmerowski, S.J.; Jones, D.L.; Kalkstein, S.; Greene, J.L.; Gehrman, P. Development and Clinical Evaluation of an mHealth Application for Stress Management. *Front. Psychiatry* **2016**, *7*, 130. [CrossRef] [PubMed]
27. Lee, R.A.; Jung, M.E. Evaluation of an mHealth App (DeStressify) on university students' mental health: Pilot trial. *JMIR Ment. Health* **2018**, *5*, e2. [CrossRef]
28. Flett, J.A.; Hayne, H.; Riordan, B.C.; Thompson, L.M.; Conner, T.S. Mobile mindfulness meditation: A randomised controlled trial of the effect of two popular apps on mental health. *Mindfulness* **2019**, *10*, 863–876. [CrossRef]

29. Hwang, W.J.; Jo, H.H. Evaluation of the Effectiveness of Mobile App-Based Stress-Management Program: A Randomized Controlled Trial. *Int. J. Environ. Res. Public Health* **2019**, *16*, 4270. [CrossRef] [PubMed]
30. Miralles, I.; Granell, C.; Díaz-Sanahuja, L.; Van Woensel, W.; Bretón-López, J.; Mira, A.; Casteleyn, S. Smartphone apps for the treatment of mental disorders: Systematic review. *JMIR Mhealth Uhealth* **2020**, *8*, e14897. [CrossRef] [PubMed]
31. An, S.; Lee, H. Use of Mobile Mental Health Application for Mental Health Promotion: Based on the Information-Motivation-Behavioral Skills Model. *Asian Commun. Res.* **2018**, *62*, 167–194. [CrossRef]
32. Kanthawala, S.; Joo, E.; Kononova, A.; Peng, W.; Cotten, S. Folk theorizing the quality and credibility of health apps. *Mob. Media Commun.* **2019**, *7*, 175–194. [CrossRef]
33. Chung, B.Y.; Oh, E.H.; Song, S.J. Mobile Health for Breast Cancer Patients: A Systematic Review. *Asian Oncol. Nurs.* **2017**, *17*, 133–142. [CrossRef]
34. Anderson, K.; Burford, O.; Emmerton, L. Mobile Health Apps to Facilitate Self-Care: A Qualitative Study of User Experiences. *PLoS ONE* **2016**, *11*, e0156164. [CrossRef]
35. Fischer, E.H.; Farina, A. Attitudes toward seeking professional psychologial help: A shortened form and considerations for research. *J. Coll. Stud. Dev.* **1995**, *36*, 368–373.
36. Fisher, W.A.; Fisher, J.D.; Harman, J. The information-motivation-behavioral skills model: A general social psychological approach to understanding and promoting health behavior. *Soc. Psychol. Found. Health Illn.* **2003**, *22*, 82–106.
37. Linardon, J.; Cuijpers, P.; Carlbring, P.; Messer, M.; Fuller-Tyszkiewicz, M. The efficacy of app-supported smartphone interventions for mental health problems: A meta-analysis of randomized controlled trials. *World Psychiatry* **2019**, *18*, 325–336. [CrossRef] [PubMed]
38. Lecomte, T.; Potvin, S.; Corbière, M.; Guay, S.; Samson, C.; Cloutier, B.; Khazaal, Y. Mobile apps for mental health issues: Meta-review of meta-analyses. *JMIR mHealth uHealth* **2020**, *8*, e17458. [CrossRef] [PubMed]
39. Weisel, K.K.; Fuhrmann, L.M.; Berking, M.; Baumeister, H.; Cuijpers, P.; Ebert, D.D. Standalone smartphone apps for mental health—a systematic review and meta-analysis. *NPJ Digit. Med.* **2019**, *2*, 1–10. [CrossRef]
40. Deady, M.; Choi, I.; Calvo, R.A.; Glozier, N.; Christensen, H.; Harvey, S.B. eHealth interventions for the prevention of depression and anxiety in the general population: A systematic review and meta-analysis. *BMC Psychiatry* **2017**, *17*, 1–14. [CrossRef] [PubMed]
41. Stratton, E.; Lampit, A.; Choi, I.; Calvo, R.A.; Harvey, S.B.; Glozier, N. Effectiveness of eHealth interventions for reducing mental health conditions in employees: A systematic review and meta-analysis. *PLoS ONE* **2017**, *12*, e0189904. [CrossRef] [PubMed]
42. Kesiraju, L. Health and Fitness Apps Finally Take Off, Fueled by Fitness Fanatics. 2017. Available online: https://www.flurry.com/blog/post/165079311062/health-fitness-app-users-are-going-the-distance (accessed on 13 June 2020).
43. Martinez-Perez, B.; de la Torre-Diez, I.; Lopez-Coronado, M. Mobile Health Applications for the Most Prevalent Conditions by the World Health Organization: Review and Analysis. *J. Med. Internet Res.* **2013**, *15*, e120. [CrossRef] [PubMed]
44. Yasini, M.; Beranger, J.; Desmarais, P.; Perez, L.; Marchand, G. mHealth Quality: A Process to Seal the Qualified Mobile Health Apps. *Stud. Health Technol. Inform.* **2016**, *228*, 205–209. [PubMed]
45. Boulos, M.N.; Brewer, A.C.; Karimkhani, C.; Buller, D.B.; Dellavalle, R.P. Mobile medical and health apps: State of the art, concerns, regulatory control and certification. *Online J. Public Health Inform.* **2014**, *5*, 229. [CrossRef] [PubMed]
46. Loo Gee, B.; Griffiths, K.M.; Gulliver, A. Effectiveness of mobile technologies delivering Ecological Momentary Interventions for stress and anxiety: A systematic review. *J. Am. Med. Inform. Assoc.* **2016**, *23*, 221–229. [CrossRef]
47. Klasnja, P.; Pratt, W. Healthcare in the pocket: Mapping the space of mobile-phone health interventions. *J. Biomed. Inform.* **2012**, *45*, 184–198. [CrossRef] [PubMed]
48. Shoaib, M.; Bosch, S.; Incel, O.D.; Scholten, H.; Havinga, P.J. Fusion of smartphone motion sensors for physical activity recognition. *Sensor* **2014**, *14*, 10146–10176. [CrossRef] [PubMed]
49. Lee, S.-Y. Updates in management of occupational mental health problems in the clinical preactice. *J. Korean Neuropsychiatr. Assoc.* **2020**, *59*, 87. [CrossRef]
50. Larsen, M.E.; Huckvale, K.; Nicholas, J.; Torous, J.; Birrell, L.; Li, E.; Reda, B. Using science to sell apps: Evaluation of mental health app store quality claims. *NPJ Digit. Med.* **2019**, *2*, 1–6. [CrossRef] [PubMed]
51. Larsen, M.E.; Nicholas, J.; Christensen, H. A systematic assessment of smartphone tools for suicide prevention. *PLoS ONE* **2016**, *11*, e0152285. [CrossRef] [PubMed]
52. Firth, J.; Torous, J.; Nicholas, J.; Carney, R.; Rosenbaum, S.; Sarris, J. Can smartphone mental health interventions reduce symptoms of anxiety? A meta-analysis of randomized controlled trials. *J. Affect. Disord.* **2017**, *218*, 15–22. [CrossRef] [PubMed]
53. Coulon, S.M.; Monroe, C.M.; West, D.S. A Systematic, Multi-domain Review of Mobile Smartphone Apps for Evidence-Based Stress Management. *Am. J. Prev. Med.* **2016**, *51*, 95–105. [CrossRef] [PubMed]
54. Ernsting, C.; Dombrowski, S.U.; Oedekoven, M.; LO, J.; Kanzler, M.; Kuhlmey, A.; Gellert, P. Using smartphones and health apps to change and manage health behaviors: A population-based survey. *J. Med. Internet Res.* **2017**, *19*, e101. [CrossRef] [PubMed]

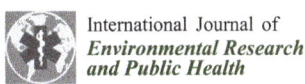

*Review*

# Neurophysiological Approach by Self-Control of Your Stress-Related Autonomic Nervous System with Depression, Stress and Anxiety Patients

**Kees Blase [1,\*], Eric Vermetten [2], Paul Lehrer [3] and Richard Gevirtz [4]**

1. National Centre Stress Management, Innovational and Educational Centre HartFocus, 1231 NC78 Loosdrecht, The Netherlands
2. Department Psychiatry, Leiden University Medical Center, 2333 ZA Leiden, The Netherlands; h.g.j.m.vermetten@lumc.nl
3. Rutgers Medical School, Rutgers University, Monmouth Junction, NJ 08852, USA; lehrer@rwjms.rutgers.edu
4. California School of Professional Psychology, Alliant International University, San Diego, CA 92131, USA; rgevirtz@alliant.edu
* Correspondence: k.blase@hartfocus.nl

**Abstract:** Background: Heart Rate Variability Biofeedback (HRVB) is a treatment in which patients learn self-regulation of a physiological dysregulated vagal nerve function. While the therapeutic approach of HRVB is promising for a variety of disorders, it has not yet been regularly offered in a mental health treatment setting. Aim: To provide a systematic review about the efficacy of HRV-Biofeedback in treatment of anxiety, depression, and stress related disorders. Method: Systematic review in PubMed and Web of Science in 2020 with terms HRV, biofeedback, Post-Traumatic Stress Disorder (PTSD), depression, panic disorder, and anxiety disorder. Selection, critical appraisal, and description of the Random Controlled Trials (RCT) studies. Combined with recent meta-analyses. Results: The search resulted in a total of 881 studies. After critical appraisal, nine RCTs have been selected as well as two other relevant studies. The RCTs with control groups treatment as usual, muscle relaxation training and a "placebo"-biofeedback instrument revealed significant clinical efficacy and better results compared with control conditions, mostly significant. In the depression studies average reduction at the Beck Depression Inventory (BDI) scale was 64% (HRVB plus Treatment as Usual (TAU) versus 25% (control group with TAU) and 30% reduction (HRVB) at the PSQ scale versus 7% (control group with TAU). In the PTSD studies average reduction at the BDI-scale was 53% (HRV plus TAU) versus 24% (control group with TAU) and 22% (HRVB) versus 10% (TAU) with the PTSD Checklist (PCL). In other systematic reviews significant effects have been shown for HRV-Biofeedback in treatment of asthma, coronary artery disease, sleeping disorders, postpartum depression and stress and anxiety. Conclusion: This systematic review shows significant improvement of the non-invasive HRVB training in stress related disorders like PTSD, depression, and panic disorder, in particular when combined with cognitive behavioral therapy or different TAU. Effects were visible after four weeks of training, but clinical practice in a longer daily self-treatment of eight weeks is more promising. More research to integrate HRVB in treatment of stress related disorders in psychiatry is warranted, as well as research focused on the neurophysiological mechanisms.

**Keywords:** self-control; HRV; HRV-Biofeedback; PTSD; depression; anxiety; sleeping disorder; stress; psychophysiology; neurophysiology; Vagal Tone; coronary artery disease

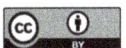

## 1. Introduction

Heart Rate Variability (HRV) is a neurobiological marker of the autonomic nervous system (ANS) with decreased HRV indices being associated with a variety of negative physical and psychological outcomes [1–5]. Heart Rate Variability Biofeedback (HRVB) is a non-invasive treatment, in which patients are assumed to self-regulate a physiological dysregulated vagal nerve function by restoring the autonomic homeostasis [6–8]. This is relevant for stress-related disorders such as sleep disorders, anxiety, asthma, fibromyalgia, recovery of heart failure, and others. In this time of COVID-19 more knowledge about self-control, Digital Health and a balance in the Autonomic Nervous System (ANS) is relevant.

HRVB affects cardiovascular homeostatic reflexes by increasing flexibility and recovery from fight or flight adaptive situations [9]. Thousands of studies have been published about HRV and HRVB. Most of the studies are focused on HRV as marker for instance as predictor of physical outcomes anxiety disorders and PTSD, cancer recovery [10–13]. HRVB has been characterized as making visible the neurophysiological effect of meditation [14]. Work-related stress develops gradually and effects both the physical and mental health of those experiencing it, which can eventually lead to burnout. Work related stress symptoms include insomnia, sleep disturbances, menstrual disorders, irritation, and depression [2]. HRV represents the ability to adapt to stress and is a marker of physiological stress [1]. Higher HRV amplitude indicates better self-regulation and is associated with lower cardiovascular risk and alleviating symptoms of stress, anxiety [15–17]. A recent meta-analysis affirms the efficacy of HRVB with wearable devices on self-reported stress [18].

In this study different HRV-Biofeedback devices are reported like StressEraser, Infinity HRV-Biofeedback and Balance Manager. In this study we will focus on HRV-Biofeedback studies as additional treatment in clinical practice.

In 1996, the Taskforce of the European Society of Cardiology and the North American Society of Pacing and Electrophysiology formulated definitions of the various HRV metrics [1]. These international standards: High Frequency(HF), Very Low Frequency(VLF), and Low Frequency(LF) are derived by spectral analysis of the interbeat interval (RR).

VLF (very low frequency = 0.003–0.04 Hz), when measured over long time frames, has been interpreted as reflecting sympathetic activity (Action); LF (low frequency = 0.04–0.15 Hz) reflects the combination of sympathetic and vagal balance (Balance), though recent studies have questioned this interpretation, and HF (high frequency = 0.15–0.4 Hz) is interpreted as reflecting vagal activity (Calm/sleepy) (see Figure 2).

We can describe this as ABC: Action, Balance, or Calm/Sleepy, where A indicates dominance of VLF (Action in the mind or body)

B indicates Balance between sympathetic and vagal activity or LF, and C indicates dominance of HF (Calm/sleepy) (see Figure 1).

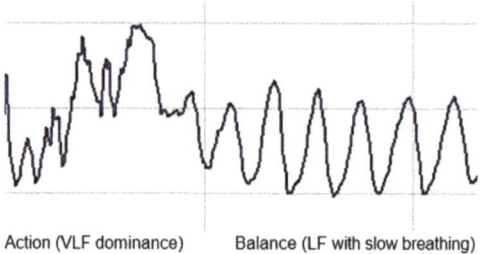

Action (VLF dominance)    Balance (LF with slow breathing)

**Figure 1.** HRV (Heart Rate Variability) patterns (tachogram).

Autonomic Balance is the marker of the state of the ANS. Unconscious perception of safety is reflected in higher HF values, while threat produces HF (vagal) withdrawal and sympathetic activation. Autonomic balance is defined in terms of complex heart rate (HR) patterns that increase and decrease in response to respiratory fluctuations (Figure 2).

| Oscillator | Frequency | Function | Process |
|---|---|---|---|
| Primary oscillator BREATH Respiratory Sinus Arrhythmia (RSA) | HF = High Frequency 0.15 Hz – 0.40 Hz | 'Vagal Brake': braking of sympathetic nerve facilitated by exhalation | 'Vagal Brake': exhalation is slowing down heart rhythm, inhalation is speeding up heart rhythm. |
| Secundary oscillator BLOODPRESSURE | LF = Low Frequency 0.04 Hz – 0.15 Hz | Baroreceptors send information to sinus node to bring homeostasis in blood pressure. | Alternately amplifying and contracting of aorta and carotids. Lowering bloodpressure activates baroreceptors sending a signal to speed up heart rhythm. |
| Tertiary oscillator VASCULAR RHYTHM | VLF = Very Low Frequency 0.003 Hz – 0.04 Hz | Activation of sympathetic nervous system (SNS) | Muscle activation and mental hyperactivity activate SNS |

Figure 2. HRV as composition of 3 oscillation processes [7]

However, when clients shift to slow effortless breathing patterns (as shown above), they stimulate reflexes in the Autonomous Nervous System (ANS) and Central Nervous system (CNS) that, over time, "rewire" these systems so as to enhance ANS flexibility. This formula, during slow effortless breathing, LF: (VLF+LF+HF) can be used as an index of the client's success in achieving their training goals. This formula is used in HRV-Biofeedback instruments Balance Manager and StressEraser Pro. After 20 years of research and clinical work, this formula was maybe more effective than LF:HF.

HRVB is a natural oscillation between the breathing cycle and heartrate. Inhalation temporarily suppresses vagal activity, causing a decrease in the inter-beat interval and an increase in heart rate; exhalation activates vagal activity, causing an increase in the inter-beat interval and a decrease in heart rate [19]. Heart rate is a dynamic function that varies in each moment. An HRV pattern (tachogram) is a composition of three oscillation processes: Respiratory Sinus Arrhythmia (RSA), baroreflex, and vascular rhythm [19].

Until 1996, HRV was primarily used as marker of the autonomic nervous system, but in 1996 Paul Lehrer (in collaboration with Evgeny Vaschillo) reported the observation that if you breath in the frequency of the baroreceptor and you slow down the tertiary oscillator (quietly not moving too much) than the ANS come into autonomic balance.

The body can be brought into the state of autonomic balance through guided breathing with HRV-Biofeedback. Breathing in the resonance frequency (between 0.05 and 0.15 Hz, which is the same as 4–7 breaths per minute) can be compared to guiding someone on a swing by pushing the swing at the correct moment to optimize their swing (resonance). Breathing at resonance frequency trains the reflexes of the cardiovascular system, in particular the baroreflex [19]. Breathing in the resonance frequency (resonance between respiratory and baroreflex rhythms) and using HRV-Biofeedback creates autonomic balance in the ANS and in this study we will show the effects of training Autonomic Balance with HRVB.

Long standing stress, PTSD and traumatic incidents can disturb stability of the Vagus nerve and create complex disturbances in heartbeat, HRV and hyperarousal, allowing overactivation in the Sympathetic Nervous System [6,20,21]. Our nervous system is continuously evaluating risk in the environment through an unconscious process of neuroception [22]. That is why it is innovative and important to integrate neurophysiological body-focused and self-regulating methods like HRVB in treatment of depression, trauma, and anxiety [23,24]. Reduced HRV amplitude has been found in patients with major depression disorder (MDD) [25]. HRV is a biological marker of the autonomic nervous system with decreased HRV indices being associated with MDD patients and probably being a biomarker of depression [26].

## 2. Method

In 2016, we published a systematic review and we now present an updated systematic review [7]. This review is based on searches in PubMed and Web of Science with an evidence-based critical review based on the GRADE method [27]. GRADE means Grades of Recommendation Assessment, Development and Evaluation. GRADE can be compared to the Prisma Statement with search terms: HRV (and synonyms) combined with PTSD, combat disorder, depression, depressed mood, anxiety, panic disorder (Figure 3).

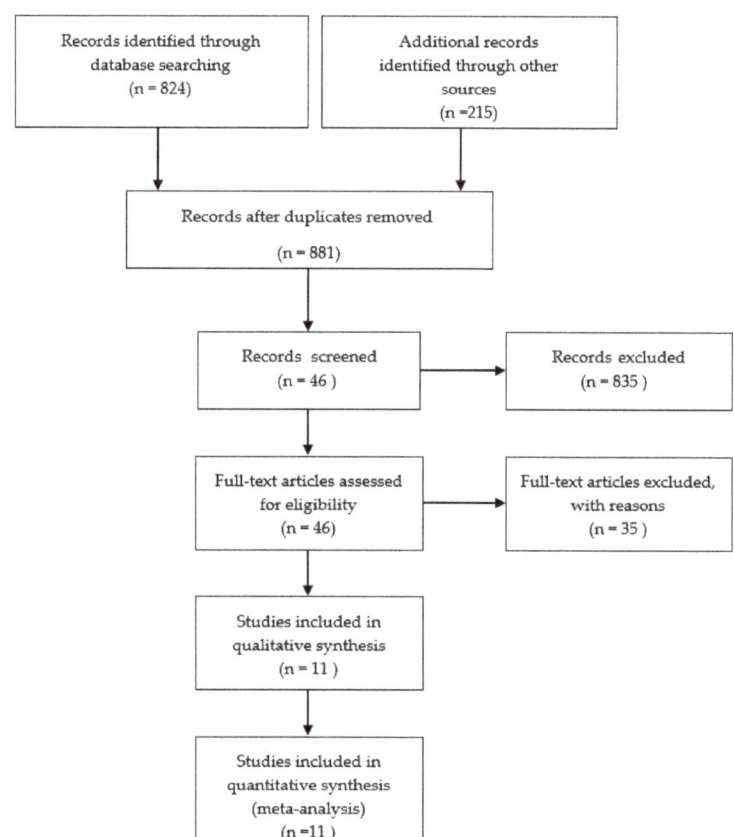

**Figure 3.** Flow diagram (for the selection of review articles).

Studies were screened by title and summary. This produced 881 articles. These articles have been judged by two raters with GRADE criteria, based on relevance (design, validation, setting, period, protocol, scale) and results (starting measures, result, significance, and missing data). The 46 selected articles have been screened again and the 11 selected studies are described in Table 1 in next chapter. Inclusion criteria were HRVB as clinical intervention of depression, PTSD and anxiety disorder with adults. Exclusion criteria: observational studies, anxiety studies with persons without disorders, children, other languages than English and German. Other meta-analyses of HRVB were added to find the evidence-based effects of HRVB treatment.

Table 1. The results of the selected studies.

| | RCT Studies HRVB for Treatment PTSD and Depression | | | | | | | | | | |
|---|---|---|---|---|---|---|---|---|---|---|---|
| | RELEVANCE | | | | | | | RESULTS | | | |
| Autor | Design | n | Domain | Setting | Period | Scale | Pre | Post | Reduction | | Signif. |
| | RCT/SGT | | | | | | Exp | Exp | Exp | Cont | Pre-Post |
| Zucker (2009)[28] | RCT HRVB vs. PMR | 38 | PTSD | 1e line | 4 weeks daily | PCL | 52.6 | 38.6 | 27% | 18% | p < 0.05 |
| | | | | | | BDI-II | 26.4 | 12.3 | 53% | 24% | p < 0.05 |
| Tan (2011) [29] | RCT HRVB vs. TAU | 20 | PTSD | Veteran hosp | 8 weeks daily | PCL-S | 64.8 | 54.4 | 16% | 2% | p < 0.05 |
| | | | | | | CAPS | 86.4 | 71.2 | 18% | 9% | p < 0.001 |
| Rene (2008) [30] | RCT HRVB vs. PMR | 46 | Depression | 1e line | 8 weeks daily | BDI-II | 35.0 | 7.8 | 78% | 44% | p < 0.005 |
| Chaudhri (2008) [31] | RCT HRVB+DBT vs sertraline | 60 | Depression | univ.hos | 12 weeks daily | BDI-II | 31.0 | 7.5 | 76% | 29% | p < 0.001 |
| | | | | | | DERS | 123.1 | 64.2 | 48% | 8% | p < 0.001 |
| Patron (2013) [32] | RCT HRVB vs. TAU | 26 | Depression after infarct | univ.hos | 2 weeks daily | CES-D | 15.3 | 8.9 | 42% | 1% | p = 0.02 |
| Van der Zwan (2019) [33] | RCT HRVB vs. waitinglist | 50 | Depression Anxiety Stress | University pregnant Women | 5 weeks daily | DASS | 5.45 | 2. | 49% | 35% | p = 0.039 |
| | | | | | | PSQI | 6.55 | 84.7 | 21% | 10% | p = 0.063 |
| Karavidas (2007) [34] | SGT | 11 | Depression | univ.hos | 10 weeks | BDI | 26.0 | 12.5 | 52% | - | p < 0.001 |
| Siepman (2008) [35] | HRVB vs. healthy | 38 | Depression | univ.h vs. stud | 4 weeks 3× a Week | BDI | 21.5 | 5.5 | 74% | - | p < 0.05 |
| Thode (2019) [36] | RCT HRVB vs. TAU | 37 | MDD | LatinoHealth center | 4 weeks | PHQ-9 | 16.42 | 10.85 | 40% | 7% | p < 0.05 |
| | | | | | | GAD-7 | 11.08 | 6.50 | 41% | 9% | p < 0.05 |
| Lin (2016)[37] | Case control study | 9 | MDD Depression | Heroin users | 5weeks 1× a week | BDI-II | 23 | 18.3 | 20% | - | p > 0.05 |
| | | | | | | BDI cogn | 19 | 14.3 | 25% | | |
| Lin (2019) [38] | RCT HRVB vs. med.care | 48 | MDD | 3 hospitals | 6 weeks | BDI-II | 24.25 | 15.04 | 38% | 1% | p = 0.007 |
| | | | | | | PSQI | 12.42 | 8.92 | 28% | 5% | p = 0.012 |

RCT: Randomized controlled trial; SGT: Single Group Trial; PMR = progressive muscle relaxation; DBT = dialectical behavioral therapy; PPD: postpartum depression; univ.hos = university hospital; BDI: Beck Depression Inventory; PCL: PTSD Check-List; CAPS: Clinical Administered PTSD Scale; CES-D: Centre Epidemiological Study-Depression; DERS: Difficulty in Emotion Regulation Scale; STAI: State-Trait Anxiety Inventory; PHQ-9: Patient Health Questionnaire; GAD-7: Generalized Anxiety Disorder.

## 3. Results

Most studies were single blind studies except for studies of Karavidas and Siepman [35,39]. Double blind study is not possible in biofeedback studies. Al studies had a high validity in presenting starting description and quality of outcome data.

*3.1. HRVB as Additional Treatment of Depression*

One of the first single blind RCT HRVB studies was focused on 46 female depressed welfare-to-work recipients in California. The HRVB-group ($n = 20$) and the control group treated by progressive muscle relaxation ($n = 26$) received antidepressant medicine [30,40].

The HRVB group showed significant reduction in the Beck Depression Inventory (BDI) score from 35.0 (SD 8.0) towards 17, (SD 12.6) in the first 4 weeks and after 8 weeks even towards 7.8. In the control group, reduction was smaller: from 30.1 (SD 10.2) towards 16.9 (SD 13.3) in 8 weeks. Reduction of 78% HRVB, versus 44% in the control group.

Another early RCT study with StressEraser focused on 60 patients after myocard infarct [31]. HRVB was integrated with dialectic behavioral therapy in conjunction with sertraline medication. The control group only used sertraline medication. The reduction on BDI scale was 76% after 12 weeks daily exercising 20 min with HRVB (BDI from 30.9 towards 7.5) versus 29% reduction in control group (BDI from 30.5 towards 22.0).

A third RCT as a bio behavioral intervention for depressive symptoms in patients after cardiac surgery was in Italy [32]. HRVB group and control group, TAU group, received both TAU that consisted of daily counseling sessions such as dietary and smoking cessation counseling, weight management, and stress-management according to the guidelines of the American Heart Association and the American Association of Cardiovascular and Pulmonary Rehabilitation. The HRVB group added 2 weeks of daily 45 min biofeedback. The significant reduction measured by CES-D (Centre Epidemiological Study-Depression) scale after 2 weeks was 42% compared with the control group's 1% reduction.

The psychophysiological mechanisms underlying depression as a risk factor for cardiovascular disease, cardiac morbidity, and fatal cardiac events after surgery are still debated. In the Netherlands, a scientific clinical consortium called Benefit is focusing on cardiac rehabilitation and prevention of cardiac diseases using lifestyle interventions and self-regulation programs such as non-smoking programs, personal lifestyle coaching, blended care with eHealth, HRV-Biofeedback, and mindfulness.

Another study in the Netherlands (University of Amsterdam), in cooperation with Paul Lehrer (USA), is a randomized controlled trial with 20 pregnant and 30 non-pregnant women, mean age 31.6 years [33,41]. The intervention consisted of a 5-week HRVB training with weekly 60–90 min sessions and daily exercises with StressEraser. Research has convincingly shown that high levels of maternal stress, anxiety, and depression during pregnancy are not only harmful for the women herself, but may also affect the child she is carrying. The control group was a wait-list group. The Depression Anxiety Stress Scale (DASS) and Pittsburg Sleep Quality Index (PSQI) were administered pre- and post-intervention. Effect sizes were larger in the HRVB group on all scales. The DASS depression scale women started with a score of 5.45 and after 5 weeks went down to 2.8 (reduction 49%). The wait-list reduction was 35%.

In total, two studies of the Kaohsiung Medical University in Taiwan were selected for review: HRVB with heroin users with depressive symptoms and patients with Major Depression Disorder [37,38]. The prevalence of major depressive episodes among heroin users has been found to be 25%. The nine participants had weekly sessions with HRVB software. They had a reduction of 20% on the BDI depression scale, and 25% on the BDI cognitive depression scale.

In 2019, at Kaohsiung Medical University, there was a RCT study with 48 participants with MDD depression and insomnia [38]. The HRVB group received weekly 60-min sessions for 6 weeks, and the control group received medical care only. The significant reduction at the BDI-II scale was 38 versus 1% in the control group. The significant reduction on the sleep disorder scale (PSQI) was 28% in the HRVB group and 5% in the control group. In 2019, at Alliant University in San Diego USA, a dissertation was presented with 37 participants with MDD and a Latino background [36]. There are different factors that appear to limit the access and quality of mental health care for Latinos, including lack of insurance, cultural barriers, stigma, distrust of medical providers, expression of distress, and fear of deportation. The HRVB participants received four HRV-Biofeedback sessions, were trained in diafragmatic breathing and finding their personal resonance frequency. They were provided with an app to be used as a pacer for daily exercising 10–20 min during 4 weeks in addition to sessions with their psychotherapist.

TAU participants completed four consecutive weeks of psychotherapy. Pre- and post-tests show 39.9% reduction in the Patient Health Questionnaire (PHQ-9): from 16.42 (SD2.93) towards 10.85 (SD6.81). With the TAU group reduction was 6.6% from 17.70 (SD 4.61) towards 16.52 (SD 6.57). In the Anxiety test (GAD-7) reduction was 41.3%: from 11.08 (SD3.40) towards 6.50 (SD3.37) versus TAU 8.8% reduction: from 15.36 (SD 4.41) towards 14.00 (SD4.56).

### 3.2. HRVB as Additional Treatment of PTSD

Although the connection between HRV and PTSD was already well-known the first RCT study of HRVB and PTSD was reported in 2009 [28,42–44]. In total, 76 participants were recruited from an urban residential therapeutic community program for the treatment of PTSD with comorbid substance use disorder. After randomization, 38 participants joined the 4 weeks daily program. The HRVB group trained 20 min daily with the StressEraser and the control group received daily 20 min Progressive Muscle Relaxation (PMR). The HRVB group had significantly ($p = 0.001$) greater reductions in depression scores compared to PMR (Progressive Muscle Relaxation) In HRVB group BDI-II reduced 53% (from 26.4 to 12.3) and 24% (from 25.95 to 19.47). On the scale, 29–63 = severe depression; 20–28 = moderate depression; 14–19 = mild depression; 0–13 = minimal depression. Reduction on PCL scale was 27% (HRVB) compared to 18% (PMR).

A second RCT study, with PTSD and HRVB, was focused on participants of US Department of Veteran Affairs—MEDVAMC [29]. In an 8 weeks program of weekly sessions with the Resonance Frequency protocol of Lehrer et al., veterans were trained in autonomic balance.

PCL score reduced significantly by 16% with HRVB while the TAU control group (only TAU) reduction after 8 weeks was 9% (not significant). Patients reported a satisfaction score of 8 (scale 1–10) and more than 50% wanted to continue using breathing in resonance frequency.

In 2014 a systematic review for psychiatric disorders with integration of treatment with HRVB was published [45]. In 2020, a systematic review and meta-analysis was published showing HRVB improves emotional and physical health, and performance [46]. Their initial review yielded 1868 papers from which 58 met inclusion criteria. HRVB has the largest effect sizes for depression (Hedge $g = -0.72$ and $p < 0.0005$), anger ($g = -0.54$ and $p < 0.02$), emotion regulation ($g = -0.34$ and $p < 0.0005$), asthma ($g = -1.357$), and athletic performance ($g = -90$), and smaller effect sizes on PTSD ($g = 0.29$) and quality of life ($g = 0.14$). The average effect size of the 58 studies for HRVB and paced breathing versus control conditions was found to be small to medium Hedge $g = 0.37$. High effect size $g = -0.8$ medium effect size: $g = -0.5$ and small effect size: $g = -0.2$.

In our study, we focalized on Depression, PTSD and Anxiety and with the GRADE method we got a smaller selection of 10 studies. Most of the selected studies showed a large effect size [46]: [28] PTSD study: $g = -0.739$ [29] PTSD study: $g = -0.296$ [30] Depression: $g = -0.748$ [32] Depression: $g = -0.958$

## 4. Discussion

In the first review of RCT studies of Heart Rate Variability Biofeedback the conclusion was: "a number of research studies have given at least tentative support for the effectiveness of HRVB for a wide range of medical and emotional disorders." [19].

Below you can see the summary, with addition of the RCT studies after 2014 (Table 2):

**Table 2.** Search HRVB RCT studies.

| Condition | n | p | Country |
|---|---|---|---|
| Asthma [47] | n = 64 | p < 0.003 | USA |
| Angina Pectoris [48] | n = 63 | p < 0.001 | Canada |
| Angina Pectoris [11] | n = 154 | sig | Taiwan |
| Anxiety [49] | n = 15 | sig | South Korea |
| Anxiety [50] | n = 40 | p < 0.05 | USA |
| Cancer [51] | n = 5 | p < 0.06 | Belgium |
| Chronic fatigue syndrome [52] | n = 28 | sig | Germany |
| Chronic Pain [53] | n = 20 | p < 0.001 | USA |
| Coronary artery disease [54] | n = 63 | p < 0.001 | USA |
| Coronary artery disease [55] | n = 210 | p = 0.001 | Taiwan |
| Depression (see Table 1) | n = 230 | sig | USA, Italy, Taiwan, Netherlands |
| Emotion regulation [56] | n = 58 | sig | Australia |
| Sleep apnea [57] | n = 853 | sig | Brazil |
| Sleep [58] | n = 69 | p = 0.001 | Japan |
| Selfcontrol Psychotic sympt [59] | n = 84 | p = 0.006 | Germany |
| Stress and anxiety [18] | n = 484 | Hedges g = 0.81 | USA |
| Stressreduction [60] | n = 23 | sig | Netherlands |
| Pediatric Irritable Bowel Syndr [61] | n = 24 | sig | USA |
| Postpartum depression [62] | n = 55 | p < 0.001 | Japan |
| PTSD (see Table 1) | n = 97 | p < 0.05 | USA |
| Trait Anxiety [49] | n = 15 | sig | South Korea |

While the first studies and RCTs were mostly done in USA, you can see the emergence of high quality studies from all over the world (Germany, the Netherlands, Belgium and the UK, South Korea, Taiwan, Japan, Brazil, and Australia).

In our manuscript the systematic review is focused on depression, PTSD, and anxiety. Effects were visible after 4 weeks of HRVB-training, but clinical practice in a longer daily self-treatment of 8 weeks showed more reduction on the BDI. Daily HRV-Biofeedback was more effective than weekly training, as we see in the studies of Rene and Chaudri with the StressEraser [31,40]. Perhaps three 8 min a day or two 10 min a day sessions are the most effective7.

Interestingly, in the systematic review it was stated: "an interesting implication of our findings is that length of treatment and home practice does not influence the effect size. Perhaps learning how to breathe at resonance frequency provides a sufficient method for most of the beneficial effects."(p. 125) [46].

The StressEraser, used in many of the HRVB studies was a noninvasive portable handheld device attempting to increase RSA using a respiratory training system. A highly sensitive infrared light sensor detects tiny changes in the rate at which blood pulses through the fingertip. The finger sensor has a photoplethysmograph to identify every pulse. The StressEraser (Figure 4a) was a very effective device, because the resonance frequency (resonance between heart rhythm and breathing rhythm) was automatically seen on the screen. StressEraser is not any more available since 2015. However, the StressEraser Pro (Figure 4b) has been developed for iPhone with more detailed information of HRV patterns:

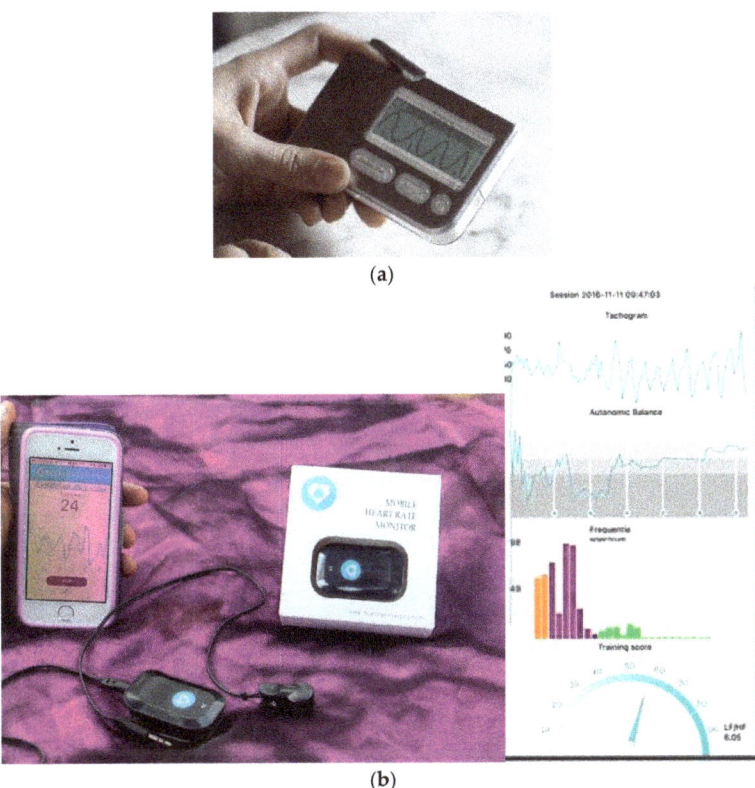

**Figure 4.** (**a**) StressEraser. (**b**) StressEraser Pro.

In this StressEraser Pro, you can read the tachogram, the frequency spectre with VLF (Orange), LF (purple), and HF (green) and the training effect score: LF/(VLF+ LF + HF).

For Samsung phones the HRV biofeedback device ResCalm (Figure 5) has been developed in South Korea with 10 playful wave patterns like hills, mountains, and motivating wave movements. Data definition is the same as the Balance Manager (Figure 6) for Windows computer.

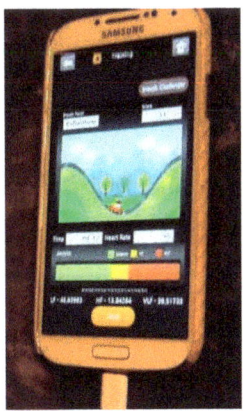

**Figure 5.** ResCalm.

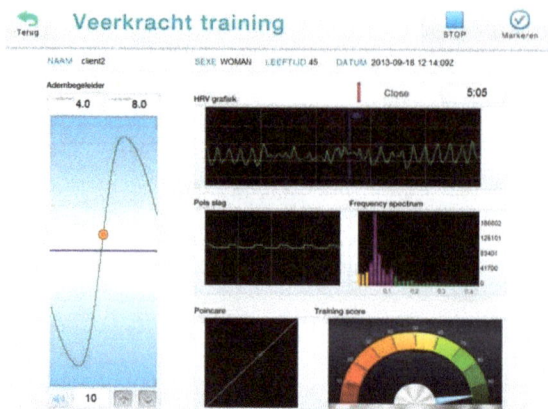

**Figure 6.** Balance Manager.

Additionally, in the Infinity HRV biofeedback devices (Figure 7), playful pictures are effective in the treatment.

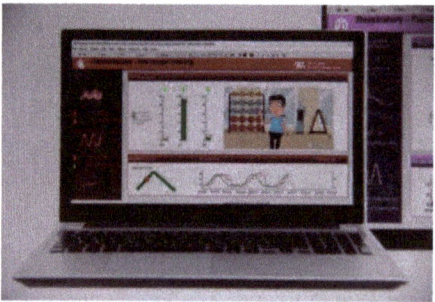

**Figure 7.** Infinity biofeedback.

All these devices were very effective, because users can install their personal frequency and their preferred rate of inhalation–exhalation. While searching for different systematic reviews, we also found a study that used HRV-Biofeedback devices that only used the frequency of 0.1 Hz [63]. That study did not show significant results compared with the devices where a client can install a personal breathing frequency like Balance Manager, StressEraser Pro, and Infinity.

In spite of the significance and efficacy of HRVB showed in this systematic review HRVB is not yet integrated into standard treatment. One of the most popular therapies is Acceptance and Commitment Therapy (ACT) [64]. In most trials ACT is reported to be superior or equally effective as cognitive behavioral therapy [65].Maybe it would be more efficient for our health system to integrate psychophysiology like ACT, HRV-Biofeedback and mindfulness in treatment of depression, PTSD, and anxiety disorders, because of the efficacy, more self-control of the client, and lowering the cost of treatment [66].

*Limitations*

The search strategy was bias-free but limited to articles published in English.

## 5. Conclusions

More than 4000 studies that investigated HRV, show the relevance of HRV in neuroscience related to a range of medical and emotional disorders and especially stress related disorders. Stress related disorders have a connection to a disturbance of the Autonomic Nervous System and a dysregulated Vagus nerve.

This systematic review shows significant improvement of the non-invasive HRVB training in stress related disorders like PTSD, depression and panic disorder, in particular when combined with cognitive behavioral therapy or other TAU.

After critical appraisal from the 881 studies about depression, PTSD and anxiety, eight RCT studies and two related studies have been selected. The RCTs with control groups treatment as usual combined with muscle relaxation training, and a "placebo"-biofeedback instrument revealed significant clinical efficacy and better results compared with control conditions, mostly significant ($p < 0.001$).

In the depression studies average reduction at the Beck Depression Inventory scale was 64% (HRVB plus TAU) versus 25% (control group with TAU) and 30% reduction (HRVB) at the PSQ scale versus 7% (control group with TAU).

In the PTSD studies average reduction at the BDI scale was 53% (HRVB plus TAU) versus 24% (control group with TAU) and 22% (HRVB) versus 10% (TAU) with the PCL scale. Even with studies with groups from 26 to 60 participants there is significance efficacy, so the effect size is very interesting.

In the different meta-analyses, significant effects have been shown of HRVB in treatment of asthma, angina pectoris, coronary artery disease, sleeping disorders, prevention of postpartum depression, and stress and anxiety.

More research on the integration of HRVB in the treatment of stress related disorders in psychiatry is warranted. In addition, research focused on the neurophysiological mechanisms will solidify the scientific basis of HRVB.

Nevertheless, because financial support for behavioral research has not reached the level necessary to test thousands of, meta-analysis may be the best alternative for evaluating these effects.

**Author Contributions:** Conceptualization, K.B., E.V. and R.G.; formal analysis, K.B. and E.V.; resources, K.B., P.L. and R.G.; writing—original draft preparation, K.B.; writing—review and editing, E.V., R.G. and P.L.; project administration, K.B.; All authors have read and agreed to the published version of the manuscript.

**Funding:** This research received no external funding.

**Institutional Review Board Statement:** Not applicable.

**Informed Consent Statement:** Not applicable.

**Conflicts of Interest:** The authors declare no conflict of interest.

# References

1. Taskforce of the European Society of Cardiology and the North American Society of Pacing and Electrophysiology. Heart Rate Variability, Standards of measurement, physiological interpretation and clinical use. *Eur. Heart J.* **1996**, *17*, 354–381. [CrossRef]
2. Lin, I.M.; Fan, S.Y.; Lu, H.C.; Lin, T.H.; Chu, C.S.; Kuo, H.F.; Lee, C.S.; Lu, Y.H. Randomized controlled trial of heart rate variability biofeedback in cardiac autonomic and hostility among patients with coronary artery disease. *Behav. Res. Ther.* **2015**, *70*, 38–46. [CrossRef]
3. Agelink, M.; Boz, C.; Ullrich, J. Relationship between major depressive disorder and heart rate variability. Clinical consequences and implications for antidepressive treatment. *Psychiatry Res.* **2002**, *113*, 139–149. [CrossRef]
4. Berntson, G.G.; Bigger, J.T.; Eckberg, D.L.; Grossman, P. HRV: Origins, methods and interpretive caveats. *J. Psychophysiol.* **1997**, *34*, 623–648. [CrossRef] [PubMed]
5. Gevirtz, R.; Lehrer, P. Resonance frequency heart rate feedback. In *Biofeedback, a Practitioner's Guide*, 3rd ed.; Schwartz, M.S., Andrasik, F., Eds.; Guilford: New York, NY, USA, 2003; pp. 245–264.
6. Porges, S.W. *The Polyvagal Theory; Neuropsychological Foundations of Emotions, Attachment, Communication and Selfregulation*; Norton: New York, NY, USA; London, UK, 2011.
7. Blase, K.; van Dijke, A.; Cluitmans, P.; Vermetten, E. Effectiviteit van hartritme variabiliteit biofeedback als aanvulling bij behandeling van depressie en posttraumatische stressstoornis. *Tijdschr. Voor Psychiatr.* **2016**, *4*, 293–300.
8. Gevirtz, R. Autonomic nervous system markers for psychophysiological, anxiety and physical disorders. *Integr. Neurosci. Pers. Med.* **2010**, 164–180.

9. Gevirtz, R. The promise of Heart Rate Variability Biofeedback: Evidence-based application. *Biofeedback* **2013**, *41*, 110–120. [CrossRef]
10. Sloan, R.; Shapiro, P.A.; Gorenstein, E.E.; Tager, F.A.; Monk, C.E.; McKinley, P.S.; Myers, M.M.; Bagiella, E.; Chen, I.; Steinman, R.; et al. Cardiac autonomic control and treatment of hostility: A randomized contolled trial. *Psychosom. Med.* **2010**, *72*, 1–8. [CrossRef]
11. Lin, S.L.; Huang, C.Y.; Shiu, S.P.; Yeh, S.H. Effects of yoga on stress, stress adaptation and Heart Rate Variability among mental health professionals. *Worldviews Evid. Based Nurs.* **2015**, *12*, 236–245. [CrossRef]
12. Chalmers, J.A.; Quintana, D.S.; Abbott, M.J.; Kemp, A.H. Anxiety disorders are associated with reduced heart rate variability. *Front. Psychiatry* **2014**, *5*, 80. [CrossRef]
13. Larkey, L.; Kim, W.; James, D. Mind-body and psychosocial interventions may similarly affect Heart Rate Variability patterns in cancer recovery. *Integr. Cancer Ther.* **2019**, *19*, 1–10.
14. Blase, K.; van Waning, A. Heart Rate Variability, cortisol and attention focus during Shamatha quiescence meditation. *Appl. Psychophysiol. Biofeedback* **2019**, *44*, 331–342. [CrossRef]
15. Kiviniemi, A.M.; Hautala, A.J.; Kinnunen, H.; Nissilä, J.; Virtanen, P.; Karjalainen, J.; Tulppo, M.P. Daily exercise prescription on the basis of HRV among men and women (Randomied Controlled Trial). *Med. Sci. Sports Exerc.* **2010**, *42*, 1355–1363. [CrossRef]
16. Prinsloo, G.; Derman, W.; Lambert, M.; Rauch, H. The effect of a single session of short duration biofeedback induced deep breathing on measures of HRV during laboratory induced cognitive stress. *Appl. Psychophysiol. Biofeedback* **2013**, *38*, 81–90. [CrossRef]
17. Lewis, G.; Hourani, L.; Tueller, S.; Weimer, B. Relaxation training assisted by HRVB: Implication for a military predeployment stress inoculation protocol. *Psychophysiology* **2015**, *52*, 1167–1174. [CrossRef]
18. Goessl, V.; Curtiss, J.; Hofmann, S. The effect of HRV biofeedback training on stress and anxiety: A meta-analysis. *Psychol. Med.* **2017**, *47*, 2578–2586. [CrossRef]
19. Lehrer, P.; Gevirtz, R. Heart Rate Variability biofeedback: How and why does it work? *Front. Psychol.* **2014**, *5*, 756. [CrossRef]
20. Carney, R.M.; Freedland, K.E.; Skala, E.A.; Jaffe, A.S. Change in heart rate and heart rate variability during treatment for depression in patients with coronary heart disease. *Psychosom Med.* **2000**, *62*, 639–647. [CrossRef] [PubMed]
21. Cohen, H.J.; Benjamin, J.; Matar, M.A.; Kaplan, Z. Autonomic dysregulation in panic disorder and in posttraumatic stress disorder: Application of power spectrum analysis of heart rate variability at rest and in response to recollection of trauma or attacks. *Psychiatry Res.* **2000**, *96*, 1–13. [CrossRef]
22. Porges, S.W.; Dana, D.A. *Clinical Applications of the Polyvagal Theory: The Emergence of Polyvagal-Informed Therapies*; Norton Series on Interpersonal Neurobiology; WW Norton & Company: New York, NY, USA, 2018.
23. Van der Kolk, B. *Clinical Implications of Neuroscience Research in PTSD. Psychobiology of Posttraumatic Stress Disorders*; Annals of the New York Academy of Sciences; Blackwell Publishing: Oxford, UK, 2006; Volume 1071, pp. 277–293.
24. Lanius, R.; Vermetten, E.; Pain, C. *The Hidden Epidemic; the Impact of Early Life Trauma on Health and Disease*; Cambridge University Press: Cambridge, UK, 2010.
25. Licht, C.; de Geus, E.; Zitman, F.; Hoogendijk, W.; van Dijck Penninx, B. Association between major depression disorder and HRV in the Netherlands Study of Depression and Anxiety (NESDA). *Arch. Gen. Psychiatry* **2008**, *65*, 1358–1367. [CrossRef] [PubMed]
26. Sgoifo, A.; Carnevali, I.; Alfonso, M.; Amore, M. Autonomic dysfunction and heart rate variability in depression. *Stress* **2015**, *18*, 343–352. [CrossRef]
27. GRADE Working Group. Grading quality of evidence and strength of recommandations. *BMJ* **2004**, *328*, 1490. [CrossRef]
28. Zucker, T.L.; Samuelson, K.W.; Muench, F.; Gevirtz, R.N. The effects of respiratory sinus arrhythmia biofeedback on heart rate variability and posttraumatic stress disorder symptoms. *Appl. Psychophysiol. Biofeedback* **2009**, *34*, 135–143. [CrossRef]
29. Tan, G.; Dao, T.K.; Farmer, L.; Sutherland, R.J.; Gevirtz, R. Heart Rate Variability and Posttraumatic Stress Disorder: A pilot study. *Appl. Psychophysiol. Biofeedback* **2011**, *36*, 27–35. [CrossRef] [PubMed]
30. Rene, R. The efficacy of a portable HRV feedback device in conjunction with mental health treatment of clients with major depressive disorder enrolled in a country welfare-to-work program. *Diss. Abstr. Int. Sect. B Sci. Eng.* **2008**, *69*, 2000.
31. Chaudhri, P. *The Effects of Cardiorespiratory Biofeedback and Dialectical Behavioral Skills Training with Sertraline on Post Myocardial Infarction Major Depression and Low Heart Rate Variability*; Alliant University: San Diego, CA, USA, 2008.
32. Patron, E.; Benvenutti, G.F.; Palomba, D. Biofeedback assisted control of RSA as a biobehavioral intervention for depressive symptoms in patients after cardiac surgery: A preliminary study. *Appl. Psychophysiol. Biof.* **2013**, *38*, 1–9. [CrossRef] [PubMed]
33. Van der Zwan, J.; Huizink, A.; Lehrer, P.; Koot, H.; Vente, W. The effect of Heart Rate Variability Biofeedback training on mental health of pregnant and non-pregnant women: A randomized contolled trial. *Int. J. Environ. Res. Public Health* **2019**, *16*, 1051. [CrossRef] [PubMed]
34. Karavidas, M.; Lehrer, P.; Vaschillo, E.; Vaschillo, B.; Marin, H.; Buyske, S. Preliminary results of an open label study of heart rate variability biofeedback for the treatment of major depression. *Appl. Psychophysiol. Biofeedback* **2007**, *32*, 19–30. [CrossRef] [PubMed]
35. Siepman, M.; Aykac, V.; Unterdorfer, J.; Mueck-Weymann, M. A pilot study on the effects of heart rate variability biofeedback in patients with depression and in healthy subjects. *Appl. Psychophysiol. Biofeedback* **2008**, *33*, 195–201. [CrossRef] [PubMed]
36. Thode, L. *Heart Rate Variability Biofeedback as a Complementary Treatment for Depression in Latinos*; Alliant International University: San Diego, CA, USA, 2019.

37. Lin, I.M.; Ko, J.M.; Fan, S.Y.; Yen, C.F. Heart Rate Variability and the efficacy of biofeedback in heroin users with depressive symptoms. *Clin. Psychopharmacol. Neurosci.* **2016**, *14*, 168–176. [CrossRef]
38. Lin, I.M.; Fan, S.Y.; Yen, C.F.; Yeh, Y.C.; Tang, T.C.; Huang, M.F.; Liu, T.L.; Wang, P.W.; Lin, H.C.; Tsai, H.Y.; et al. Heart Rate Variability biofeedback increased autonomic activation and improved symptoms of depression and insomnia among patients with Major Depression Disorder. *Clin. Psychopharmacol. Neurosci.* **2019**, *17*, 222–232. [CrossRef]
39. Karavidas, M.K. Heartrate variability biofeedback for major depression. *Biofeedback* **2008**, *36*, 18–21.
40. Rene, R. *The Efficacy of a Portable Heart Rate Variability Feedback Device in Conjunction with Mental Health Treatment of Clients with Major Depressive Disorder Enrolled in a County Welfare-to-Work Program*; Alliant University: San Diego, CA, USA, 2011.
41. De Bruin, E.; Van der Zwan, J.; Bogels, S. A RCT Compairing Daily Mindfulness meditations, Biofeedback Exercises and Physical Exercise on Attention Control, Executive Functioning, Mindful Awareness, SelfCompassion and Worrying in Stressed Young Adults. *Mindfullness* **2016**, *7*, 1182–1192. [CrossRef] [PubMed]
42. Porges, S. Respiratory sinus arrhythmia: Physiological basis, quantitative methods and clinical implications. In *Cardiorespiratory and Cardiosomatic Psychophysiology*; Plenum Press: New York, NY, USA, 1986; pp. 101–115.
43. Blanchard, E. Elevated basal level of cardiovascular responses in Vietnam veterans with PTSD: a health problem I the making? *J. Anxiety Disord.* **1990**, *4*, 233–237. [CrossRef]
44. Cohen, H.; Kotler, M.; Matar, M.; Kaplan, Z. Power spectral analysis of heart rate variability in posttraumatic stress disorder patients. *Biol. Psychiatry* **1997**, *41*, 627–629. [CrossRef]
45. Schoenberg, P.L.; David, A.S. Biofeedback for psychiatric disorders: A systematic review. *Appl. Psychophysiol. Biofeedback* **2014**, *39*, 109–135. [CrossRef]
46. Lehrer, P.; Kaur, K.; Sharma, A.; Shah, K.; Huseby, R.; Bhavsar, J.; Zhang, Y. Heart Rate Variability Biofeedback Improves Emotional and Physical Health and Performance: A Systematic Review and Meta Analysis. *Appl. Psychophysiol. Biofeedback* **2020**, *45*, 109–129. [CrossRef] [PubMed]
47. Lehrer, P.; Vaschillo, E.; Vaschillo, B.; Habib, H. Biofeedback treatment for asthma. *Chest* **2004**, *126*, 352–361. [CrossRef]
48. Nolan, R.P.; Kamath, M.V.; Floras, J.S.; Picton, P. Heart Rate Variability biofeedback as a behavioral neurocardiac intervention to enhance vagal heart rate control. *Am. Heart J.* **2005**, *149*, 1137.e1–1137.e7. [CrossRef] [PubMed]
49. Lee, J.; Kim, J.; Wachholtz, A. The benefit of heart rate variability biofeedback and relaxation training in reduction trait anxiety. *Hanguk Simni Hakhoe Chi. Kongang* **2015**, *20*, 391–408.
50. Henriques, G.; Keffer, S.; Abrahamson, C.; Horst, S.J. Exploring the effectiveness of a computer-based HRV biofeedback program in reducing anxiety in college students. *Appl. Psychophysiol. Biofeedback* **2011**, *36*, 101–112. [CrossRef]
51. De Couck, M.; de Leeuw, I.; Blase, K.; Gidron, Y. Effects of heart rate variability biofeedback on the tumor marker CEA in metastatic colon cancer. *J. Immunol. Res.* **2018**, *79*, A18.
52. Windthorst, P.; Mazurak, N.; Kuske, M.; Hipp, A.; Giel, K.E.; Enck, P.; Nieß, A.; Zipfel, S.; Teufel, M. Heart Rate Variability biofeedback therapy and graded exercise training in management of chronic fatigue syndrome. *J. Psychosom. Res.* **2017**, *93*, 6–13. [CrossRef]
53. Berry, M.; Ginsberg, J.; Nagpal, M. Non-pharmalogical intervention for chronic pain in veterans: A pilot study of HRV. *Glob. Adv. Health Med.* **2014**, *3*, 28–33. [PubMed]
54. Del Pozo, J.M.; Gevirtz, R.N.; Scher, B.; Guarneri, E. Biofeedback treatment increases heart rate variability in patients with known coronary artery disease. *Am. Heart J.* **2004**, *147*, 545. [CrossRef]
55. Yu, L.C.; Lin, I.M.; Fan, S.Y.; Chien, C.L.; Lin, T.H. One year cardiovascular prognosis of the randomized controlled short term HRV biofeedback among patients with coronary artery disease. *Int. J. Behav. Med.* **2018**, *25*, 271–282.
56. Francis, H.; Penglis, K.; Mc Donald, S. Manipulation of heart rate variability can modify response to anger-inducing stimuli. *Soc. Neurosci.* **2016**, *11*, 545–552. [CrossRef]
57. Sequeira, V.; Bandeira, P.; Azevedo, J. Heart Rate Variability in adults with obstructive sleep apnea: A systematic review. *Sleep Sci.* **2019**, *12*, 214–221. [CrossRef] [PubMed]
58. Hasuo, H.; Kanbara, K.; Fukunaga, M. Effect of Heart Rate Variability biofeedback sessions with resonant breathing on sleep. *Sci. Rep.* **2020**, *10*, 7417.
59. Clamor, A.; Koenig, J.; Thayer, J.; Lincoln, T. A randomized-controlled trial of heart rate variability for psychotic symptoms. *Behav. Res.* **2016**, *87*, 207–215. [CrossRef]
60. Van der Zwan, J.; de Vente, W.; Huizink, A.; Bögels, S.; de Bruin, E. Physical activity, mindfulness meditation, or HRVbiofeedback for stress reduction: a randomized contolled trial. *Appl. Psychophysiol Biofeedback* **2015**, *40*, 257–268. [CrossRef]
61. Stern, M.; Guilles, R.; Gevirtz, R. HRVBiofeedback for Pedriatic Irritable Bowel Syndrome and Functional Abdominal Pain: a clinical replication series. *Appl. Psychophysiol. Biofeedback* **2014**, *39*, 3–4. [CrossRef] [PubMed]
62. Kudo, N.; Shinohara, H.; Kodama, H. Heart Rate Variability biofeedback intervention for reduction of psychological stress during the early postpartum period. *Appl. Psychophysiol. Biofeedback* **2014**, *39*, 203–211. [CrossRef]
63. Lande, R.G.; Williams, L.B.; Marin, M.L. Efficacy of biofeedback for post-traumatic stress disorder. *Complement. Med.* **2010**, *18*, 256–259. [CrossRef] [PubMed]
64. Hayes, S.; Strosahl, K.; Wilson, K. *Acceptance and Commitment Therapy: An Experiential Approach to Behavior Change*; Guilford Press: New York, NY, USA, 1999.

65. Gevirtz, R. Incorporating HRV biofeedback info Acceptance and Commitment Therapy. *Biofeedback* **2020**, *48*, 16–19. [CrossRef]
66. Brinkman, A.; Press, S.; Helmert, E.; Hautzinger, M.; Khazan, I.; Vagedes, J. Comparing effectiveness of HRVB and mindfulness for workplace stressreduction: A Randomized controlled trial. *Appl. Psychophysiol. Biofeedback* **2020**, *45*, 307–322. [CrossRef]

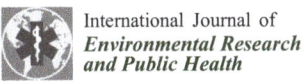

## Article

# Work-Related Stress, Health Status, and Status of Health Apps Use in Korean Adult Workers

Won Ju Hwang [1] and Minjeong Kim [2,*]

[1] College of Nursing Science, East-West Nursing Research Institute, Kyung Hee University, Seoul 02447, Korea; hwangwj@khu.ac.kr
[2] School of Nursing, San Diego State University, San Diego, CA 92182, USA
* Correspondence: minjeong.kim@sdsu.edu

**Abstract:** Although health apps have been developed and utilized in many countries, there is no baseline study about what percentage of Korean workers use these types of health apps. Therefore, the purpose of this study was to describe the work-related stress, health status, and utilization of health apps of Korean adult workers. This descriptive study included 95 adults in South Korea. Demographic variables, work-related stress, health status, and utilization of health apps were obtained using an online self-reported survey. Descriptive analyses were used to explore prevalence of each variable. This study found that almost 65% of the participants fell into the higher work-related stress group. About 41.6% of the participants in this sample evaluated their general health status as fair to poor with 26.8% being overweight to obese and 11.6% having hypertension. However, only about 33.7% of the sample have used health apps. Therefore, utilization of health apps as health and stress management tools should be encouraged at a public health level.

**Keywords:** Koreans; mobile applications; occupational stress

## 1. Introduction

Mental health promotion in adults has great public health concerns and social significance [1]. According to the results of the Korean Working Conditions Survey (KWCS), the number of workers who experienced depression and anxiety in the past 12 months was 1.6% in 2010, 1.5% in 2011, and 1.4% in 2014. Considering the reluctance to expose mental symptoms due to stigma at work and difficulties in returning to work after treatment, it is expected that the number of workers will continue to increase in the future [2].

As of 2021, the number of Korean workers was 18,945 thousand, which is 36.7% of the total population in Korea. According to classification of industries, the number of workers in manufacture was the largest (n = 3675 thousands), followed by sales (n = 2286 thousands), health and social work service (n = 2045 thousands), education service (n = 1677 thousands), and construction (n = 1378 thousands). Korean workers reported that they worked 149 h per month and their monthly income was around $3075 [3].

### 1.1. Work-Realted Stress and Health Status of Korean Adult Workers

Recent studies of Korean workers' stress found that Korean workers have experienced high levels of stress at work [2–5]. Park, Kook [2] found that over-time working significantly increased stress levels in Korean young adult workers. Job insecurity, a lack of reward, and uncomfortable organizational environment have also been reported as work-related stressors in Korean workers, which are typical Asian work environment which place a heavy emphasis on diligence and senior authority [6,7]. More specifically, studies of health care workers' stress found that professional burnout was related to higher work-related stress in medical doctors [8] and high emotional labor was one of the stressors in interpersonal service workers in hospitals [9].

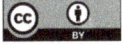

Relationships between work-related stress and health problems have already established in numerous studies. Some studies found that over-time working, job insecurity, a lack of reward, and uncomfortable organizational environment significantly increased the risk of depression, suicidal ideation, and musculoskeletal disease in Korean workers [2,6,7,10]. In regards to specific types of job, work-related stress significantly increased depression, anxiety, and sleep problems in Korean dentists [11] and suicidal ideation in Korean firefighters [12]. Emotional labor and job insecurity also significantly increased the risk of depression in female call center workers [13].

Similar relationships between work-related stress and health problems have also been found in studies with Asian and various populations. Higher levels of over-commitment and less organizational support significantly increased the risk of chronic fatigue syndrome in Chinese nurses [14]. Higher stress significantly increased the risk of hypertension in 530 Asian Americans [15], and alterations in circadian rhythm increased systolic and diastolic blood pressure in night shift workers in airline companies [16]. Two studies of diabetes found that work-related stress significantly increased blood glucose level (HbA1C) [17] and the incidence of both prediabetes and diabetes [18].

Although Korean adult workers experience work-related stress and even stress-related health problems, very few of them have utilized professional mental health service [19,20], which might be due to a lack of knowledge on self-care including stress management and not enough available resources in Korea. Since the onset of the COVID-19 pandemic, public health orders including stay-at-home and physical distancing measures have put people in more stressful situations, such as financial difficulties and changes from in-person to online work environments. It is also evident that people have been reluctant to see a doctor for the management of their current health conditions due to the fear of getting infected with COVID-19 in health care settings, resulting in undermanaged health problems [21].

*1.2. Status of Health Apps Use of Korean Adult Workers*

Very recently, various health apps have been developed and utilized to help track their blood pressure, blood sugar, food, exercise, weight, and even medications for prevention and self-care purposes in Korea as well as other countries. Examples of health apps that are widely used in Korea include "WishCare" [22], "MyTherapy" [23], and "HeLpy" [24]. In addition to physical health apps, stress care apps have also been developed to manage their stress and anxiety, featuring recommendations for mindfulness-based breathing techniques, meditation, and healing sounds based on their stress and anxiety level (in mind [25], KLAR [26], and "MindHealer" [27]).

Recently, studies of effects and efficacy of the health apps have been conducted in other countries. Specifically, mindfulness meditation apps significantly decreased perceived stress level in 88 medical students in the Unites States (Happy Healers) [28] and in 74 adults in the United Kingdom (Headspace) [29], and significantly decreased job strain, distress, and systolic blood pressure in 238 healthy employees in the United Kingdom [30]. Music-based emotion regulation apps (Music eScape) was also effective in improvement of emotional regulation skills and well-being in 169 young people with mild mental distress [31]. A study of effectiveness of an integrated health apps which offers diet, physical activity, sleeping habits, stress, and alcohol use, is ongoing in 209 Sweden adult workers [32]. Although many clinical trials about the effectiveness of health apps have been emerged in many countries and found their effectiveness on health, there is no baseline study about what percentage of Korean workers use these types of health apps. Therefore, this baseline descriptive study looking at work-related stress and health status and status of health apps use in Korean workers, is needed first.

*1.3. Purpose of the Present Study*

Therefore, the purpose of the present study was (1) to describe work-related stress and health status in a sample of Korean adult workers and (2) describe status of health apps use in this sample.

## 2. Methods

### 2.1. Study Design

This descriptive study used a cross-sectional design to describe work-related stress and health status, and status of health apps use in the Korean adult workers.

### 2.2. Participants and Setting

This web-based survey study included 95 adult workers in South Korea between November 2018 and December 2018. The inclusion criteria were: (1) self-identified as Korean; (2) between 18 and 65 years old; (3) able to communicate in Korean; (4) has an electronic device, such as a cellphone, tablet, or PC; (5) understands the purpose of this study. All participants who did not meet the inclusion criteria were excluded.

### 2.3. Procedure

Potential participants were reached out using social media in Seoul, South Korea. A convenience sampling method was employed. A 4-part, web-based self-report survey was developed using the Survey Monkey software and a survey link was sent to potential participants. Potential participants were also asked to share this study information with their friends if they are eligible for this study. A potential participant proceeded with this study if s/he was interested.

### 2.4. Measures

#### 2.4.1. Demographic Questionnaire

A 6-item investigator-developed demographic questionnaire was used. The items included questions on gender (male and female), age (in years), educational level (high school or below, college or Bachelor degree, and above graduate school), marriage status (single, married, and others), types of job (white-collar, blue-collar, and others), and monthly family income ($1809.00 or below, $1809.00–$3617.00, and above $3617.00).

#### 2.4.2. Work-Related Stress

A short version of the Effort–Reward Imbalance Questionnaire (ERIQ) is a self-report, 4-point Likert scale to measure participants' effort, reward, and over commitment at work: Effort Scale (ES, 3 items), Reward Scale (RS, 7 items), and Over Commitment (OC, 4 items). A sum of each subscale ranges from 3–12 for the ES, 7–28 for the RS, and 4–16 for the OC. The Effort/Reward(ER) ratio was computed by placing the effort score in the enumerator and the reward score in the denominator. The latter score was multiplied by a correction factor prior to being placed in the denominator to adjust for the unequal number of items. Correction factor was 0.4286 when the enumerator contained 3 items and the denominator contained 7 items. An ER ratio higher than 1.0 indicates an imbalance between high effort and low reward [33]. Cronbach alphas for our sample of Korean adults were 0.68 for the ES, 0.80 for the RS, and 0.83 for the OC.

#### 2.4.3. Health Status

Participants' health status was assessed by three measures: general health status, Body Mass Index (BMI), and health problems. To assess the participants' evaluation of their overall health, one question was answered on a five-point scale consisting of the answers excellent, very good, good, fair, and poor. BMI was computed by putting weight in kilograms in the enumerator and height in meters squared in the denominator. Scores below 18.5 are considered underweight, scores between 18.5 and 24.99 for normal, scores between 25.0 and 29.99 for overweight, and scores above 30.0 for obese [34]. Health problems were noted as yes/no for hypertension, hyperlipidemia, and diabetes.

2.4.4. Status of Health Apps Use

A 1-item investigator-developed questionnaire was used. The item asked if what types of health apps has been ever used at work or at home: overall health, mental health-focused, or physical health-focused apps.

2.5. Data Analysis

SPSS 26.0 version (IBM, Armonk, NY, US)program was used to analyze the data in this study. Descriptive statistics were used to examine demographic characteristics, including frequency and percent for gender, educational level, marriage status, types of job, and monthly family income, and mean (M) and standard deviations (SD) for age. M and SD were also calculated for the work-related stress, and frequency and percent for general health status, BMI, health problems, and types of health apps use.

3. Results

Participants consisted of 32 males (38.1%) and 52 females (61.9%). The mean age of the participants was 40.3 years (32–47 years, SD = 7.4). About 92.9% had college or higher education levels. About 71.4% of the participants were married. About 79.1% of the participants reported that they were white-collar workers. About 57.8% of the participants reported that "their family earns higher than $3617.00 monthly" and 38.6% reported that "their family earns between $1809.00 and $3617.00 monthly" (Table 1).

**Table 1.** Demographic characteristics of Korean workers (n = 95, valid case only).

| Variable | n (%)/M (SD) |
| --- | --- |
| Gender | |
| Male | 32 (38.1) |
| Female | 52 (61.9) |
| Age | 40.3 (7.4) |
| Educational level | |
| High school or below | 6 (7.1) |
| College or Bachelor degree | 42 (49.4) |
| Graduate school or higher | 37 (43.5) |
| Marriage status | |
| Single | 21 (25.0) |
| Married | 60 (71.4) |
| Others (divorce, etc.) | 3 (3.6) |
| Types of job | |
| White-collar | 68 (79.1) |
| Blue-collar | 4 (4.7) |
| Others | 7 (8.1) |
| Unemployed | 7 (8.1) |
| Monthly family income | |
| $1809.00 or below | 3 (3.6) |
| $1809.00–$3617.00 | 32 (38.6) |
| $3617.00 or higher | 48 (57.8) |

Participants' levels of work-related stress are presented in Table 2. The mean score of the ES was 9.0 (SD = 1.9) and 19.1 (SD = 4.4) for the RS. The ER ratio was 1.2 (SD = 0.6), which indicated that about 64.8% of the participants fell into a higher work-related stress group and the other 35.2% of the participants fell into a lower work-related stress group. The mean score of the OC was 10.0 (SD = 3.3).

Table 2. Levels of work-related stress of Korean workers (n = 95, valid case only).

| Variable | M (SD)/n (%) |
|---|---|
| Effort-Reward Imbalance Questionnaire (ERIQ) | |
| Effort Scale (ES) | 9.0 (1.9) |
| Reward Scale (RS) | 19.1 (4.4) |
| Effort-Reward (ER) ratio | 1.2 (0.6) |
| ≥1.0 (higher stress group) | 57 (64.8) |
| <1.0 (lower stress group) | 31 (35.2) |
| Over Commitment (OC) | 10.0 (3.3) |

As shown in Table 3, about 41.6% of the participants fell into either the "fair" or "poor" health status groups, whereas only 19.1% of the participants fell into either the "excellent" or "very good" health status groups. About 26.8% of the participants were in either the "overweight" or "obese" group. Among health problems, the prevalence of hypertension was the greatest (n = 11, 11.6%), followed by hyperlipidemia (n = 6, 6.3%) and diabetes (n = 4, 4.2%).

Table 3. Health status of Korean workers (n = 95).

| Variable | n (%) |
|---|---|
| General health status | |
| Excellent | 3 (3.4) |
| Very good | 14 (15.7) |
| Good | 35 (39.3) |
| Fair | 29 (32.6) |
| Poor | 8 (9.0) |
| Body Mass Index (BMI) | |
| 18.5 or below (underweight) | 5 (5.8) |
| 18.5–24.9 (normal) | 58 (67.4) |
| 25.0–29.9 (overweight) | 22 (25.6) |
| 30.0 or higher (obese) | 1 (1.2) |
| Health problems (multiple response) | |
| Hypertension | 11 (11.6) |
| Hyperlipidemia | 6 (6.3) |
| Diabetes | 4 (4.2) |

Participants' status of health apps use are presented in Table 4. About 33.7% of the participants reported that they have ever used health apps. More specifically, about 10.1% (n = 9) of the participants have ever used mental health-focused apps, and only 4.5% (n = 4) for physical health-focused apps.

Table 4. Status of health Apps use of Korean workers (n = 95).

| Variable | n (%) |
|---|---|
| Types of health apps use (multiple response) | |
| Overall health | 30 (33.7) |
| Mental health-focused | 9 (10.1) |
| Physical health-focused | 4 (4.5) |

## 4. Discussion

This study explored Korean adult worker's work-related stress, health status, and status of health apps use. Of demographic variables, most of our study participants (79.1%) fell into a white-collar employee group. Moreover, about half of our study participants had a graduate school or higher educational level (43.5%) and earned $3617.00 or higher per month (57.8%), which may be due to a selection bias of a convenience sampling. Therefore, repeated studies with more representative samples of Korean adult workers including those with low socio-economic status or vulnerable population, are needed.

Higher work-related stress was reported by 64.8% of the participants in this study, which was similar or quite higher than those from other studies that reported Korean workers reported higher work-related stress [2–5]. This finding indicated that Korean workers have put a lot of effort, energy, and commitment towards their accomplishments at work, but have received quite less rewards than they deserve, considering the negative adverse work environments typically seen in Asian culture [6,7].

The study findings about the prevalence of hypertension (11.6%) was inconsistent with those from other reports which showed 3.3% of hypertension rate among 4865 employed pregnant women from the Amsterdam Born Children and their Development data [35], 5.5% in Chinese patients [36], 19.4% in Chinese petroleum workers [37], and 33.3% in Egyptian bus drivers [38]. The prevalence of 4.2% of diabetes rate in this study was comparable to those from other studies which found 2.2% of diabetes rate from the Brazilian Longitudinal Study of Adult Health [18] and 3.4% of cardio-metabolic disease rate (coronary heart disease, stroke, or diabetes) from the European Work Consortium data [39]. Although there were some inconsistent findings regarding participants' health status, our understanding is that our participants' sedentary lifestyle might contribute to increased hypertension and diabetes rate [2,6,7,40,41]. This study did not look at the relationships among types of jobs, work-related stress, and health status, therefore, further analyses are needed.

Our participants in this study reported use of overall health apps (33.7%), mental health-focused apps (10.1%), and physical health-focused apps (4.5%). Study findings about the utilization of health apps were hard to compare with those from other studies because of a lack of studies on the prevalence of health apps use in the adult worker populations [28–32]. This underutilization of health apps might be due to a lack of health apps available in the Korea, a lack of research study about the effectiveness of health apps as health and stress management tools, and a lack of public awareness about the importance of health apps use in improving their health status. Further analyses are also needed to identify factors that may contribute to the lower use of health apps. Since the COVID-19 pandemic, the need for self-care and stress managements has significantly increased. Therefore, the utilization of health apps should be encouraged at public health level.

Limitations of this study should be noted. Due to a convenience sampling method, our study findings may not be generalized to all Korean adult workers. This study used a self-report online survey for work-related stress and health status that might be often under-reported due to stigma around stress and health issues. Moreover, this study did not analyze the relationships among work-related stress, health status, and health apps use so causal relationship cannot be guaranteed. Despite the study limitations, this study is significant in that this study was the very first study that addressed work-related stress and health apps use in Korean adult workers.

## 5. Conclusions

This study found that Korean adult workers experienced higher levels of work-related stress, fair to poor health status, overweight, and hypertension. Participants underutilized health apps. Health apps use which help tracking and managing their stress and health should be encouraged for Korean adult workers.

**Author Contributions:** M.K. and W.J.H. developed the study design and drafted the manuscript. M.K. performed data collection & analysis. W.J.H. supervised overall study and reviewed the manuscript. All authors have read and agreed to the published version of the manuscript.

**Funding:** This research was supported by a grant from the Korea Health Technology R&D Project through the Korea Health Industry Development Institute (KHIDI), and it was funded by the Ministry of Health & Welfare, Republic of Korea (grant number: HI18C1317). The funding agencies had no role in the study design, the collection, analysis, or interpretation of data, the writing of the report, or the decision to submit the article for publication.

**Institutional Review Board Statement:** The study was conducted according to the guidelines of the Declaration of Helsinki, and approved by the Institutional Review Board of University (project identification code: 20181687). The overall study was registered at the Kyung Hee University for clinical trials (registration no.: 18-077).

**Informed Consent Statement:** Informed consent was obtained from all subjects involved in the study.

**Data Availability Statement:** Please contact the corresponding author for data availability.

**Conflicts of Interest:** The authors declare that the research was conducted in the absence of any commercial or financial relationships that could be construed as a potential conflict of interest.

## References

1. Ministry of Employment and Labor. *Report on Labor Force Survey at Establishments*; Ministry of Employment and Labor: Sejong, Korea, 2021.
2. Park, S.; Kook, H.; Seok, H.; Lee, J.H.; Lim, D.; Cho, D.-H.; Oh, S.-K. The negative impact of long working hours on mental health in young Korean workers. *PLoS ONE* **2020**, *15*, e0236931. [CrossRef] [PubMed]
3. Lim, S.; Chi, S.; Lee, J.D.; Lee, H.-J.; Choi, H. Analyzing psychological conditions of field-workers in the construction industry. *Int. J. Occup. Environ. Health* **2017**, *23*, 261–281. [CrossRef] [PubMed]
4. Ryu, S. Turnover Intention among Field Epidemiologists in South Korea. *Int. J. Environ. Res. Public Health* **2020**, *17*, 949. [CrossRef] [PubMed]
5. Yim, H.-Y.; Seo, H.-J.; Cho, Y.; Kim, J. Mediating Role of Psychological Capital in Relationship between Occupational Stress and Turnover Intention among Nurses at Veterans Administration Hospitals in Korea. *Asian Nurs. Res.* **2017**, *11*, 6–12. [CrossRef]
6. Kim, S.-Y.; Shin, Y.-C.; Oh, K.-S.; Shin, D.-W.; Lim, W.-J.; Cho, S.J.; Jeon, S.-W. Gender and age differences in the association between work stress and incident depressive symptoms among Korean employees: A cohort study. *Int. Arch. Occup. Environ. Health* **2019**, *93*, 457–467. [CrossRef]
7. Kim, S.-Y.; Shin, Y.-C.; Oh, K.-S.; Shin, D.-W.; Lim, W.-J.; Cho, S.J.; Jeon, S.-W. Association between work stress and risk of suicidal ideation: A cohort study among Korean employees examining gender and age differences. *Scand. J. Work. Environ. Health* **2019**, *46*, 198–208. [CrossRef]
8. Lee, Y.-G.; Maeng, C.H.; Kim, D.Y.; Kim, B.-S. Perspectives on Professional Burnout and Occupational Stress among Medical Oncologists: A Cross-sectional Survey by Korean Society for Medical Oncology (KSMO). *Cancer Res. Treat.* **2020**, *52*, 1002–1009. [CrossRef]
9. Sohn, B.K.; Park, S.M.; Park, I.-J.; Hwang, J.Y.; Choi, J.-S.; Lee, J.-Y.; Jung, H.-Y. The Relationship between Emotional Labor and Job Stress among Hospital Workers. *J. Korean Med. Sci.* **2018**, *33*, 246. [CrossRef]
10. Kim, Y.M.; Cho, S.I. Work-Life Imbalance and Musculoskeletal Disorders among South Korean Workers. *Int. J. Environ. Res. Public Health* **2017**, *14*, 1331. [CrossRef]
11. Song, K.-W.; Choi, W.-S.; Jee, H.-J.; Yuh, C.-S.; Kim, Y.-K.; Kim, L.; Lee, H.-J.; Cho, C.-H. Correlation of occupational stress with depression, anxiety, and sleep in Korean dentists: Cross-sectional study. *BMC Psychiatry* **2017**, *17*, 1–11. [CrossRef]
12. Park, H.; Kim, J.I.; Min, B.; Oh, S.; Kim, J.-H. Prevalence and correlates of suicidal ideation in Korean firefighters: A nationwide study. *BMC Psychiatry* **2019**, *19*, 1–9. [CrossRef] [PubMed]
13. Cho, S.S.; Kim, H.; Lee, J.; Lim, S.; Jeong, W.C. Combined exposure of emotional labor and job insecurity on depressive symptoms among female call-center workers: A cross-sectional study. *Medicine* **2019**, *98*, e14894. [CrossRef] [PubMed]
14. Li, M.; Shu, Q.; Huang, H.; Bo, W.; Wang, L.; Wu, H. Associations of occupational stress, workplace violence, and organizational support on chronic fatigue syndrome among nurses. *J. Adv. Nurs.* **2020**, *76*, 1151–1161. [CrossRef] [PubMed]
15. Lu, X.; Juon, H.S.; He, X.; Dallal, C.M.; Wang, M.Q.; Lee, S. The Association Between Perceived Stress and Hypertension Among Asian Americans: Does Social Support and Social Network Make a Difference? *J. Community Health* **2019**, *44*, 451–462. [CrossRef]
16. Morris, C.J.; Purvis, T.E.; Mistretta, J.; Hu, K.; Scheer, F.A.J.L. Circadian Misalignment Increases C-Reactive Protein and Blood Pressure in Chronic Shift Workers. *J. Biol. Rhythm.* **2017**, *32*, 154–164. [CrossRef]
17. Walker, R.J.; Garacci, E.; Campbell, J.A.; Egede, L.E. The influence of daily stress on glycemic control and mortality in adults with diabetes. *J. Behav. Med.* **2019**, *43*, 723–731. [CrossRef]
18. Santos, R.D.S.; Griep, R.H.; Fonseca, M.D.J.M.D.; Chor, D.; Santos, I.D.S.; Melo, E.C.P. Combined Use of Job Stress Models and the Incidence of Glycemic Alterations (Prediabetes and Diabetes): Results from ELSA-Brasil Study. *Int. J. Environ. Res. Public Health* **2020**, *17*, 1539. [CrossRef]

19. Park, S.; Lee, Y.; Seong, S.J.; Chang, S.M.; Lee, J.Y.; Hahm, B.J.; Hong, J.P. A cross-sectional study about associations between personality characteristics and mental health service utilization in a Korean national community sample of adults with psychiatric disorders. *BMC Psychiatry* **2017**, *17*, 170. [CrossRef]
20. Arnault, D.M.S.; Gang, M.; Woo, S. Factors Influencing on Mental Health Help-seeking Behavior Among Korean Women: A Path Analysis. *Arch. Psychiatr. Nurs.* **2018**, *32*, 120–126. [CrossRef]
21. CDC. COVID-19. 2021. Available online: https://www.cdc.gov/coronavirus/2019-ncov/prevent-getting-sick/prevention.html (accessed on 7 June 2021).
22. Tastylife. WishCare. Available online: https://apkcombo.com/de/wisikeeo-hyeoldang-dangnyo-imdang-hyeol-ab-gwanli-doumi/com.tastylife.wishcare/ (accessed on 7 June 2021).
23. MyTherapy. MyTherapy. Available online: https://www.tech-wonders.com/2017/10/mytherapy-medication-reminder-app-review.html (accessed on 7 June 2021).
24. EISAIKOREA. HeLpy. Available online: https://play.google.com/store/apps/details?id=com.helpy.mobile&hl=ko&gl=US (accessed on 7 June 2021).
25. Demand. in Mind. Available online: http://www.demand.co.kr/app_inmind (accessed on 7 June 2021).
26. Piaw, C.Y. Establishing a Brain Styles Test: The YBRAINS Test. *Procedia-Soc. Behav. Sci.* **2011**, *15*, 4019–4027. [CrossRef]
27. Hwang, W.J.; Jo, H.H. Evaluation of the Effectiveness of Mobile App-Based Stress-Management Program: A Randomized Controlled Trial. *Int. J. Environ. Res. Public Health* **2019**, *16*, 4270. [CrossRef] [PubMed]
28. Yang, E.; Schamber, E.; Meyer, R.M.L.; Gold, J.I. Happier Healers: Randomized Controlled Trial of Mobile Mindfulness for Stress Management. *J. Altern. Complement. Med.* **2018**, *24*, 505–513. [CrossRef] [PubMed]
29. Champion, L.; Economides, M.; Chandler, C. The efficacy of a brief app-based mindfulness intervention on psychosocial outcomes in healthy adults: A pilot randomised controlled trial. *PLoS ONE* **2018**, *13*, e0209482. [CrossRef] [PubMed]
30. Bostock, S.; Crosswell, A.D.; Prather, A.A.; Steptoe, A. Mindfulness on-the-go: Effects of a mindfulness meditation app on work stress and well-being. *J. Occup. Health Psychol.* **2019**, *24*, 127–138. [CrossRef]
31. Hides, L.; Dingle, G.; Quinn, C.; Stoyanov, S.R.; Zelenko, O.; Tjondronegoro, D.; Johnson, D.; Cockshaw, W.; Kavanagh, D.J. Efficacy and Outcomes of a Music-Based Emotion Regulation Mobile App in Distressed Young People: Randomized Controlled Trial. *JMIR Mhealth Uhealth* **2019**, *7*, e11482. [CrossRef]
32. Bonn, S.E.; Löf, M.; Östenson, C.-G.; Lagerros, Y.T. App-technology to improve lifestyle behaviors among working adults—The Health Integrator study, a randomized controlled trial. *BMC Public Health* **2019**, *19*, 273. [CrossRef]
33. Siegrist, J.; Li, J.; Montano, D. Psychometric Properties of the Effort-Reward Imbalance Questionnaire. 2014. Uniklinik Düsseldorf Web Site. Available online: https://www.uniklinik-duesseldorf.de/fileadmin/Fuer-Patienten-und-Besucher/Kliniken-Zentren-Institute/Institute/Institut_fuer_Medizinische_Soziologie/Dateien/ERI/ERI_Psychometric-New.pdf (accessed on 7 June 2021).
34. CDC. Body Mass Index (BMI). Available online: https://www.cdc.gov/healthyweight/assessing/bmi/index.html (accessed on 7 June 2021).
35. Vrijkotte, T.; Brand, T.; Bonsel, G. First trimester employment, working conditions and preterm birth: A prospective population-based cohort study. *Occup. Environ. Med.* **2021**, *78*, 654–660. [CrossRef]
36. Lu, W.-H.; Zhang, W.-Q.; Zhao, Y.-J.; Gao, Y.-T.; Tao, N.; Ma, Y.-T.; Liu, J.-W.; Wulasihan, M. Case–Control Study on the Interaction Effects of rs10757278 Polymorphisms at 9p21 Locus and Traditional Risk Factors on Coronary Heart Disease in Xinjiang, China. *J. Cardiovasc. Pharmacol.* **2020**, *75*, 439–445. [CrossRef]
37. Tao, N.; Ge, H.; Wu, W.; An, H.; Liu, J.; Xu, X. Association of glucocorticoid receptor gene polymorphism and occupational stress with hypertension in desert petroleum workers in Xinjiang, China. *BMC Med. Genet.* **2018**, *19*, 213. [CrossRef]
38. Mohsen, A.; Hakim, S.A. Workplace stress and its relation to cardiovascular disease risk factors among bus drivers in Egypt. *East. Mediterr. Health J.* **2019**, *25*, 878–886. [CrossRef]
39. Kivimäki, M.; Pentti, J.; Ferrie, J.E.; Batty, G.; Nyberg, S.T.; Jokela, M.; Virtanen, M.; Alfredsson, L.; Dragano, N.; Fransson, E.I.; et al. Work stress and risk of death in men and women with and without cardiometabolic disease: A multicohort study. *Lancet Diabetes Endocrinol.* **2018**, *6*, 705–713. [CrossRef]
40. Hallgren, M.; Vancampfort, D.; Owen, N.; Rossell, S.; Dunstan, D.W.; Bellocco, R.; Lagerros, Y.T. Prospective relationships of mentally passive sedentary behaviors with depression: Mediation by sleep problems. *J. Affect. Disord.* **2019**, *265*, 538–544. [CrossRef] [PubMed]
41. Vancampfort, D.; Stubbs, B.; Firth, J.; Hagemann, N.; Myin-Germeys, I.; Rintala, A.; Probst, M.; Veronese, N.; Koyanagi, A. Sedentary behaviour and sleep problems among 42,489 community-dwelling adults in six low- and middle-income countries. *J. Sleep Res.* **2018**, *27*, e12714. [CrossRef] [PubMed]

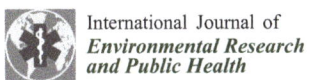 

Article

# The Association between Insulin Resistance and Cardiovascular Disease Risk: A Community-Based Cross-Sectional Study among Taiwanese People Aged over 50 Years

Mei-Chun Lu [1,2,3], Wei-Ching Fang [1], Wen-Cheng Li [1,3,4], Wei-Chung Yeh [1], Ying-Hua Shieh [5] and Jau-Yuan Chen [1,3,*]

1. Department of Family Medicine, Chang-Gung Memorial Hospital, Linkou Branch, Taoyuan City 33305, Taiwan; b101092026@tmu.edu.tw (M.-C.L.); winds75526@gmail.com (W.-C.F.); wcl20130714@gmail.com (W.-C.L.); sendoh777777@gmail.com (W.-C.Y.)
2. Department of Family Medicine, Chang Gung Memorial Hospital, Taoyuan Branch, Taoyuan City 33378, Taiwan
3. College of Medicine, Chang Gung University, Taoyuan City 33302, Taiwan
4. Department of Health Management, Xiamen Chang-Gung Hospital, Xiamen 361000, China
5. Department of Family Medicine, New Taipei Municipal TuCheng Hospital, New Taipei City 23652, Taiwan; tony470120@gmail.com
* Correspondence: welins@cgmh.org.tw; Tel.: +886-975362672; Fax: +886-3-3287715

Received: 22 August 2020; Accepted: 29 September 2020; Published: 1 October 2020

**Abstract:** Background and Aims: Previous studies have implied that insulin resistance (IR) could represent a major underlying abnormality leading to cardiovascular disease (CVD). The aim of this study was to evaluate the relationships between IR (estimated by the homeostasis model assessment of IR (HOMA-IR) index) and CVD risk among middle-aged and elderly Taiwanese individuals. Methods: In this cross-sectional, community-based study, a total of 320 participants were interviewed to collect demographical parameters and blood samples. The recruited participants were divided into tertiles according to their levels of HOMA-IR. The Framingham risk score (FRS) was calculated according to the 2008 general CVD risk model from the Framingham Heart Study. Results: The HOMA-IR index was significantly correlated with the FRS, with a Pearson's coefficient of 0.22. In the multiple logistic regression model, a higher HOMA-IR level was significantly associated with a high FRS (FRS ≥ 20%) (highest tertile vs. lowest tertile of HOMA-IR, crude OR = 3.69; 95% CI = 1.79–7.62), even after adjusting for smoking, fasting plasma glucose (FPG), and systolic blood pressure (SBP) (highest tertile vs. lowest tertile of HOMA-IR, adjusted OR = 11.51; 95% CI = 2.55–51.94). The area under the receiver operating characteristic curve for the HOMA-IR index as the predictor of high FRS was 0.627, and the optimal HOMA-IR cutoff value was 1.215 (sensitivity = 83.6%, specificity – 42.9%). Conclusions: We considered that HOMA-IR is an independent factor but that it cannot be used solely for evaluating the CVD risk due to the low AUC value. Further prospective cohort studies are warranted to better assess the relationship between CVD risk and insulin resistance.

**Keywords:** insulin resistance; HOMA-IR; prediction; CVD; Framingham risk score

## 1. Introduction

Insulin resistance (IR) is thought to be the key mechanism of metabolic syndrome, a cluster of cardiovascular risk factors [1–6]. Previous studies have shown that hyperinsulinemia was an independent predictor of incident myocardial ischemic events in a non-diabetic population [7]. IR is also an independent risk factor for various chronic diseases, such as hypertension [8], hepatic steatosis and steatohepatitis [9], chronic kidney disease [10], and even lung cancer [11] and Alzheimer's disease [12].

Overnutrition, obesity, and specific dietary components can trigger IR [9,13]. Excess daily calories, fructose, and saturated fatty acid intake; a lack of n-3 polyunsaturated fatty acids and antioxidants; as well as intestinal microbiome imbalance can increase the oxidative stress in the liver and lead to IR and non-alcoholic hepatic steatosis and steatohepatitis [9].

The hyperinsulinemic–euglycemic clamp technique is the gold standard for evaluating insulin resistance, but it is impractical in clinical practice. Thus, surrogate markers such as the homeostasis model assessment of IR (HOMA-IR) have been developed to assess IR [14]. In Taiwan, the 2008 version of Framingham risk score (FRS) is frequently used by clinicians to estimate a person's risk of cardiovascular disease (CVD) in the next 10 years. Additionally, previous studies have shown that the FRS is applicable in Asian populations [15]. However, only limited studies have discussed the association of HOMA-IR with FRS [16,17]. For example, obese children with an increased HOMA-IR have a higher CVD risk [17].

Therefore, the aim of the current study was to investigate the associations between the HOMA-IR index and FRS and evaluate the ability of HOMA-IR to identify community residents with a high FRS (FRS ≥ 20%) in middle-aged and elderly Taiwanese individuals.

## 2. Materials and Methods

### 2.1. Participants

This was a cross-sectional study. The participants were recruited through a community health promotion project in Linkou Chang Gung Memorial Hospital in Taiwan from February 2014 to August 2014. The project was approved by the Institutional Review Board (102-2304B) of Linkou Chang Gung Memorial Hospital, and informed consent was signed by all the participants before enrollment.

A total of 400 participants aged over 50 years living in Guishan district (a rural district in northeastern Taiwan) were recruited. General information, including medical history and lifestyle, was obtained by appropriately trained interviewers. Participants with a history of CVD ($n$ = 19), aged 75 years and above ($n$ = 56), or with incomplete data ($n$ = 3) were excluded. Extreme outliers of HOMA-IR ($n$ = 2) were excluded. Finally, 320 participants were included in this study.

### 2.2. Anthropometric

Detailed anthropometric measurements, such as height, weight, waist circumference (WC), and blood pressure, were conducted by trained research assistants or nurses under the supervision of a medical doctor. The measurement of heights was carried out with the subjects standing with their feet together. Body mass index (BMI) was calculated by dividing weight by the square of the height (kg/m$^2$). Blood pressure (BP) was measured using an automated sphygmomanometer after the participants were relaxed and seated for more than 10 min. The WC was measured halfway between the iliac crest and the lowest rib at the end of a relaxed expiration. The height meter and weight scale were calibrated once per day.

### 2.3. Laboratory Examinations

Participants were requested to fast for at least 12 h and avoid a high-fat diet or alcohol consumption before blood sampling. Blood samples were stored in a refrigerator at 4 °C and then sent to the hospital laboratory. Clinical biochemistry tests were performed in a hospital laboratory accredited by the College of American Pathologists. The fasting plasma glucose (FPG); fasting insulin; alanine aminotransferase (ALT); creatinine; uric acid; and fasting lipid profiles, such as triglyceride (TG), high-density lipoprotein cholesterol (HDL-C), and low-density lipoprotein cholesterol (LDL-C), were measured.

### 2.4. Assessment of Insulin Resistance

We assessed insulin resistance by HOMA-IR [14], which is expressed as:

$$\mathrm{HOMA-IR} = \frac{\text{fasting glucose (in mmol/L)} \times \text{fasting insulin (in mU/ml)}}{22.5}$$

Subjects were divided into tertiles based on the HOMA-IR index:
Low HOMA-IR group: HOMA-IR ≤ 1.15;
Middle HOMA-IR group: 1.15 < HOMA-IR ≤ 1.93;
High HOMA-IR group: HOMA-IR > 1.93.

### 2.5. Cardiovascular Risk Assessments

We used the 2008 Framingham risk score (FRS) assessments to determine the risk of CVD [18]. The risk factors and the equations used to calculate the FRS are listed below:

Women

$$\text{Risk Factors} = (\ln(\text{Age}) \times 2.32888) + (\ln(\text{Total cholesterol}) \times 1.20904)$$
$$- (\ln(\text{HDL Cholesterol}) \times 0.70833)$$
$$+ (\ln(\text{Systolic blood pressure}) \times \text{blood pressure medication factor})$$
$$+ \text{Cigarette smoker factor} + \text{Diabetes present factor} - 26.1931$$
$$\text{FRS} = 100 \times \left((1 - 0.95012)^r\right)$$
$$r = e^{(\text{Risk factors})}$$

Men

$$\text{Risk Factors} = (\ln(\text{Age}) \times 3.06117) + (\ln(\text{Total cholesterol}) \times 1.12370)$$
$$- (\ln(\text{HDL Cholesterol}) \times 0.93263)$$
$$+ (\ln(\text{Systolic blood pressure}) \times \text{blood pressure medication factor})$$
$$+ \text{Cigarette smoker factor} + \text{Diabetes present factor} - 23.9802$$
$$\text{FRS} = 100 \times \left((1 - 0.88936)^r\right)$$
$$r = e^{(\text{Risk factors})}$$

A high FRS was defined as an FRS ≥ 20%.

### 2.6. Statistical Analysis

Demographics and clinical characteristics are presented as means with standard deviations and counts with percentages for continuous and discrete variables, respectively. Descriptive statistics were presented, and differences between groups with different HOMA-IR levels were compared using one-way ANOVA for continuous data and the chi-square test for categorical data. The correlation of cardiovascular disease risk factors and HOMA-IR levels was assessed using Pearson's analysis. Multiple logistic regression analysis was used to adjust for covariates. A receiver operating characteristic (ROC) curve was constructed to assess the performance of the HOMA-IR to predict a high FRS. Youden's index, which maximizes the sum of sensitivity and specificity (max (sensitivity+ specificity-1)), was used to determine the optimal cutoff point, and the corresponding sensitivity, specificity, and area under the receiver operating characteristic curve (AUC) were calculated. All the statistical tests were regarded as statistically significant, with a $p$-value less than 0.05 (two-sided). Data were analyzed using the Statistical Package for the Social Sciences software, version 22.0 (SPSS Inc., Chicago, IL, USA).

## 3. Results

### 3.1. Baseline Characteristics of the Patient Population

The general characteristics of the participants according to the tertile of the HOMA-IR level are summarized in Table 1. Overall, the mean age was 61.88 ± 6.21 years, and the mean FRS was 14.31 ± 11.47%. There were no significant differences between the three groups concerning age, creatinine, smoking, alcohol drinking, and regular exercise. However, the mean FRS was significantly higher in the groups with higher HOMA-IR levels. The mean FRS were 10.95 ± 7.85% (low HOMA-IR group), 13.94 ± 10.21% (middle HOMA-IR group), and 18.04 ± 14.33% (high HOMA-IR group), respectively. Other parameters with significant differences between the three groups with $p$-values lower than 0.05 were SBP, BMI, WC, ALT, FPG, HDL-C, TG, LDL-C, and uric acid. Figure 1 shows that the prevalence of high FRS was higher among the high HOMA-IR tertile than among the two lower tertiles (*p*-value for the Cochran–Armitage trend test of <0.001).

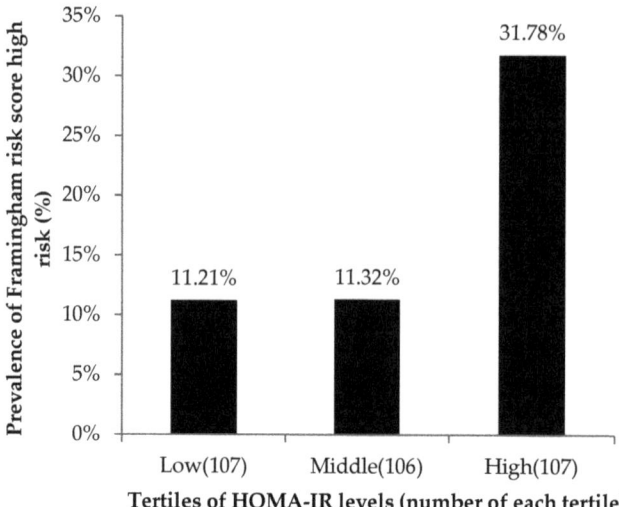

**Figure 1.** Prevalence of high FRS (FRS ≥ 20%) according to the tertiles of the HOMA-IR index levels. The prevalence of high FRS was higher among the high HOMA-IR tertile than among the two lower tertiles.

Table 1. General characteristics of the study population according to the tertiles of the HOMA-IR levels.

| Variables | Total (n = 320) | | Low (HOMA-IR ≤ 1.15) (n = 107) | | Middle (1.15 < HOMA-IR ≤ 1.93) (n = 106) | | High (HOMA-IR > 1.93) (n = 107) | | p-value |
|---|---|---|---|---|---|---|---|---|---|
| Age (year) | 61.88 | ±6.21 | 61.38 | ±6.13 | 61.72 | ±6.54 | 62.53 | ±5.93 | 0.38 |
| SBP (mmHg) | 128.76 | ±16.09 | 124.52 | ±16.77 | 129.20 | ±14.41 | 132.56 | ±16.11 | 0.001 |
| DBP (mmHg) | 78.12 | ±10.80 | 76.80 | ±11.56 | 78.01 | ±9.97 | 79.55 | ±10.72 | 0.176 |
| BMI (kg/m$^2$) | 24.61 | ±3.52 | 22.95 | ±2.99 | 24.55 | ±2.82 | 26.32 | ±3.84 | <0.001 |
| Waist circumference (cm) | 84.54 | ±9.37 | 80.31 | ±7.52 | 83.62 | ±8.04 | 89.68 | ±9.89 | <0.001 |
| ALT (U/L) | 22.89 | ±12.89 | 19.61 | ±7.49 | 22.18 | ±11.71 | 26.89 | ±16.75 | <0.001 |
| Creatinine (mg/dL) | 0.72 | ±0.28 | 0.69 | ±0.16 | 0.73 | ±0.32 | 0.74 | ±0.34 | 0.37 |
| eGFR (ml/min/1.73m$^2$) | 117.43 | ±30.65 | 121.03 | ±28.94 | 116.23 | ±31.53 | 115.01 | ±31.37 | 0.32 |
| FPG (mg/dL) | 95.33 | ±21.96 | 85.065 | ±8.44 | 92.113 | ±12.37 | 108.77 | ±30.49 | <0.001 |
| HDL-C (mg/dL) | 54.96 | ±13.83 | 61.037 | ±14.67 | 54.472 | ±12.36 | 49.36 | ±11.84 | <0.001 |
| HOMA-IR index | 1.85 | ±1.36 | 0.80 | ±0.23 | 1.51 | ±0.23 | 3.24 | ±1.52 | <0.001 |
| LDL-C (mg/dL) | 120.20 | ±31.85 | 121.77 | ±34.23 | 124.78 | ±30.51 | 114.10 | ±29.96 | 0.04 |
| Triglyceride (mg/dL) | 123.37 | ±65.14 | 93.97 | ±41.90 | 119.44 | ±54.73 | 156.66 | ±77.71 | <0.001 |
| Uric Acid (mg/dL) | 5.71 | ±1.41 | 5.39 | ±1.30 | 5.71 | ±1.41 | 6.03 | ±1.45 | 0.003 |
| Framingham risk score (%) | 14.31 | ±11.47 | 10.95 | ±7.85 | 13.94 | ±10.21 | 18.04 | ±14.33 | <0.001 |
| Current smoking, n (%) | 35 | (10.9) | 13 | (12.1) | 10 | (9.4) | 12 | (11.2) | 0.81 |
| Alcohol drinking ≥ 2 times/week, n (%) | 62 | (19.4) | 26 | (24.3) | 21 | (19.8) | 15 | (14.0) | 0.16 |
| Regular exercise, n (%) | 259 | (80.9) | 92 | (86.0) | 87 | (82.1) | 80 | (74.8) | 0.11 |
| HTN, n (%) | 152 | (47.5) | 40 | (37.4) | 42 | (39.6) | 70 | (65.4) | <0.001 |
| DM, n (%) | 54 | (16.9) | 2 | (1.9) | 13 | (12.3) | 39 | (36.4) | <0.001 |
| Hyperlipidemia, n (%) | 211 | (65.9) | 60 | (56.1) | 70 | (66.0) | 81 | (75.7) | 0.01 |

Notes: Clinical characteristics are expressed as the mean ± SD for continuous variables and n (%) for categorical variables. p-values were derived from a one-way analysis of variance (one-way ANOVA) for continuous variables and chi-square tests for categorical variables. Abbreviations: BMI, body mass index; SBP, systolic blood pressure; DBP, diastolic blood pressure; ALT, alanine aminotransferase; FPG, fasting plasma glucose. HDL-C, high-density lipoprotein cholesterol; LDL-C, low-density lipoprotein cholesterol; TG, triglyceride; HTN, hypertension.

## 3.2. Correlation Analysis

The correlations of the HOMA-IR levels with the CVD risk factors are shown in Table 2. The factors with significant positive correlations with IR were SBP, BMI, FRS, WC, FPG, TG, and uric acid, while HDL-C and LDL-C showed significant negative correlations with IR. Among them, BMI, WC, FPG, and TG showed a stronger correlation with IR than the correlation of the FRS with IR. Considering that the negative correlation of LDL-C was very weak (Pearson's coefficient -0.11), we did not involve LDL-C in the subsequent multiple logistic regression analysis. Figure 2 demonstrates the correlation of FRS and IR with a Pearson's coefficient of 0.22.

**Table 2.** Pearson correlation coefficient of the HOMA-IR levels with the cardiovascular disease risk factors.

| Variables | HOMA-IR Index ($n = 320$) | |
|---|---|---|
| | Pearson's coefficient | p-value |
| Age (year) | 0.02 | 0.68 |
| SBP (mmHg) | 0.16 | 0.005 |
| DBP (mmHg) | 0.09 | 0.126 |
| BMI (kg/m$^2$) | 0.46 | <0.001 |
| Framingham risk score (%) | 0.22 | <0.001 |
| Waist circumference (cm) | 0.45 | <0.001 |
| FPG (mg/dL) | 0.58 | <0.001 |
| HDL-C (mg/dL) | −0.32 | <0.001 |
| TG (mg/dL) | 0.34 | <0.001 |
| LDL-C (mg/dL) | −0.11 | 0.04 |
| Uric Acid (mg/dL) | 0.16 | 0.003 |

Abbreviations: SBP, systolic blood pressure; DBP, diastolic blood pressure; BMI, body mass index; FPG, fasting plasma glucose; HDL-C, high-density lipoprotein cholesterol; LDL-C, low-density lipoprotein cholesterol; TG, triglyceride.

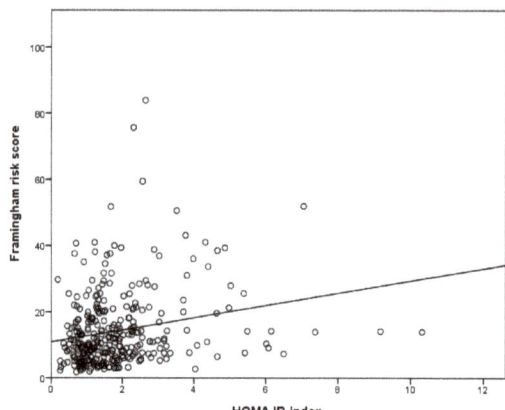

**Figure 2.** Correlation coefficients between the HOMA-IR levels and the Framingham risk score.

## 3.3. Association between the Tertiles of HOMA-IR Levels and the Framingham Risk Factors

Table 3 shows the results of the multiple logistic regression analyses in comparing the risk of high FRS between subjects with different HOMA-IR levels (with the low HOMA-IR level group as the reference group). In Model 1 (unadjusted), the odds ratios (ORs) for the middle and high HOMA-IR groups were 2.71 (95% CI: 1.29–5.69, p-value 0.009) and 3.69 (95% CI: 1.79–7.62, p-value < 0.001), respectively. In Model 2, the ORs (95% CI) were determined after further adjustment for gender. In Model 3, the ORs (95% CI) were determined after further adjustment for gender, age, and BMI. In Model 4, the HOMA-IR level remained significantly correlated with high FRS after adjustment for covariates, including age, gender, BMI, smoking status, SBP, and FPG. The adjusted ORs for the middle

HOMA-IR and high HOMA-IR groups were 11.31 (95% CI: 2.94–43.52, *p*-value < 0.001) and 11.51 (95% CI: 2.55–51.94, *p*-value = 0.001), respectively.

*3.4. ROC Analysis*

The AUC for the HOMA-IR index as a predictor of high FRS was 0.627, as shown in Table 4 and Figure 3. According to Youden's index, the optimal cutoff point for the HOMA-IR index for predicting a high FRS was 1.215, with a sensitivity and a specificity of 83.6% and 42.9%, respectively.

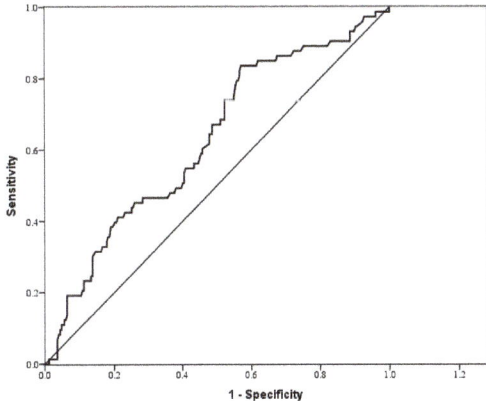

**Figure 3.** ROC curve for the HOMA-IR index as a predictor of the Framingham risk score.

Table 3. Association between the tertiles of the HOMA-IR levels and a high FRS (FRS ≥ 20%).

| Variables | Model 1 | | | Model 2 | | | Model 3 | | | Model 4 | | |
|---|---|---|---|---|---|---|---|---|---|---|---|---|
| | OR | (95% CI) | p-value | OR | (95% CI) | p-value | OR | (95% CI) | p-value | OR | (95% CI) | p-value |
| Low | 1.00 | | | 1.00 | | | 1.00 | | | 1.00 | | |
| Middle | 2.71 | (1.29–5.69) | 0.009 | 5.16 | (2.12–12.57) | <0.001 | 5.66 | (2.17–14.78) | <0.001 | 11.31 | (2.94–43.52) | <0.001 |
| High | 3.69 | (1.79–7.62) | <0.001 | 9.67 | (3.83–24.37) | <0.001 | 9.01 | (3.14–25.81) | <0.001 | 11.51 | (2.55–51.94) | 0.001 |
| p-value for trend | | | <0.001 | | | <0.001 | | | <0.001 | | | 0.002 |

Model 1: unadjusted; Model 2: adjusted for sex; Model 3: adjusted for factors in model 2 plus age and BMI; Model 4: adjusted for factors in model 3 plus smoking. FPG, SBP. Abbreviations: BMI, body mass index; FPG, fasting plasma glucose; SBP, systolic blood pressure; CI, confidence interval.

Table 4. The areas under the ROC curve (AUC), sensitivity, and specificity of the optimized cut-off points for the HOMA-IR index in predicting high FRS (FRS ≥ 20%).

| Variables | AUC (95% CI) | p Value | Cut-off point | Sensitivity | Specificity |
|---|---|---|---|---|---|
| HOMA-IR index | 0.627 | 0.001 | 1.215 | 0.836 | 0.429 |

Abbreviations: ROC curve, receiver operating characteristic curve; CI, confidence interval.

## 4. Discussion

Our study objective was to investigate the associations between IR and future CVD risk. In this community-based cross-sectional study among Taiwanese people aged over 50 years, the level was positively associated with the FRS after adjusting for potential confounders. Several studies have reported a positive correlation between CVD risk and IR [19–22], which is consistent with our findings.

HOMA-IR is a frequently used tool to estimate IR. However, there are only limited studies focusing on the use of the HOMA-IR level for predicting high FRS. In our study, participants with high HOMA-IR levels had a higher prevalence of high FRS compared with those with lower HOMA-IR levels (Figure 1). After adjusting for other risk factors, including sex, age, BMI, current smoking status, FPG, and SBP through multiple logistic regression models, the HOMA-IR level was still significantly associated with high FRS. These results reinforce that HOMA-IR is an independent risk factor for high FRS. We then evaluated the ability of HOMA-IR to identify community residents with a high FRS. However, due to the low specificity and low AUC value, HOMA-IR cannot be used as the sole predictor of high FRS.

The recent studies have revealed that there are several mechanisms to induce IR, such as genetic defects, overnutrition, obesity, and inflammation [13,23]. In overnutrition status, the excess intra-cellular free fatty acids will lead to the activation of PKC and NFκB, then induce serine 307 phosphorylation for IRS-1, which inhibits the insulin signal pathway and eventually results in IR in the skeleton muscle and hepatocytes. The PKC activation and increased free fatty acid flux to the liver results in hepatosteatosis [13,24,25].

Excess free fatty acids in cardiomyocytes and endothelial cells also cause serine 307 phosphorylation for IRS-1, then inhibit the insulin signaling pathway [23,26]. An inhibited insulin signaling pathway results in increased free fatty acid oxidation and decreased glucose oxidation in cardiomyocyte and causes cell death [23]. In the endothelial cells, IR causes an imbalance between the production of eNO and the secretion of endothelin-1, resulting in endothelial dysfunction [26].

The early detection of IR, as well as interventions in lifestyle and dietary components, could decrease the development and progression of IR and reverse further damage to the liver, heart, and endothelium. In Taiwan, free adult health exams offered by the Health Promotion Administration cover all the needed parameters for FRS calculation and fasting glucose, but not fasting insulin. Besides, clinicians do not routinely check HOMA-IR. For individuals with diabetes or obesity, it is easy to link their condition with insulin resistance. However, for high FRS individuals who are elderly, smokers, or have hypertension, it is harder for clinicians to think about IR. This study revealed that HOMA-IR is an independent risk factor for high FRS. Clinicians should be more alert for IR in high-FRS individuals, and offer lifestyle and dietary interventions earlier for better prognosis.

Lifestyle interventions and dietary interventions are reported to improve IR, the lipid profile, and liver function enzymes [9,13]. Lifestyle interventions include body weight loss of over 5% of the initial weight, physical activity for 150 min/week or more, training exercises for four weeks, or a regular exercise program. Dietary interventions include daily calorie restriction by reducing 500 Kcal from usual food consumption, a high-protein diet, fructose restriction, and choosing a Mediterranean diet. Supplementation with anti-oxidatives, amino acids, vitamins, n-3 polyunsaturated fatty acids, and prebiotics/probiotics may have potential benefits, but lack sufficient evidence [9].

This study still has some limitations. First, the study was cross-sectional; therefore, it is unable to explore the cause–effect relationship between FRS and IR. Second, we do not have a direct outcome measure of CVD. Third, we did not check Hba1c, a more reliable marker for identifying pre-diabetic and diabetic individuals. Finally, our sample size was relatively small. Further studies are warranted with unknown confounders.

## 5. Conclusions

In conclusion, a high FRS (FRS ≥ 20%) was significantly associated with IR in the middle-aged and elderly population in Taiwan. HOMA-IR is an independent risk factor for high FRS, but cannot be used as the sole predictor due to its low specificity. Further prospective cohort studies are warranted to better assess the relationship between CVD risk and insulin resistance in middle-aged and elderly Taiwanese populations.

**Author Contributions:** Conceptualization, W.-C.L. and J.-Y.C.; methodology, J.-Y.C.; software, J.-Y.C.; validation, J.-Y.C.; formal analysis, J.-Y.C.; investigation, M.-C.L., W.-C.F., and J.-Y.C.; resources, Y.-H.S. and J.-Y.C.; data curation, M.-C.L. and J.-Y.C.; writing—original draft preparation, M.-C.L.; writing—review and editing, M.C.L.; visualization, W.-C.F. and J.-Y.C.; supervision, W.-C.L. and J.-Y.C.; project administration, W.-C.Y. and J.-Y.C.; funding acquisition, J.-Y.C. All authors have read and agreed to the published version of the manuscript.

**Funding:** This study was supported by Chang Gung Memorial Hospital (grants CORPG3C0171, CORPG3C0172, CZRPG3C0053, CORPG3G0021, CORPG3G0022, and CORPG3G0023).

**Conflicts of Interest:** The authors declare no conflict of interest.

## Abbreviations

| | |
|---|---|
| HOMA-IR | homeostasis model assessment of insulin resistance |
| IR | insulin resistance |
| CVD | cardiovascular disease |
| CKD | chronic kidney disease |
| WC | waist circumference |
| FRS | Framingham risk score |
| BMI | body mass index |
| BP | blood pressure |
| FPG | fasting plasma glucose |
| HDL-C | high-density lipoprotein cholesterol |
| LDL-C | low-density lipoprotein cholesterol |
| TG | triglyceride |
| ALT | alanine aminotransferase |
| eGFR | estimated glomerular filtration rate |
| ROC | receiver operating characteristic |
| AUC | area under the ROC curve |
| OR | odds ratio |
| aOR | adjusted odds ratio |

## References

1. DeFronzo, R. Insulin resistance: a multifaceted syndrome responsible for NIDDM, obesity, hypertension, dyslipidaemia and atherosclerosis. *Neth. J. Med.* **1997**, *50*, 191–197. [CrossRef]
2. Beilby, J.P. Definition of Metabolic Syndrome: Report of the National Heart, Lung, and Blood Institute/American Heart Association Conference on Scientific Issues Related to Definition. *Clin. Biochem. Rev.* **2004**, *25*, 195–198.
3. Girman, C.J.; Rhodes, T.; Mercuri, M.; Pyörälä, K.; Kjekshus, J.; Pedersen, T.R.; A Beere, P.; Gotto, A.M.; Clearfield, M. The metabolic syndrome and risk of major coronary events in the Scandinavian Simvastatin Survival Study (4S) and the Air Force/Texas Coronary Atherosclerosis Prevention Study (AFCAPS/TexCAPS). *Am. J. Cardiol.* **2004**, *93*, 136–141. [CrossRef] [PubMed]
4. Lakka, H.-M.; Laaksonen, D.E.; Lakka, T.; Niskanen, L.K.; Kumpusalo, E.; Tuomilehto, J.; Salonen, J.T. The metabolic syndrome and total and cardiovascular disease mortality in middle-aged men. *JAMA* **2002**, *288*, 2709–2716. [CrossRef] [PubMed]
5. Eckel, R.; Alberti, K.; Grundy, S.M.; Zimmet, P. The metabolic syndrome. *Lancet* **2010**, *375*, 181–183. [CrossRef]
6. Reaven, G.M. Banting lecture 1988. Role of insulin resistance in human disease. *Diabetes* **1988**, *37*, 1595–1607. [CrossRef]
7. Després, J.-P.; Lamarche, B.; Mauriège, P.; Cantin, B.; Dagenais, G.R.; Moorjani, S.; Lupien, P.-J. Hyperinsulinemia as an Independent Risk Factor for Ischemic Heart Disease. *New Engl. J. Med.* **1996**, *334*, 952–958. [CrossRef]
8. Wang, F.; Han, L.; Hu, D. Fasting insulin, insulin resistance and risk of hypertension in the general population: A meta-analysis. *Clin. Chim. Acta* **2017**, *464*, 57–63. [CrossRef]
9. Hernandez-Rodas, M.C.; Valenzuela, R.; A Videla, L. Relevant Aspects of Nutritional and Dietary Interventions in Non-Alcoholic Fatty Liver Disease. *Int. J. Mol. Sci.* **2015**, *16*, 25168–25198. [CrossRef]

10. E Kosmas, C.; Silverio, D.; Tsomidou, C.; Salcedo, M.D.; Montan, P.D.; Guzman, E. The Impact of Insulin Resistance and Chronic Kidney Disease on Inflammation and Cardiovascular Disease. *Clin. Med. Insights: Endocrinol. Diabetes* **2018**, *11*. [CrossRef]
11. Petridou, E.T.; Sergentanis, T.; Antonopoulos, C.N.; Dessypris, N.; Matsoukis, I.L.; Aronis, K.N.; Efremidis, A.; Syrigos, C.; Mantzoros, C.S. Insulin resistance: an independent risk factor for lung cancer? *Metab.* **2011**, *60*, 1100–1106. [CrossRef] [PubMed]
12. Ma, L.; Wang, J.; Li, Y. Insulin resistance and cognitive dysfunction. *Clin. Chim. Acta* **2015**, *444*, 18–23. [CrossRef] [PubMed]
13. Valenzuela, R.; Videla, L.A. The importance of the long-chain polyunsaturated fatty acid n-6/n-3 ratio in development of non-alcoholic fatty liver associated with obesity. *Food Funct.* **2011**, *2*, 644–648. [CrossRef]
14. Matthews, D.R.; Hosker, J.P.; Rudenski, A.S.; Naylor, B.A.; Treacher, D.F.; Turner, R.C. Homeostasis model assessment: insulin resistance and ?-cell function from fasting plasma glucose and insulin concentrations in man. *Diabetol.* **1985**, *28*, 412–419. [CrossRef] [PubMed]
15. Selvarajah, S.; Kaur, G.; Haniff, J.; Cheong, K.C.; Hiong, T.G.; Van Der Graaf, Y.; Bots, M.L. Comparison of the Framingham Risk Score, SCORE and WHO/ISH cardiovascular risk prediction models in an Asian population. *Int. J. Cardiol.* **2014**, *176*, 211–218. [CrossRef] [PubMed]
16. Li, X.; Wang, F.; Xu, H.; Qian, Y.; Zou, J.; Yang, M.; Zhu, H.; Yi, H.; Guan, J.; Yin, S. Interrelationships among common predictors of cardiovascular diseases in patients of OSA: A large-scale observational study. *Nutr. Metab. Cardiovasc. Dis.* **2020**, *30*, 23–32. [CrossRef]
17. Ferreira, A.P.; Oliveira, C.E.R.; De França, N.M. Metabolic syndrome and risk factors for cardiovascular disease in obese children: the relationship with insulin resistance (HOMA-IR). *J. de Pediatr.* **2007**, *83*, 21–26. [CrossRef]
18. D'Agostino, R.B.; Vasan, R.S.; Pencina, M.J.; Wolf, P.A.; Cobain, M.; Massaro, J.; Kannel, W.B. General Cardiovascular Risk Profile for Use in Primary Care: The Framingham Heart Study. *Circulation* **2008**, *117*, 743–753. [CrossRef]
19. Stern, M.P.; Williams, K.; Gonzalez-Villalpando, C.; Hunt, K.J.; Haffner, S.M. Does the Metabolic Syndrome Improve Identification of Individuals at Risk of Type 2 Diabetes and/or Cardiovascular Disease? *Diabetes Care* **2004**, *27*, 2676–2681. [CrossRef]
20. McNeill, A.M.; Rosamond, W.D.; Girman, C.J.; Golden, S.H.; Schmidt, M.I.; East, H.E.; Ballantyne, C.M.; Heiss, G. The Metabolic Syndrome and 11-Year Risk of Incident Cardiovascular Disease in the Atherosclerosis Risk in Communities Study. *Diabetes Care* **2005**, *28*, 385–390. [CrossRef]
21. Hu, G.; Qiao, Q.; Tuomilehto, J.; Balkau, B.; Borch-Johnsen, K.; Pyorala, K. Prevalence of the Metabolic Syndrome and Its Relation to All-Cause and Cardiovascular Mortality in Nondiabetic European Men and Women. *Arch. Intern. Med.* **2004**, *164*, 1066–1076. [CrossRef] [PubMed]
22. Wannamethee, S.G.; Shaper, A.G.; Lennon, L.T.; Morris, R. Metabolic Syndrome vs Framingham Risk Score for Prediction of Coronary Heart Disease, Stroke, and Type 2 Diabetes Mellitus. *Arch. Intern. Med.* **2005**, *165*, 2644–2650. [CrossRef] [PubMed]
23. Ormazabal, V.; Nair, S.; Elfeky, O.; Aguayo, C.; Salomon, C.; Zúñiga, F.A. Association between insulin resistance and the development of cardiovascular disease. *Cardiovasc. Diabetol.* **2018**, *17*, 122. [CrossRef] [PubMed]
24. Ragheb, R.; Shanab, G.M.; Medhat, A.M.; Seoudi, D.M.; Adeli, K.; Fantus, I. Free fatty acid-induced muscle insulin resistance and glucose uptake dysfunction: Evidence for PKC activation and oxidative stress-activated signaling pathways. *Biochem. Biophys. Res. Commun.* **2009**, *389*, 211–216. [CrossRef]
25. Roden, M.; Price, T.B.; Perseghin, G.; Petersen, K.F.; Rothman, D.L.; Cline, G.W.; Shulman, G.I. Mechanism of free fatty acid-induced insulin resistance in humans. *J. Clin. Investig.* **1996**, *97*, 2859–2865. [CrossRef]
26. Muniyappa, R.; Sowers, J.R. Role of insulin resistance in endothelial dysfunction. *Rev. Endocr. Metab. Disord.* **2013**, *14*, 5–12. [CrossRef] [PubMed]

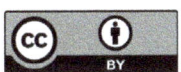

© 2020 by the authors. Licensee MDPI, Basel, Switzerland. This article is an open access article distributed under the terms and conditions of the Creative Commons Attribution (CC BY) license (http://creativecommons.org/licenses/by/4.0/).

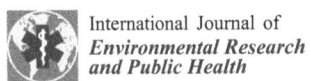 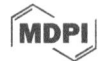

Article

# The Association between Metabolic Syndrome and Related Factors among the Community-Dwelling Indigenous Population in Taiwan

Yu-Chung Tsao [1,2], Wen-Cheng Li [2,3,4], Wei-Chung Yeh [3], Steve Wen-Neng Ueng [2,5,*], Sherry Yueh-Hsia Chiu [6,7] and Jau-Yuan Chen [2,3,*]

1. Department of Occupational Medicine, Chang Gung Memorial Hospital, Linkou Branch, Taoyuan City 33305, Taiwan; eusden@gmail.com
2. College of Medicine, Chang Gung University, Taoyuan City 33302, Taiwan; wcl20130714@gmail.com
3. Department of Family Medicine, Chang-Gung Memorial Hospital, Linkou Branch, Taoyuan City 33305, Taiwan; sendoh777777@gmail.com
4. Department of Health Management, Xiamen Chang-Gung Hospital, Xiamen 361028, China
5. Department of Orthopedics, Chang Gung Memorial Hospital, Linkou Branch, Taoyuan City 33305, Taiwan
6. Department of Health Care Management, College of Management, Chang Gung University, Taoyuan City 33302, Taiwan; sherrychiu@mail.cgu.edu.tw
7. Department of Internal Medicine, Kaohsiung Chang Gung Memorial Hospital, Kaohsiung Branch 83301, Taiwan
* Correspondence: wenneng@cgmh.org.tw (S.W.-N.U.); welins@cgmh.org.tw (J.-Y.C.); Tel.: +886-9-75362672 (J.-Y.C.); Fax: +886-3-3287715 (J.-Y.C)

Received: 20 October 2020; Accepted: 28 November 2020; Published: 2 December 2020

**Abstract:** The aim of this study was to conduct a community-based study with a view to construct a detailed analysis about metabolic syndrome and the related risk factors of the indigenous population. This was an observational, population-based and cross-sectional study that was conducted in remote villages of an indigenous community in northern Taiwan between 2010 and 2013. A total of 586 participants, 275 men and 311 women, were eligible for analysis. The participants underwent a questionnaire survey that included demographic and health behavior issues. An anthropometric assessment and measurements of blood pressure were carried out including serum biochemical variables. Metabolic syndrome (MetS) was defined by following the criteria provided by the modified Adult Treatment Panel III (ATP III) criteria of the National Cholesterol Education Program (NCEP). Univariate and multiple logistic regressions were used to identify the risk factors for metabolic syndrome. The standardized prevalence rates of substance use (cigarette smoking, alcohol drinking and betel nut chewing) were significantly higher than the general population regardless of whether it was northern, central or southern Taiwan and this was especially the case with betel nut chewing in women. The prevalence rate of metabolic syndrome was 42.9% in the indigenous population with 41.3% in men and 44.4% in women, which was higher than for urban Taiwanese. In the multiple logistic regression models, we found that the significant associated factors for metabolic syndrome were older age, lower education level, high levels of uric acid, alanine transaminase (ALT), gamma-glutamyl transferase ($\gamma$-GT) and creatinine. A higher prevalence rate of metabolic syndrome and substance use were observed in the indigenous population compared with urban Taiwanese, especially in women.

**Keywords:** metabolic syndrome; substance usage indigenous people; rural health

## 1. Introduction

Metabolic syndrome is a complex of interrelated risk factors for cardiovascular disease (CVD) and diabetes (DM). These factors include dysglycemia, raised blood pressure, elevated triglyceride levels, low high-density lipoprotein cholesterol levels and obesity (particularly central adiposity) [1,2].

Individuals with metabolic syndrome are associated with approximately five and two-fold increased risk for type 2 DM and CVD, respectively [3], as well as a risk factor for all-cause mortality [4]. Recent interest has focused on the possible involvement of insulin resistance as a linking factor although the pathogenesis remains unclear. With these risk factors, it has been demonstrated clearly that the syndrome is common and that it has a rising prevalence worldwide, which relates largely to increasing obesity and sedentary lifestyles. As a result, metabolic syndrome is now both a public health and a clinical problem. In the public health arena, more attention must be given to modification of lifestyles of the general public of all nations to reduce obesity and to increase physical activity. At a clinical level, individual patients with metabolic syndrome need to be identified so that their multiple risk factors, including lifestyle risk factors, can be reduced [1].

The prevalence of metabolic syndrome in Taiwan had been well described in recent studies [5,6]. The comparison between Taiwan and other Asian countries was also described [7]. In other countries, a higher prevalence among the indigenous population is one of the greatly emphasized public health issues [8]. However, there have been only scanty studies with small sample sizes [9,10] or a few hospital-based studies [11] that focused on the health issue of metabolic syndrome of the indigenous population in Taiwan. We aimed to conduct a community-based study with a view to constructing a detailed analysis about metabolic syndrome and related factors among an indigenous population in Taiwan. Therefore, our findings hopefully may provide valuable information for the prevention of metabolic syndrome (MetS) by further health promoting programs or intervention in this population.

## 2. Materials and Methods

### 2.1. Participants

We conducted a cross-sectional study with a design based on the annual health checkup service to collect associated information between October 2010 and February 2013 from three remote villages in the Fuxing District, Taoyuan City, Taiwan (as shown in Figure 1). Participants were informed about this study and voluntarily agreed to participate. The study was approved by the Chang Gung Medical Foundation 74 Institutional Review Board (99-0231B, 101-4156A3). Participants were recruited if they were over the age of 18 and had lived in this area for more than six months. A total of 2309 residents met our inclusion criteria.

We distributed questionnaires that included basic information about personal history, occupation, substance use and exercise habits. We also arranged free health checks that included basic laboratory data. According to the data from Fuxing District Health Station, the number of actual residents who lived in the three remote villages was around 1850. Therefore, after the exclusion of potential participants with incomplete data, we had a coverage rate of 42.1% over laboratory data ($n = 778$) and 50.7% over complete questionnaires ($n = 938$). With a view to evaluating the prevalence of metabolic syndrome and related factors, we excluded those who could not be identified with the criteria of metabolic syndrome due to missing data. With these exclusion criteria, we had a coverage rate of 31.7% ($n = 586$).

Figure 1 outlines the geographic location of the mountainous area (Fuxing District) in Taoyuan city. Gaoyi, Hualing and Sanguang were the three indigenous villages where we performed the integrated delivery system. Local medical care resources and local churches were marked on the map.

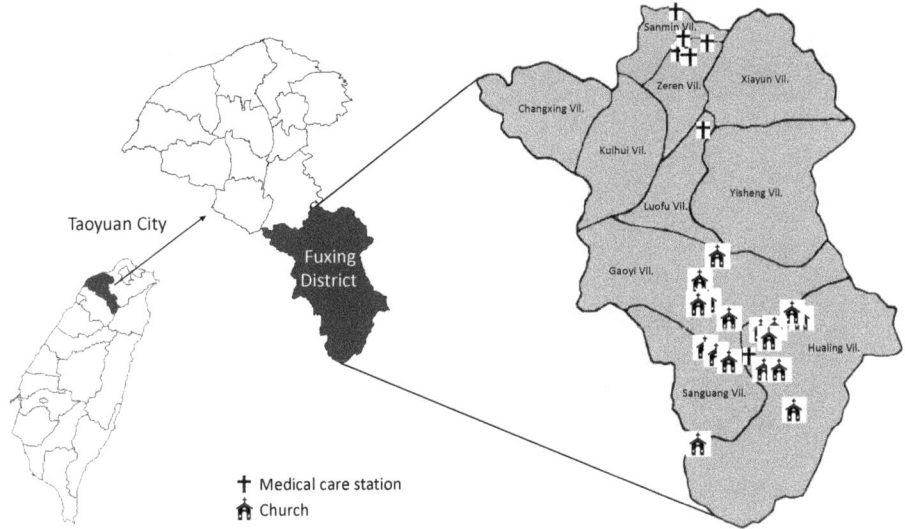

**Figure 1.** Geographical information of the remote area of the Fuxing District.

*2.2. Questionnaire*

A questionnaire was used to obtain socio-demographic data (i.e., race, gender, age, education level, religion, marital status, occupation and income) as well as information on tobacco, alcohol, betel quid usage and physical activity status. Smoking, drinking and betel nut usage were categorized as either current, never or past user. Smoking and betel nut usage were defined as at least three days a week in the recent month. An alcohol drinking habit was defined as more than three times a week.

Definitions of Metabolic Syndrome and Measurements

Metabolic syndrome was defined by following the criteria provided by the modified Adult Treatment Panel III (ATP III) criteria of the National Cholesterol Education Program (NCEP) [3]. The presence of any three of the following five factors was required for a diagnosis of metabolic syndrome: abdominal obesity (90 cm for Asian men and 80 cm for Asian women), hypertriglyceridemia (triglycerides $\geq$ 150 mg/dl or current use of triglycerides-lowering drugs), low high-density lipoprotein cholesterol (HDL) (HDL cholesterol < 40 mg/dL for men and <50 mg/dL for women), elevated blood pressure (systolic blood pressure $\geq$ 130 mmHg and/or diastolic blood pressure $\geq$ 85 mmHg or current use of anti-hypertensive drugs) and impaired fasting glucose (fasting plasma glucose $\geq$ 100 mg/dL or current use of anti-diabetic drugs).

Blood samples were drawn from the antecubital vein following a 12-h overnight fast. After centrifugation at standard conditions, plasma samples were frozen and transported immediately to our laboratory where they were analyzed. Participants' medical history on using anti-hypertensive and anti-diabetic medication and participants with high blood pressure or DM were recorded.

The waist circumference was measured midway between the iliac and costal margin whilst the participant was standing. The procedure used for blood pressure measurements was in agreement with the recommendations of the American Society of Hypertension, where all blood pressure measurements were conducted on the upper arm of the subject with an automatic blood pressure recorder after a 5 min resting period.

All blood analyses were performed at the clinical laboratory department of the Linkou Chang Gung Memorial Hospital and certified by the College of American Pathologists (CAP). Biochemical parameters, including high-density lipoprotein cholesterol (HDL-C), triglycerides, fasting glucose, alanine transaminase (ALT gamma-glutamyl transferase), aspartate transaminase (AST), gamma-glutamyl transferase ($\gamma$-GT), high sensitive C-reactive protein (HS-CRP), glycohemoglobulin

(HbA1c), uric acid, urinary microalbumin, creatinine, low-density lipoprotein cholesterol (LDL-C) and very-low-density lipoprotein cholesterol (VLDL-C) were analyzed on a Hitachi 7600–210 autoanalyzer (Hitachi, Tokyo, Japan). Blood tests were carried out in accordance with the hospital's laboratory standard operating procedure that was accredited by the CAP. The aforementioned biomarkers related to metabolic syndrome were selected according to previous studies [12].

### 2.3. Statistical Analysis

Descriptive statistics for demographic and biochemical variables were computed separately for male and female genders. The differences between the two groups were analyzed by t-tests or Mann–Whitney U tests of independent samples. We performed a standardized method using the WHO 2000 population [13] for prevalence comparison. The univariate and multiple logistic regressions were used for risk factor investigations. All statistical analyses were performed using SAS software version 9.4 (SAS Institute Inc., Cary, NC, USA). All tests were two tailed and a $p$-value of <0.05 was considered statistically significant.

## 3. Results

### 3.1. Metabolic Syndrome

Under the definition of the modified ATP III criteria [3], the prevalence rate of metabolic syndrome was 42.9% in the indigenous group we observed, with 41.3% in males and 44.4% in females (Table 1).

**Table 1.** Background analysis of basic information, biomarkers and the prevalence of metabolic syndrome of the male and female population ($n = 586$).

| Variables | | Total ($n = 586$) | | Male ($n = 275$) | | Female ($n = 311$) | | $p$-Value ($\alpha = 0.05$) |
|---|---|---|---|---|---|---|---|---|
| Age | | 49.3 | ±15.8 | 50.4 | ±16.9 | 48.4 | ±14.8 | 0.1217 |
| Age | | | | | | | | 0.1361 |
| | <30 | 65 | (11.1) | 33 | (12.0) | 32 | (10.3) | |
| | 30–39 | 115 | (19.6) | 45 | (16.4) | 70 | (22.5) | |
| | 40–49 | 118 | (20.1) | 53 | (19.3) | 65 | (20.9) | |
| | 50–59 | 116 | (19.8) | 53 | (19.3) | 63 | (20.3) | |
| | 60–69 | 104 | (17.8) | 50 | (18.2) | 54 | (17.4) | |
| | >70 | 68 | (11.6) | 41 | (14.9) | 27 | (8.7) | |
| Income (NTD, New Taiwan Dollars) | | | | | | | | 0.0028 * |
| | <10,000 | 295 | (61.3) | 114 | (53.8) | 181 | (67.3) | |
| | 10,000–29,999 | 140 | (29.1) | 69 | (32.6) | 71 | (26.4) | |
| | >30,000 | 46 | (9.6) | 29 | (13.7) | 17 | (6.3) | |
| | Unknown | 105 | | 63 | | 42 | | |
| Education | | | | | | | | 0.0382 * |
| | ≤6 grade | 222 | (45.9) | 94 | (43.9) | 128 | (47.4) | |
| | 7–9 grade | 135 | (27.9) | 51 | (23.8) | 84 | (31.1) | |
| | 10–12 grade | 98 | (20.3) | 55 | (25.7) | 43 | (15.9) | |
| | College or higher | 29 | (6.0) | 14 | (6.5) | 15 | (5.6) | |
| | Unknown | 102 | | 61 | | 41 | | |
| Current cigarette smoker | | | | | | | | <0.0001 |
| | No | 351 | (73.6) | 134 | (63.2) | 217 | (81.9) | |
| | Yes | 126 | (26.4) | 78 | (36.8) | 48 | (18.1) | |
| | Unknown | 109 | | 63 | | 46 | | |
| Alcohol drinking habit | | | | | | | | 0.0513 |
| | No | 320 | (66.7) | 132 | (62.0) | 188 | (70.4) | |
| | Yes | 160 | (33.3) | 81 | (38.0) | 79 | (29.6) | |
| | Unknown | 106 | | 62 | | 44 | | |
| Betel nut chewing habit | | | | | | | | <0.0001 |
| | No | 410 | (86.0) | 166 | (78.7) | 244 | (91.7) | |
| | Yes | 67 | (14.1) | 45 | (21.3) | 22 | (8.3) | |
| | Unknown | 109 | | 64 | | 45 | | |

**Table 1.** Cont.

| Variables | | Total (n = 586) | | Male (n = 275) | | Female (n = 311) | | p-Value (α = 0.05) |
|---|---|---|---|---|---|---|---|---|
| DM | | | | | | | | 0.1210 |
| | No | 488 | (83.3) | 236 | (85.8) | 252 | (81.0) | |
| | Yes (FG ≥ 126 or with history) | 98 | (16.7) | 39 | (14.2) | 59 | (19.0) | |
| Hypertension | | | | | | | | 0.9494 |
| | No | 281 | (50.6) | 131 | (50.8) | 150 | (50.5) | |
| | Yes (SBP ≥ 140 or DBP ≥ 90 or with history) | 274 | (49.4) | 127 | (49.2) | 147 | (49.5) | |
| | Unknown | 31 | | 17 | | 14 | | |
| Metabolic syndrome | | | | | | | | 0.4728 |
| | No | 299 | (57.1) | 141 | (58.8) | 158 | (55.6) | |
| | Yes (ATP III Asian criteria) | 225 | (42.9) | 99 | (41.3) | 126 | (44.4) | |
| | Unknown | 62 | | 35 | | 27 | | |
| Uric acid | | | | | | | | <0.0001 |
| | Normal | 475 | (81.1) | 198 | (72.0) | 277 | (89.1) | |
| | Abnormal (>8 mg/dL) | 111 | (18.9) | 77 | (28.0) | 34 | (10.9) | |
| Total cholesterol | | | | | | | | 0.0672 |
| | Normal | 326 | (55.6) | 142 | (51.6) | 184 | (59.2) | |
| | Abnormal (≥200 mg/dL) | 260 | (44.4) | 133 | (48.4) | 127 | (40.8) | |
| High-density lipoprotein cholesterol (HDL-C) | | | | | | | | 0.0075 * |
| | Normal | 385 | (65.7) | 196 | (71.3) | 189 | (60.8) | |
| | Abnormal (male < 40 or female < 50 mg/dL) | 201 | (34.3) | 79 | (28.7) | 122 | (39.2) | |
| Triglyceride | | | | | | | | 0.0453 * |
| | Normal | 345 | (58.9) | 150 | (54.6) | 195 | (62.7) | |
| | Abnormal (≥150 mg/dL) | 241 | (41.1) | 125 | (45.5) | 116 | (37.3) | |
| Aspartate transaminase (AST) | | | | | | | | 0.2833 |
| | Normal | 463 | (79.0) | 212 | (77.1) | 251 | (80.7) | |
| | Abnormal (>34 U/L) | 123 | (21.0) | 63 | (22.9) | 60 | (19.3) | |
| Alanine transaminase (ALT) | | | | | | | | 0.1390 |
| | Normal | 463 | (79.0) | 210 | (76.4) | 253 | (81.4) | |
| | Abnormal (>36 U/L) | 123 | (21.0) | 65 | (23.6) | 58 | (18.7) | |
| Gamma-Glutamyl Transferase (γ-GT) | | | | | | | | 0.0019 * |
| | Normal | 443 | (75.6) | 224 | (81.5) | 219 | (70.4) | |
| | Abnormal (Male > 71 or female > 42 U/L) | 143 | (24.4) | 51 | (18.6) | 92 | (29.6) | |
| Creatinine | | | | | | | | 0.2333 |
| | Normal | 566 | (96.6) | 263 | (95.6) | 303 | (97.4) | |
| | Abnormal (Male > 1.27 or female > 1.02 mg/dL) | 20 | (3.4) | 12 | (4.4) | 8 | (2.6) | |
| Hepatitis B surface antigen (HBsAg) | | | | | | | | 0.6558 |
| | Negative | 452 | (82.0) | 208 | (81.3) | 244 | (82.7) | |
| | Positive | 99 | (18.0) | 48 | (18.8) | 51 | (17.3) | |
| | Unknown | 35 | | 19 | | 16 | | |
| Anti-HCV antibody | | | | | | | | 0.2646 |
| | Negative | 520 | (94.6) | 245 | (95.7) | 275 | (93.5) | |
| | Positive | 30 | (5.5) | 11 | (4.3) | 19 | (6.5) | |
| | Unknown | 36 | | 19 | | 17 | | |

* p-Value < 0.05.

### 3.2. Substance Use

The overall crude prevalence rate of smoking was 26.4%, with 36.8% in males and 18.1% in females. The prevalence rate of alcohol drinking was 33.3%, with males 38.0% and females 29.6%. The prevalence rate of betel quid chewing was 14.1%, with males 21.3% and females 8.3%. The standardized prevalence rate of smoking, alcohol drinking and betel quid chewing were 33.3% (male 45.3%, female 25.9%), 36.7% (male 39.1%, female 35.0%) and 18.0% (male 31.9%, female 10.0%), respectively (Table 2). We chose three urban areas in Taiwan for comparison and found that the prevalence rates of substance usage were higher than in the urban area especially in alcohol drinking and betel nut chewing. The relatively higher prevalence rates of substance usage among the indigenous female population were also observed, with 25.9% smoking (9.4%, 2.5% and 2.7% in urban areas), 35.0% alcohol drinking (9.4%, 1.7% and 1.7% in urban areas) and 10.0% betel nut chewing (7.2%, 6.5% and 5.4% in urban areas) [14,15].

**Table 2.** Crude and standardized prevalence of substance usage compared with other parts of Taiwan.

| Substance Use | Subjects | Fuxing District | | Northern Taiwan [1] | Central Taiwan [1] | Southern Taiwan [1] |
| --- | --- | --- | --- | --- | --- | --- |
| | | Prevalence | Standardized Prevalence [1] | | | |
| Cigarette smoking | Total | 26.4 | 33.3 | 28.6 | 14.0 | 16.0 |
| | Male | 36.8 | 45.3 | 59.1 | 53.7 | 52.3 |
| | Female | 18.1 | 25.9 | 9.4 | 2.5 | 2.7 |
| Alcohol drinking | Total | 33.3 | 36.7 | 24.1 | 6.8 | 8.4 |
| | Male | 38.0 | 39.1 | 47.6 | 23.7 | 27.9 |
| | Female | 29.6 | 35.0 | 9.4 | 1.7 | 1.7 |
| Betel nut chewing | Total | 14.1 | 18.0 | 7.2 | 6.5 | 5.4 |
| | Male | 21.3 | 31.9 | 18.1 | 28.9 | 23.3 |
| | Female | 8.3 | 10.0 | 0.8 | 0.3 | 0.4 |

[1] Standardized using the WHO 2000 world population, http://www.who.int/healthinfo/paper31.pdf. Total subjects: 586; male: 275, female: 311.

*3.3. Regression Models*

We built single and multiple regression models (Table 3) to discuss the related factors that are associated with metabolic syndrome. The crude odds ratio (OR) and adjusted OR are listed in Table 3. The crude ORs that were significant for metabolic syndrome were 1.03 (95% CI: 1.02, 1.04) in older age; 0.47 (95% CI: 0.31, 0.73) and 0.44 (95% CI: 0.22, 0.88) in better income; 0.48 (95% CI: 0.30, 0.76), 0.32 (95% CI: 0.19, 0.54) and 0.33 (95% CI: 0.14, 0.79) in better education; 1.93 (95% CI: 1.24, 3.02) in abnormal uric acid; 1.85 (95% CI: 1.21, 2.83) in abnormal ALT and 6.55 (95% CI: 1.86, 23.06) in abnormal creatinine. After adjusting for age and sex, the odds ratios that were significant for metabolic syndrome were 0.60 (95% CI: 0.38, 0.94) in better income, 0.46 (95% CI: 0.26, 0.83) in better education, 2.21 (95% CI: 1.22, 4.00) in betel nut chewing, 2.31 (95% CI: 1.43, 3.74) in abnormal uric acid, 1.68 (95% CI: 1.09, 2.61) in abnormal AST, 2.32 (95% CI: 1.65, 3.97) in abnormal ALT, 2.56 (95% CI: 1.65, 3.97) in abnormal $\gamma$-GT and 4.82 (95% CI: 1.33, 17.40) in abnormal creatinine. We built multiple logistic regression models and found that the models showed ORs that were significant for metabolic syndrome were 1.03 (95% CI: 1.01, 1.04) in older age, 0.44 (95% CI: 0.24, 0.83) in better education, 2.06 (95% CI: 1.22, 3.48) in abnormal uric acid, 2.02 (95% CI: 1.24, 3.29) in abnormal ALT, 1.86 (95% CI: 1.13, 3.07) in abnormal $\gamma$-GT and 5.38 (95% CI: 1.25, 23.10) in abnormal creatinine.

Table 3. Results of univariate and multivariate regression models on possible variants comparing those with and without metabolic syndrome.

| Variables | Model 1 Univariate Regression | | | Model 2 Univariate Regression, Adjusted for Age and Gender | | | Model 3 Multivariate Regression, Adjusted for Age and Gender | | |
|---|---|---|---|---|---|---|---|---|---|
| | OR | (95% CI) | p-Value | aOR | (95% CI) | p-Value | aOR (n = 524) | (95% CI) | p-Value |
| Gender | | | | | | | | | |
| Female | 1.00 | Ref. | | 1.00 | Ref. | | 1.00 | Ref. | |
| Male | 0.88 | (0.62, 1.25) | 0.4728 | 0.81 | (0.57, 1.17) | 0.2587 | 0.76 | (0.50, 1.16) | 0.2029 |
| Age | 1.03 | (1.02, 1.04) | <0.0001 | 1.03 | (1.02, 1.04) | <.0001 | 1.03 | (1.01, 1.04) | 0.0006 * |
| Age (years old) | | | | | | | | | |
| <30 | 1.00 | Ref. | | | | | | | |
| 30–39 | 2.12 | (0.96, 4.71) | 0.0648 | | | | | | |
| 40–49 | 4.99 | (2.29, 10.90) | <0.0001 | | | | | | |
| 50–59 | 5.99 | (2.74, 13.11) | <0.0001 | | | | | | |
| 60–69 | 7.47 | (3.39, 16.48) | <0.0001 | | | | | | |
| ≥70 | 4.52 | (1.96, 10.45) | 0.0004 * | | | | | | |
| Income (NTD, New Taiwan Dollars) | | | | | | | | | |
| <10,000 | 1.00 | Ref. | | 1.00 | Ref. | | | | |
| 10,000–29,999 | 0.47 | (0.31, 0.73) | 0.0006 * | 0.60 | (0.38, 0.94) | 0.0254 * | | | |
| >30,000 | 0.44 | (0.22, 0.88) | 0.0207 * | 0.58 | (0.28, 1.17) | 0.1273 | | | |
| Education | | | | | | | | | |
| ≤6 years | 1.00 | Ref. | | 1.00 | Ref. | | 1.00 | Ref. | |
| 7–9 years | 0.48 | (0.30, 0.76) | 0.0018 * | 0.68 | (0.40, 1.15) | 0.1538 | 0.59 | (0.34, 1.04) | 0.0676 |
| 10–12 years | 0.32 | (0.19, 0.54) | <0.0001 | 0.46 | (0.26, 0.83) | 0.0100 * | 0.44 | (0.24, 0.83) | 0.0103 * |
| >12 years | 0.33 | (0.14, 0.79) | 0.0126 * | 0.55 | (0.21, 1.41) | 0.2127 | 0.73 | (0.27, 1.97) | 0.5380 |

Table 3. Cont.

| Variables | Model 1 Univariate Regression | | | Model 2 Univariate Regression, Adjusted for Age and Gender | | | Model 3 Multivariate Regression, Adjusted for Age and Gender | | |
|---|---|---|---|---|---|---|---|---|---|
| | OR | (95% CI) | p-Value | aOR | (95% CI) | p-Value | aOR (n = 524) | (95% CI) | p-Value |
| Current cigarette smoker | | | | | | | | | |
| No | 1.00 | Ref. | | 1.00 | Ref. | | | | |
| Yes | 1.03 | (0.66, 1.61) | 0.9000 | 1.39 | (0.86, 2.23) | 0.1806 | | | |
| Alcohol drinking habit | | | | | | | | | |
| No | 1.00 | Ref. | | 1.00 | Ref. | | | | |
| Yes | 1.30 | (0.86, 1.96) | 0.2081 | 1.51 | (0.99, 2.31) | 0.0558 | | | |
| Betel nut chewing habit | | | | | | | | | |
| No | 1.00 | Ref. | | 1.00 | Ref. | | 1.00 | Ref. | |
| Yes | 1.52 | (0.87, 2.65) | 0.1432 | 2.21 | (1.22, 4.00) | 0.0087 * | 1.64 | (0.86, 3.13) | 0.1358 |
| Uric acid | | | | | | | | | |
| Normal | 1.00 | Ref. | | 1.00 | Ref. | | 1.00 | Ref. | |
| Abnormal (>8 mg/dL) | 1.93 | (1.24, 3.02) | 0.0039 * | 2.31 | (1.43, 3.74) | 0.0007 * | 2.06 | (1.22, 3.48) | 0.0071 * |
| Total cholesterol | | | | | | | | | |
| Normal | 1.00 | Ref. | | 1.00 | Ref. | | | | |
| Abnormal (≥200 mg/dL) | 1.65 | (1.16, 2.34) | 0.0052 * | 1.47 | (1.02, 2.12) | 0.0367 * | | | |
| AST | | | | | | | | | |
| Normal | 1.00 | Ref. | | 1.00 | Ref. | | | | |
| Abnormal (>34 U/L) | 1.47 | (0.96, 2.24) | 0.0756 | 1.68 | (1.09, 2.61) | 0.0199 * | | | |
| ALT | | | | | | | | | |
| Normal | 1.00 | Ref. | | 1.00 | Ref. | | 1.00 | Ref. | |
| Abnormal (>36 U/L) | 1.85 | (1.21, 2.83) | 0.0043 * | 2.32 | (1.49, 3.62) | 0.0002 * | 2.02 | (1.24, 3.29) | 0.0046 * |
| γ-GT | | | | | | | | | |
| Normal | 1.00 | Ref. | | 1.00 | Ref. | | 1.00 | Ref. | |
| Abnormal (Male > 71 or female > 42 U/L) | 2.06 | (1.36, 3.11) | 0.0006 * | 2.56 | (1.65, 3.97) | <0.0001 | 1.86 | (1.13, 3.07) | 0.0144 * |

Table 3. Cont.

| Variables | Model 1 Univariate Regression | | | Model 2 Univariate Regression, Adjusted for Age and Gender | | | Model 3 Multivariate Regression, Adjusted for Age and Gender | | |
|---|---|---|---|---|---|---|---|---|---|
| | OR | (95% CI) | $p$-Value | aOR | (95% CI) | $p$-Value | aOR ($n$ = 524) | (95% CI) | $p$-Value |
| Creatinine | | | | | | | | | |
| Normal | 1.00 | Ref. | | 1.00 | Ref. | | 1.00 | Ref. | |
| Abnormal (Male > 1.27 or female > 1.02 mg/dL) | 6.55 | (1.86, 23.06) | 0.0035 * | 4.82 | (1.33, 17.40) | 0.0164 * | 5.38 | (1.25, 23.10) | 0.0237 * |
| Hepatitis B surface antigen (HBsAg) | | | | | | | | | |
| Negative | 1.00 | Ref. | | 1.00 | Ref. | | | | |
| Positive | 0.77 | (0.49, 1.23) | 0.2726 | 0.79 | (0.49, 1.26) | 0.3163 | | | |
| Anti-HCV antibody | | | | | | | | | |
| Negative | 1.00 | Ref. | | 1.00 | Ref. | | | | |
| Positive | 1.75 | (0.80, 3.81) | 0.1619 | 1.52 | (0.68, 3.37) | 0.3048 | | | |

* $p$-Value < 0.05.

## 4. Discussion

### 4.1. Metabolic Syndrome

The prevalence rate of metabolic syndrome was 42.9% in the indigenous group we observed, with 41.3% in males and 44.4% in females. We performed a standardized method using the WHO 2000 population for prevalence comparison and the standardized prevalence rate of metabolic syndrome was 30.0%, with 31.9% in males and 28.3% in females. The prevalence rate was higher than that of urban Taiwanese based on recent studies with 28.6% in males and 18.8% in females [5], or similar with that of 32.4% in males and 27.8% in females [6].

A previous cross-sectional study conducted in 2008 focusing on an indigenous population ($n = 725$) in middle Taiwan showed that the prevalence rate of metabolic syndrome was 42.6%, with 41.5% in males and 43.5% in females [10]. This study showed a similar prevalence rate of metabolic syndrome with our study. Another study conducted in 2007 found that the prevalence rate of metabolic syndrome in aborigines ($n = 90$) in southern Taiwan was 83.3% (64.0% in males, 90.8% in females), which was higher than urban Taiwanese (46.6% and 40.6%, respectively) [9]. Another hospital-based study conducted in 2008 found that the prevalence rate of metabolic syndrome among indigenous people ($n = 1226$) in southeastern Taiwan was 58.7% (50.3% in males, 68.5% in females) [11].

Studies focusing on the indigenous population in other countries also showed the trend of higher prevalence rates of metabolic syndrome compared with other ethnic groups. The prevalence rate ranged from 21.4% to 37.2% in a Canadian study [8]. They suggested that the results in the indigenous community indicated that MetS was inversely associated with physical activity and fitness.

### 4.2. Substance Use

The prevalence rates for substance usage investigated by the Health Promotion Administration of Taiwan was 18.7% for smoking in 2012 and 7.8% for betel nut chewing in 2009. The prevalence rates of alcohol drinking habits among urban Taiwanese ranged from 5.6% to 8.3% [16–18]. The standardized prevalence rate of smoking, alcohol drinking and betel nut chewing in the indigenous group we addressed were 33.3% (male 45.3%, female 25.9%), 36.7% (male 39.1%, female 35.0%) and 18.0% (male 31.9%, female 10.0%), respectively, which were all higher than that in urban Taiwanese. Comparing the three studies from the urban cities of northern, middle and southern Taiwan, we found that the overall prevalence of substance usage was higher in this indigenous group, especially in the females.

The prevalence rate of smoking among the indigenous group has been described in previous studies with 71.1% in males and 25.2% in females [19], 58.7% in males [20] and 33.3% overall [21], which were similar results compared with our study.

The higher prevalence rate of alcohol drinking and alcohol drinking habits among indigenous groups was observed from previous studies. The results from a few studies even found that the overall prevalence rate of alcohol drinking was 85.5% in males and 58.0% in females in an indigenous group of northern Taiwan [19] and 78.6% in males in an indigenous group of middle Taiwan [20]. Another study showed that the prevalence rates of alcohol drinking among northern, southern and eastern indigenous groups in Taiwan were 22.1%, 20.3% and 25.8%, respectively [16]. These results varied due to a different definition of an alcohol drinking habit; however, a higher prevalence rate of alcohol drinking in indigenous groups was observed.

The prevalence rates of betel nut chewing were 49.7% in males and 6.3% in females in an indigenous group of northern Taiwan [19] and 48.9% in males in an indigenous group of middle Taiwan [20]. Another study showed that the prevalence rates of alcohol drinking among northern, southern and eastern indigenous groups in Taiwan were 24.1%, 33.0% and 54.2%, respectively [16]. It seems that the prevalence rate of betel nut chewing was lower than other indigenous groups and the possible reasons need further investigation.

Previous studies have proved that smoking is related to atherosclerotic CVD, neoplastic, respiratory, osteoporosis and all-cause mortality [22]. An increased risk of metabolic syndrome among current smokers, particularly those with a heavier consumption, has also been reported [23]. Alcohol drinking has also been reported as a significant contributing factor to medical conditions such as hepatitis, hypertension, tuberculosis, pneumonia, pancreatitis and cardiomyopathy [24]. Heavy drinking, in particular among liquor drinkers, is associated with an increased risk of metabolic syndrome by influencing its components [25]. A previous systemic review found that betel nut chewing was a significant risk factor for metabolic syndrome [26]. Another study found that both raw areca nuts and those with tobacco additives had a harmful relationship with metabolic syndrome [27]. Although the exact mechanism that links betel nut chewing with metabolic syndrome remains unclear, a meta-analysis proposed that the link might be related to the effect on inflammation, on adipogenesis and on appetite [28].

As the prevalence rates of metabolic syndrome and substance usage were higher than urban Taiwanese, we would like to know if substance usage was one of the confounding factors to metabolic syndrome in this indigenous group. Therefore, we built regression models to observe the trend. After adjusting for age and gender, we found that in this indigenous group, betel nut chewing was one of the confounding factors rather than smoking or alcohol drinking, which was different from previous studies. A better income and better education were indicators of a lower risk of suffering from metabolic syndrome. A cross-sectional study [10] that involved 725 indigenous residents in middle Taiwan conducted in 2008 showed similar results in that the significant confounding factors for metabolic syndrome were being aged 41–64 years old with OR = 1.81 (95% CI: 1.14, 2.88), education level at elementary school with OR = 1.61 (95% CI: 1.07, 2.42), an alcohol drinking habit with OR = 1.42 (95% CI: 0.99, 2.06) and a betel nut chewing habit with OR = 1.59 (95% CI: 1.03, 2.47).

*4.3. Biochemical Parameters of MetS*

With regard to biochemical parameters, the model was significant in the abnormal uric acid level with OR = 2.31 (95% CI: 1.43, 3.74), the elevated AST level with OR = 1.68 (95% CI: 1.09, 2.61), an abnormal ALT level with OR = 2.32 (95% CI: 1.65, 3.97), an abnormal $\gamma$-GT level with OR = 2.56 (95% CI: 1.65, 3.97) and an abnormal creatinine level with OR = 4.82 (95% CI: 1.33, 17.40).

Furthermore, the multiple logistic regression model was significant in older age with OR = 1.03 (95% CI: 1.01, 1.04), better education with OR = 0.44 (95% CI: 0.24, 0.83), abnormal uric acid levels with OR = 2.06 (95% CI: 1.22, 3.48), abnormal ALT levels with OR = 2.02 (95% CI: 1.24, 3.29), abnormal $\gamma$-GT levels with OR = 1.86 (95% CI: 1.13, 3.07) and abnormal creatinine levels with OR = 5.38 (95% CI: 1.25, 23.10). Aging has been suggested to be one of the major confounding factors for metabolic syndrome [29] and this was also proved to be one of the significant confounding factors in our study. The different prevalence rates of metabolic syndrome among men and women differs from studies [30–32]. Although a few studies in Taiwan have suggested a higher prevalence rate in men [33,34], we found that there was no significant difference in the indigenous population we observed. A similar finding from other indigenous populations [10] suggested that the growing prevalence among women was not only found worldwide [35] but was especially obvious in the indigenous population in Taiwan.

In this indigenous group, we observed that elevated uric acid levels, ALT levels, $\gamma$-GT levels and creatinine levels were related to metabolic syndrome. Recent studies have provided new insights into the mechanisms by which uric acid stimulates fat accumulation in the liver. Therefore, elevated serum uric acid is a strong predictor of the development of a fatty liver as well as metabolic syndrome [36]. Uric acid levels are associated with parameters of insulin resistance and indices of inflammation; however, uric acid levels do not predict the incidence of metabolic syndrome independently [37]. Another study also concluded that the elevation of ALT levels especially in obese groups reflected insulin resistance and could be a marker of metabolic syndrome [38]. A study focusing on an indigenous group also found that an elevated $\gamma$-GT level was associated with a higher waist circumference and triglyceride levels, which was also highly associated with metabolic syndrome [39]. Metabolic syndrome was suggested to be an important risk factor for chronic kidney disease [40]; however, other studies have suggested that low serum creatinine is a predictor of type 2 DM and metabolic syndrome [41].

## 5. Conclusions

Our study demonstrated that the prevalence rates of metabolic syndrome and substance use were higher in the indigenous population compared with urban Taiwanese and especially in females. Metabolic syndrome has been demonstrated to be a common precursor to the development of type 2 DM and CVD [3] as well as a risk factor for all-cause mortality [4]. We found that metabolic syndrome in this indigenous population was associated with their education level, income and biochemical parameters such as uric acid, ALT, γ-GT and creatinine levels. Therefore, we conclude that the relative lower education level, income and medical inequality could be the possible contributing factors for metabolic syndrome in this indigenous population.

This study provided us with more thorough information about the health condition and lifestyle of this indigenous group so that we can arrange further intervention programs to improve indigenous health care in clinical practice.

**Author Contributions:** Conceptualization, Y.-H.C. and J.-Y.C.; methodology, W.-C.Y. and J.-Y.C.; software, S.Y.-H.C. and J.-Y.C.; validation, S.W.-N.U. and J.-Y.C.; formal analysis, S.Y.-H.C. and J.-Y.C.; investigation, Y.-C.T., W.-C.L. and J.-Y.C.; resources, W.-C.L. and J.-Y.C.; data curation, Y.-C.T. and J.-Y.C.; writing—original draft preparation, Y.-C.T.; writing—review and editing, Y.-C.T.; visualization, J.-Y.C.; supervision, S.W.-N.U. and J.-Y.C.; project administration, S.Y.-H.C. and J.-Y.C.; funding acquisition, Y.-C.T. and J.-Y.C. All authors have read and agreed to the published version of the manuscript.

**Funding:** We appreciate Chang Gung Memorial Hospital (grants CMRPG3F0761, CMRPG3F0762, CMRPG3F0763) for supporting this study.

**Acknowledgments:** We are grateful to Yang-Wei Gao of Gao-Yang-Wei Clinic, Ting-Chih Chang, Chia-Chin Lee, Tzu-Han Lin and Cheng-Hsien Kuo for their involvement in data collection.

**Conflicts of Interest:** The authors declare no conflict of interest.

## Abbreviations

CVD, cardiovascular disease; DM, diabetes; ATP III, Adult Treatment Panel III; NCEP, National Cholesterol Education Program; CAP, College of American Pathologists; HDL, high-density lipoprotein cholesterol; ALT, alanine transaminase; AST, aspartate transaminase; γ-GT, Gamma-Glutamyl Transferase; HS-CRP, high sensitive C-reactive protein; HbA1c, glycohemoglobulin; LDL-C, low-density lipoprotein cholesterol; VLDL-C, very-low-density lipoprotein cholesterol.

## References

1. Eckel, R.H.; Alberti, K.G.; Grundy, S.M.; Zimmet, P.Z. The metabolic syndrome. *Lancet* **2010**, *375*, 181–183. [CrossRef]
2. Alberti, K.G.; Eckel, R.H.; Grundy, S.M.; Zimmet, P.Z.; Cleeman, J.I.; Donato, K.A.; Fruchart, J.C.; James, W.P.; Loria, C.M.; Smith, S.C., Jr.; et al. Harmonizing the metabolic syndrome: A joint interim statement of the international diabetes federation task force on epidemiology and prevention; national heart, lung, and blood institute; american heart association; world heart federation; international atherosclerosis society; and international association for the study of obesity. *Circulation* **2009**, *120*, 1640–1645. [PubMed]
3. Grundy, S.M.; Cleeman, J.I.; Daniels, S.R.; Donato, K.A.; Eckel, R.H.; Franklin, B.A.; Gordon, D.J.; Krauss, R.M.; Savage, P.J.; Smith, S.C., Jr.; et al. Diagnosis and management of the metabolic syndrome: An American heart association/national heart, lung, and blood institute scientific statement. *Circulation* **2005**, *112*, 2735–2752. [CrossRef]
4. Wu, S.H.; Liu, Z.; Ho, S.C. Metabolic syndrome and all-cause mortality: A meta-analysis of prospective cohort studies. *Eur. J. Epidemiol.* **2010**, *25*, 375–384. [CrossRef]
5. Lin, I.C.; Yang, Y.W.; Wu, M.F.; Yeh, Y.H.; Liou, J.C.; Lin, Y.L.; Chiang, C.H. The association of metabolic syndrome and its factors with gallstone disease. *BMC Fam. Pract.* **2014**, *15*, 138. [CrossRef]
6. Wu, T.W.; Chan, H.L.; Hung, C.L.; Lu, I.J.; Wang, S.D.; Wang, S.W.; Wu, Y.J.; Wang, L.Y.; Yeh, H.I.; Wei, Y.H.; et al. Differential patterns of effects of age and sex on metabolic syndrome in Taiwan: Implication for the inadequate internal consistency of the current criteria. *Diabetes Res. Clin. Pract.* **2014**, *105*, 239–244. [CrossRef] [PubMed]
7. Pan, W.H.; Yeh, W.T.; Weng, L.C. Epidemiology of metabolic syndrome in Asia. *Asia Pac. J. Clin. Nutr.* **2008**, *17* (Suppl. 1), 37–42. [PubMed]

8. Liu, J.; Young, T.K.; Zinman, B.; Harris, S.B.; Connelly, P.W.; Hanley, A.J. Lifestyle variables, non-traditional cardiovascular risk factors, and the metabolic syndrome in an aboriginal Canadian population. *Obesity* **2006**, *14*, 500–508. [CrossRef] [PubMed]
9. Huang, H.P.; Hsu, H.Y.; Chung, T.C.; Sun, C.A.; Chu, C.M.; Tang, T. An investigation of metabolic syndrome indicators among different ethnic groups—A case study from a health screening in Pingtung area. *Taiwan J. Public Health* **2008**, *27*, 250–258.
10. Hung, L.L.; Hsiu, H.F.; Chen, M.L.; Chang, L.C.; Chen, C.Y.; Chen, C.M. The association between health risk behavior and metabolic syndrome of aborigines in Taiwan. *Taipei City Med. J.* **2010**, *7*, 255–264.
11. Hsiao, Y.C.; Wang, K.; Bair, M.J. Prevalence of obesity and metabolic syndrome in aboriginals in Southeastern Taiwan–A hospital-based study. *J. Intern. Med. Taiwan* **2011**, *22*, 48–56.
12. Robberecht, H.; Hermans, N. Biomarkers of metabolic syndrome: Biochemical background and clinical significance. *Metab. Syndr. Relat. Disord.* **2016**, *14*, 47–93. [CrossRef] [PubMed]
13. Ahmad, O.B.; Boschi-Pinto, C.; Lopez, A.D.; Murray, C.J.; Lozano, R.; Inoue, M. Age standardization of rates: A new who standard. In *GPE Discussion Paper Series: No.31*; World Health Organization: Geneva, Switzerland, 2001.
14. Liu, Y.M.; Chen, S.L.; Yen, A.M.; Chen, H.H. Individual risk prediction model for incident cardiovascular disease: A bayesian clinical reasoning approach. *Int. J. Cardiol.* **2013**, *167*, 2008–2012. [CrossRef] [PubMed]
15. Yen, A.M.; Chen, S.L.; Chiu, S.Y.; Fann, J.C.; Wang, P.E.; Lin, S.C.; Chen, Y.D.; Liao, C.S.; Yeh, Y.P.; Lee, Y.C.; et al. A new insight into fecal hemoglobin concentration-dependent predictor for colorectal neoplasia. *Int. J. Cancer* **2014**, *135*, 1203–1212. [CrossRef]
16. Liang, C.Y.; Chou, T.M.; Ho, P.S.; Shieh, T.Y.; Yang, Y.H. Prevanlence rates of alcohol drinking in Taiwan. *Taiwan J. Oral. Med. Health Sci* **2004**, *20*, 91–104.
17. Kuo, C.J. Prevalence of alcoholism in a primary care setting. *Taiwan. J. Psychiatry* **2005**, *19*, 137–147.
18. Lin, C.Y.; Chen, K.H.; Chang, H.Y.; Tseng, F.Y.; Chen, C.Y. The relationship between the pattern of alcohol consumption and healthcare utilization in Taiwan. *Taiwan J. Public Health* **2014**, *33*, 197–208.
19. Liu, B.H.; Hsieh, S.F.; Chang, S.J.; Ko, Y.C. Prevalence of smoking, drinking and betel quid chewing and related factors among aborigines in Wufeng district. *Gaoxiong Yi Xue Ke Xue Za Zhi* **1994**, *10*, 405–411.
20. Huang, L.L.; Chang, L.C.; Chen, M.L.; Hsi, H.F.; Chen, C.Y. Exploration on health-risk behavior and its related factors in aborigines. *J. Chang Gung Inst. Technol.* **2011**, *14*, 67–77.
21. Yen, L.L.; Pan, L.Y.; Yen, H.W.; Lee, L.A. The smoking status in adults in Taiwan area: Prevalence rates and risk factors. *Chin. J. Public Health* **1994**, *13*, 371–380.
22. Jha, P.; Ramasundarahettige, C.; Landsman, V.; Rostron, B.; Thun, M.; Anderson, R.N.; McAfee, T.; Peto, R. 21st-century hazards of smoking and benefits of cessation in the United States. *N. Engl. J. Med.* **2013**, *368*, 341–350. [CrossRef] [PubMed]
23. de Oliveira Fontes Gasperin, L.; Neuberger, M.; Tichy, A.; Moshammer, H. Cross-sectional association between cigarette smoking and abdominal obesity among Austrian bank employees. *BMJ Open* **2014**, *4*, e004899. [CrossRef]
24. Zaridze, D.; Brennan, P.; Boreham, J.; Boroda, A.; Karpov, R.; Lazarev, A.; Konobeevskaya, I.; Igitov, V.; Terechova, T.; Boffetta, P.; et al. Alcohol and cause-specific mortality in Russia: A retrospective case-control study of 48,557 adult deaths. *Lancet* **2009**, *373*, 2201–2214. [CrossRef]
25. Baik, I.; Shin, C. Prospective study of alcohol consumption and metabolic syndrome. *Am. J. Clin. Nutr.* **2008**, *87*, 1455–1463. [CrossRef] [PubMed]
26. Javed, F.; Al-Hezaimi, K.; Warnakulasuriya, S. Areca-nut chewing habit is a significant risk factor for metabolic syndrome: A systematic review. *J. Nutr. Health Aging* **2012**, *16*, 445–448. [CrossRef] [PubMed]
27. Shafique, K.; Zafar, M.; Ahmed, Z.; Khan, N.A.; Mughal, M.A.; Imtiaz, F. Areca nut chewing and metabolic syndrome: Evidence of a harmful relationship. *Nutr. J.* **2013**, *12*, 67. [CrossRef]
28. Yamada, T.; Hara, K.; Kadowaki, T. Chewing betel quid and the risk of metabolic disease, cardiovascular disease, and all-cause mortality: A meta-analysis. *PLoS ONE* **2013**, *8*, e70679. [CrossRef]
29. Ford, E.S.; Giles, W.H.; Dietz, W.H. Prevalence of the metabolic syndrome among US adults: Findings from the third national health and nutrition examination survey. *JAMA* **2002**, *287*, 356–359. [CrossRef]
30. Fezeu, L.; Balkau, B.; Kengne, A.P.; Sobngwi, E.; Mbanya, J.C. Metabolic syndrome in a Sub-Saharan African setting: Central obesity may be the key determinant. *Atherosclerosis* **2007**, *193*, 70–76. [CrossRef] [PubMed]

31. He, Y.; Jiang, B.; Wang, J.; Feng, K.; Chang, Q.; Zhu, S.; Fan, L.; Li, X.; Hu, F.B. Bmi versus the metabolic syndrome in relation to cardiovascular risk in elderly Chinese individuals. *Diabetes Care* **2007**, *30*, 2128–2134. [CrossRef]
32. Regitz-Zagrosek, V.; Lehmkuhl, E.; Mahmoodzadeh, S. Gender aspects of the role of the metabolic syndrome as a risk factor for cardiovascular disease. *Gend. Med.* **2007**, *4* (Suppl. B), S162–S177. [CrossRef]
33. Chuang, S.Y.; Chen, C.H.; Chou, P. Prevalence of metabolic syndrome in a large health check-up population in Taiwan. *J. Chin. Med. Assoc.* **2004**, *67*, 611–620.
34. Hwang, L.C.; Bai, C.H.; Chen, C.J.; Chien, K.L. Gender difference on the development of metabolic syndrome: A population-based study in Taiwan. *Eur. J. Epidemiol.* **2007**, *22*, 899–906. [CrossRef] [PubMed]
35. Ford, E.S.; Giles, W.H.; Mokdad, A.H. Increasing prevalence of the metabolic syndrome among U.S. Adults. *Diabetes Care* **2004**, *27*, 2444–2449. [CrossRef] [PubMed]
36. Choi, Y.-J.; Shin, H.-S.; Choi, H.S.; Park, J.-W.; Jo, I.; Oh, E.-S.; Lee, K.-Y.; Lee, B.-H.; Johnson, R.J.; Kang, D.-H. Uric acid induces fat accumulation via generation of endoplasmic reticulum stress and SREBP-1c activation in hepatocytes. *Lab. Investig.* **2014**, *94*, 1114–1125. [CrossRef] [PubMed]
37. Ferrara, L.A.; Wang, H.; Umans, J.G.; Franceschini, N.; Jolly, S.; Lee, E.T.; Yeh, J.; Devereux, R.B.; Howard, B.V.; De Simone, G. Serum uric acid does not predict incident metabolic syndrome in a population with high prevalence of obesity. *Nutr. Metab. Cardiovasc. Dis.* **2014**, *24*, 1360–1364. [CrossRef] [PubMed]
38. Abe, Y.; Kikuchi, T.; Nagasaki, K.; Hiura, M.; Tanaka, Y.; Ogawa, Y.; Uchiyama, M. Usefulness of gpt for diagnosis of metabolic syndrome in obese Japanese children. *J. Atheroscler. Thromb.* **2009**, *16*, 902–909. [CrossRef]
39. Ho, C.I.; Tsao, Y.C.; Chen, J.Y.; Chang, K.C.; Tsai, Y.W.; Lin, J.S.; Chang, S.S. Gamma-glutamyl transpeptidase and the metabolic syndrome in a Taiwanese aboriginal population. *Int. J. Diabetes Dev. Ctries.* **2013**, *33*, 147–154. [CrossRef]
40. Chen, J.; Gu, D.; Chen, C.S.; Wu, X.; Hamm, L.L.; Muntner, P.; Batuman, V.; Lee, C.H.; Whelton, P.K.; He, J. Association between the metabolic syndrome and chronic kidney disease in Chinese adults. *Nephrol. Dial. Transpl.* **2007**, *22*, 1100–1106. [CrossRef]
41. Hjelmesaeth, J.; Roislien, J.; Nordstrand, N.; Hofso, D.; Hager, H.; Hartmann, A. Low serum creatinine is associated with type 2 diabetes in morbidly obese women and men: A cross-sectional study. *BMC Endocr. Disord.* **2010**, *10*, 6. [CrossRef]

**Publisher's Note:** MDPI stays neutral with regard to jurisdictional claims in published maps and institutional affiliations.

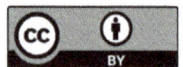

© 2020 by the authors. Licensee MDPI, Basel, Switzerland. This article is an open access article distributed under the terms and conditions of the Creative Commons Attribution (CC BY) license (http://creativecommons.org/licenses/by/4.0/).

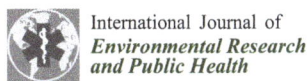 

Article

# High-Sensitivity C-Reactive Protein Elevation Is Independently Associated with Subclinical Renal Impairment in the Middle-Aged and Elderly Population—A Community-Based Study in Northern Taiwan

Hai-Hua Chuang [1,2,3,4], Rong-Ho Lin [3], Wen-Cheng Li [1], Wei-Chung Yeh [1], Yen-An Lin [1] and Jau-Yuan Chen [1,2,*]

1. Department of Family Medicine, Chang-Gung Memorial Hospital, Taipei & Linkou Branch, Taoyuan 33305, Taiwan; chhaihua@gmail.com (H.-H.C.); 620313@cgmh.org.tw (W.-C.L.); sendoh777777@gmail.com (W.-C.Y.); s19401044@gmail.com (Y.-A.L.)
2. College of Medicine, Chang Gung University, Taoyuan 33302, Taiwan
3. Department of Industrial Engineering and Management, National Taipei University of Technology, Taipei 10608, Taiwan; rhlin@mail.ntut.edu.tw
4. Obesity Institute & Genomic Medicine Institute, Geisinger, Danville, PA 17822, USA
* Correspondence: welins@cgmh.org.tw; Tel.: +886-97-536-2672

Received: 1 July 2020; Accepted: 6 August 2020; Published: 13 August 2020

**Abstract:** This cross-sectional study aimed to investigate the associations between high-sensitivity C-reactive protein (hs-CRP) and renal impairment (RI) among middle-aged and elderly people. We collected and analyzed demographic, anthropometric, metabolic, and renal function data in a community-based population in Northern Taiwan. We excluded subjects with acute inflammation from this study and defined RI as the presence of urinary albumin–creatinine ratio 30–300 mg/g or an estimated glomerular filtration rate of <60 mL/min/1.73 m$^2$. There were 131, 125, and 125 participants in the low (≤0.80 mg/L), middle (0.81–1.76 mg/L), and high (>1.77 mg/L) hs-CRP tertiles, respectively. hs-CRP exhibited significantly positive correlations with body mass index, waist circumference, systolic blood pressure, triglyceride, and fasting plasma glucose, and a negative correlation with high-density lipoprotein. The prevalence and odds ratio of RI significantly increased across hs-CRP tertiles from low to high, and this trend remained significant after adjusting for the conventional cardiometabolic risk factors. hs-CRP ≥ 1.61 mg/L in the total group and ≥2.03 mg/L in the elderly group accurately predicted RI ($p$ = 0.01 and 0.03, respectively). These findings suggest that we should carefully evaluate the renal function for at-risk individuals with hs-CRP elevation.

**Keywords:** cardiometabolic risk factors; chronic kidney disease; community medicine; high-sensitivity C-reactive protein; renal impairment

## 1. Introduction

High-sensitivity C-reactive protein (hs-CRP) is considered to be an indicator of systemic inflammation. hs-CRP is also elevated in patients with cardiometabolic risk factors such as metabolic syndrome (MetS) and its components, including obesity, elevated blood pressure, dyslipidemia, and hyperglycemia [1,2].

Renal impairment (RI) is one of the major complications in patients with the abovementioned cardiometabolic risk factors [3]. As the disease progresses, mild and subclinical RI eventually develop into chronic kidney disease (CKD) or even end-stage renal disease (ESRD), which leads to a compromised quality of life and shortened life expectancy of the patients, consequently resulting in a heavy socioeconomic burden. CKD is an increasingly prevalent condition that is estimated to affect

10–12% of the global population, and is recognized as a public health priority [4]. While the prevalence of ESRD in Taiwan is the highest in the world, the prevalence of CKD is also considerably high: 11.93% among adults of all ages (≥20 years old) and 37.2% in the elderly population (≥65 years old). Early intervention of CKD results in better health outcomes and lower medical costs. Unfortunately, most patients are not diagnosed and treated until they reach later stages of the disease.

The pathophysiology of renal function decline in patients with cardiometabolic risk factors is multifactorial, and one of the proposed mechanisms is through systemic inflammation associated with insulin resistance [5,6]. As a surrogate marker of systemic inflammation, hs-CRP is suggested to be linked to CKD in the literature [7,8]. However, the relationship between hs-CRP and subclinical RI in the middle-aged and elderly population in Taiwan is not yet well established.

We hypothesized that, in addition to being positively associated with cardiometabolic risk factors, hs-CRP was positively and independently associated with subclinical RI. The aim of the present study was to assess the associations between hs-CRP, cardiometabolic risk factors, and subclinical RI in a middle-aged and elderly population in Taiwan.

## 2. Materials and Methods

### 2.1. Study Design and Subjects

This was a cross-sectional quantitative study. Data for this study were collected from a community-based health promotion project "Health Screening in the Middle-elderly and Health Promotion Effectiveness of Intervention in Guishan Township, Taoyuan County". The project was conducted from March to August 2014 by a medical center in northern Taiwan to its nearby communities. The project was approved by Chang Gung Medical Foundation Institutional Review Board on 2013/08/16 (102-2304B). Residents older than 50 years of age were recruited and completed a questionnaire during a face-to-face interview. Each subject was enrolled voluntarily and provided written informed consent [1]. The inclusion criteria were: (a) age ≥50 years; (b) having enough ability to complete a questionnaire; and (c) residents had lived in the community for ≥6 months. The exclusion criteria were: (a) having a history of recent cardiovascular disease (CVD); (b) outliers of hs-CRP; and (c) declining to participate (Figure 1).

### 2.2. Data Collection and Parameter Measurements

Data collection included background information, medical history, anthropometric measurements, metabolic profiles, renal function studies, and inflammatory markers. Background information included age, sex, alcohol consumption, smoking status, marital status, Chinese herb use, nonsteroidal anti-inflammatory drug (NSAID) use, hypertension, diabetes mellitus, and hyperlipidemia. Anthropometric measurements included body height (BH), body weight (BW), and waist circumference (WC). Body mass index (BMI) was calculated as the ratio between BW and BH in meters squared ($kg/m^2$). Metabolic profiles included blood pressure (BP), lipid profile (total cholesterol; TC), low-density lipoprotein (LDL), high-density lipoprotein (HDL), triglycerides (TGs), and fasting plasma glucose (FPG). The renal function study measured the serum creatinine and urine albumin/creatinine ratio (ACR). The inflammatory marker was hs-CRP. To exclude acute inflammation from this study, we further excluded subjected with hs-CRP > 10 mg/L [9].

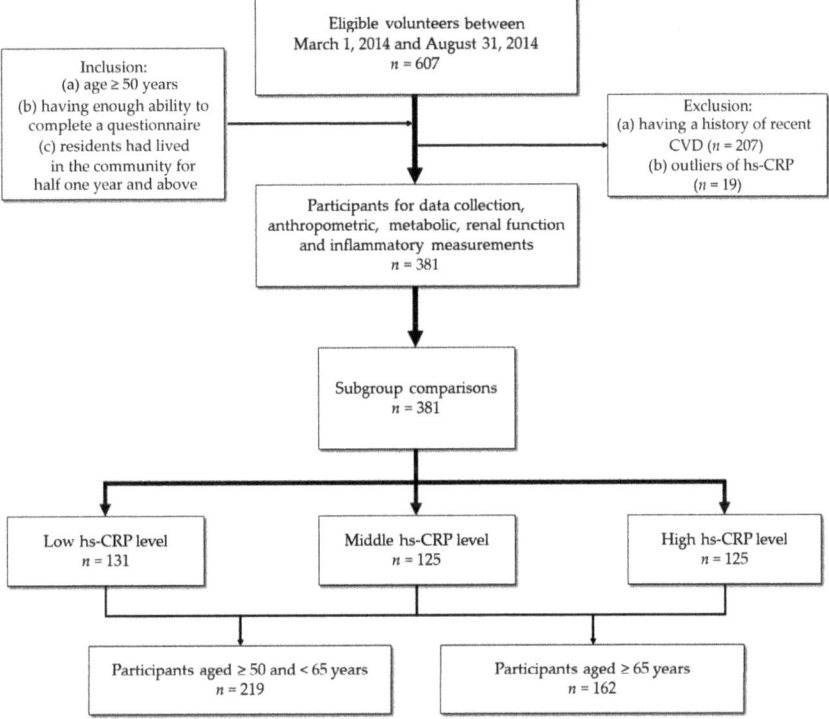

**Figure 1.** Study flow chart. Initially, we recruited 607 eligible volunteers to participate in a community health promotion project; however, we excluded 11 cases with a history of recent cardiovascular disease (CVD), 19 outliers of high-sensitivity C-reactive protein (hs-CRP) (>10 mg/L), and 196 that declined to participate; therefore, we statistically analyzed 381 participants in the present study.

### 2.3. Definition of Renal Impairment (RI)

The estimated glomerular filtration rate (eGFR) was calculated using a modified version of the Modification of Diet in Renal Disease equation for Chinese CKD patients: $175 \times (\text{creatinine})^{-1.234} \times (\text{age})^{-0.179} \times 0.79$ (for females). RI was defined as the presence of kidney damage (urine ACR ≥ 30 mg/g and <300 mg/g) or decreased renal function with eGFR < 60 mL/min/1.73 m$^2$. We chose subclinical RI as the term for our main outcome of interest instead of CKD, since this was a cross-sectional study, and it might not have been correct to make a diagnosis of CKD based on a one-time urine and blood test from the subjects.

### 2.4. Statistical Analysis

Statistical analysis was conducted using SPSS Statistics Version 22 (IBM, SPSS, Armonk, NY, USA). A $p$-value < 0.05 was considered statistically significant. Most of the distributions of the variables were non-normal, assessed using the Kolmogorov–Smirnov test.

Subjects were stratified into tertiles according to hs-CRP levels. Clinical characteristics were compared among tertiles using one-way analysis of variance (one-way ANOVA) for continuous variables and chi-square test for categorical variables. The correlation between hs-CRP and cardiometabolic risk factors was examined with Spearman's correlation test. The association between tertiles of hs-CRP and RI was analyzed using multiple logistic regression; model 1 was unadjusted; model 2 was adjusted for age and sex; and model 3 was adjusted for age, sex, smoking, BMI, systolic BP, LDL, FPG, Chinese herb use, and NSAID use. The Cochran–Armitage trend test was used to evaluate the increasing prevalence of RI as a function of hs-CRP level tertiles. Areas under the receiver operating characteristic curve (AUCs) were used to examine the ability of hs-CRP to predict RI, and the optimized cutoff points for hs-CRP, sensitivity, and specificity were acquired using the maximal Youden Index.

## 3. Results

### 3.1. General Characteristics of the Study Population according to Tertiles of hs-CRP Levels

There were 607 eligible volunteers who attended the community screening, among whom 11, 19, and 196 were excluded due to recent CVD, extreme values of hs-CRP, and declining to participate, respectively. A final total of 381 subjects, including 134 men and 247 women, with a mean age of 64.55 ± 8.48 years, were enrolled for the analysis. None of the subjects reported symptoms of advanced CKD. Subjects were categorized into tertiles based on their levels of hs-CRP. There were 131, 125, and 125 subjects in the low, middle, and high tertiles, respectively. BMI, WC, SBP, hs-CRP, HDL, LDL, TGs, urinary ACR, and RI were significantly different across the tertiles. There was no significant difference observed for other variables (Table 1).

Table 1. General characteristics of the study population according to tertiles of hs-CRP levels.

| Variables | Total | hs-CRP Levels (mg/dL) | | | p-Value |
| | | Low (≤0.80 mg/L) | Middle (0.81–1.76 mg/L) | High (>1.77 mg/L) | |
| --- | --- | --- | --- | --- | --- |
| | (n = 381) | (n = 131) | (n = 125) | (n = 125) | |
| Age (years) | 64.55 ± 8.48 | 64.47 ± 7.56 | 64.18 ± 8.20 | 65.02 ± 9.63 | 0.73 |
| Middle-aged people, n (%) | 219 (57.5) | 71 (54.2) | 73 (58.4) | 75 (60.0) | 0.62 |
| Men, n (%) | 134 (35.2) | 51 (38.9) | 41 (32.8) | 42 (33.6) | 0.53 |
| Marital status (single), n (%) | 74 (19.4) | 29 (22.1) | 19 (15.2) | 26 (20.8) | 0.33 |
| Current smoking, n (%) | 39 (10.2) | 11 (8.4) | 12 (9.6) | 16 (12.8) | 0.49 |
| BMI (kg/m$^2$) | 24.53 ± 3.52 | 23.45 ± 3.38 | 24.62 ± 3.11 [a] | 25.57 ± 3.75 [a] | <0.001 *** |
| Waist circumference (cm) | 85.04 ± 9.59 | 81.91 ± 8.98 | 85.39 ± 9.09 [a] | 87.98 ± 9.78 [a] | <0.001 *** |
| SBP (mmHg) | 129.60 ± 16.57 | 126.22 ± 16.20 | 131.08 ± 16.26 | 131.66 ± 16.85 [a] | 0.02 * |
| DBP (mmHg) | 77.00 ± 11.44 | 76.26 ± 10.65 | 77.31 ± 11.13 | 77.46 ± 12.54 | 0.66 |
| hs-CRP (mg/L) | 1.76 ± 1.72 | 0.52 ± 0.17 | 1.25 ± 0.29 [a] | 3.57 ± 1.93 [a,b] | <0.001 *** |
| HDL-C (mg/dL) | 54.83 ± 13.85 | 57.92 ± 15.33 | 55.34 ± 13.25 [a] | 51.09 ± 11.92 [a] | <0.001 *** |
| LDL-C (mg/dL) | 118.94 ± 32.04 | 111.77 ± 28.80 | 121.75 ± 32.69 [a] | 123.64 ± 33.51 [a] | 0.01 * |
| TG (mg/dL) | 121.60 ± 65.96 | 112.76 ± 65.70 | 116.11 ± 61.72 | 136.34 ± 68.32 [a,b] | 0.01 * |
| FPG (mg/dL) | 95.94 ± 24.98 | 92.26 ± 15.02 | 97.97 ± 33.45 | 97.77 ± 23.13 | 0.11 |
| Creatinine (mg/dL) | 0.77 ± 0.34 | 0.75 ± 0.31 | 0.77 ± 0.36 | 0.79 ± 0.35 | 0.63 |
| eGFR (mL/min/1.73 m$^2$) | 112.76 ± 32.90 | 115.44 ± 31.42 | 112.71 ± 32.58 | 110.00 ± 34.71 | 0.42 |
| ACR ≥ 30 mg/g, n (%) | 69 (18.1) | 16 (12.2) | 23 (18.4) | 30 (24.0) [a] | 0.05 |
| RI, n (%) | 75 (19.7) | 18 (13.7) | 24 (19.2) | 33 (26.4) [a] | 0.04 * |
| Chinese herb use, n (%) | 31 (8.14) | 14 (10.69) | 7 (5.60) | 10 (8.00) | 0.33 |
| NSAID use, n (%) | 29 (7.61) | 13 (9.92) | 7 (5.60) | 9 (7.20) | 0.42 |
| HTN, n (%) | 192 (50.39) | 62 (47.33) | 59 (47.20) | 71 (56.80) | 0.22 |
| DM, n (%) | 75 (19.69) | 18 (13.74) | 25 (20.00) | 32 (25.60) | 0.06 |
| Hyperlipidemia, n (%) | 249 (65.35) | 77 (58.78) | 83 (66.40) | 89 (71.20) | 0.11 |

Clinical characteristics are expressed as mean ± SD for continuous variables and n (%) for categorical variables. The p-values were derived from one-way analysis of variance (one-way ANOVA) for continuous variables and chi-square test for categorical variables. [a] $p < 0.05$ versus low group; [b] $p < 0.05$ versus middle group in the Bonferroni post hoc comparisons; * $p < 0.05$; *** $p < 0.001$. Abbreviations: SBP, systolic blood pressure; DBP, diastolic blood pressure; BMI, body mass index; ALT, alanine aminotransferase; eGFR, estimated glomerular filtration rate; FPG, fasting plasma glucose; HDL-C, high-density lipoprotein cholesterol; hs-CRP, high-sensitivity C-reactive protein; LDL-C, low-density lipoprotein cholesterol; TG, triglyceride; ACR, albumin to creatinine ratio; RI, renal impairment; NSAID, nonsteroidal anti-inflammatory drug.

Figure 2 demonstrates the prevalence of RI according to tertiles of hs-CRP levels. The prevalence was 13.7%, 19.2%, and 26.4% in the low, middle, and high tertiles, respectively. The trend test and chi-square ($\chi^2$) test were significant.

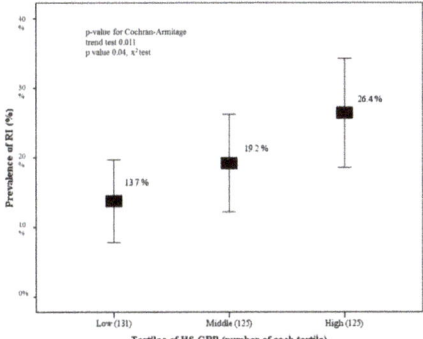

**Figure 2.** Prevalence of RI according to tertiles of hs-CRP levels. There was a modest linearly increasing trend across hs-CRP tertiles.

### 3.2. Correlations Between hs-CRP and Cardiometabolic Risk Factors

hs-CRP had a significant positive correlation with BMI, WC, SBP, FPG, LDL, and TGs. In contrast, hs-CRP and HDL were inversely correlated. After adjusting for age, the aforementioned findings remained significant (Table 2).

**Table 2.** Correlation between hs-CRP and cardiometabolic risk factors.

| | hs-CRP (n = 381) | | | |
|---|---|---|---|---|
| Variables | Unadjusted | | Adjusted for Age | |
| | Spearman's Coefficient | p-Value | Spearman's Coefficient | p-Value |
| Age (years) | −0.02 | 0.74 | NA | NA |
| BMI (kg/m$^2$) | 0.28 | <0.001 *** | 0.23 | <0.001 *** |
| Waist circumference (cm) | 0.30 | <0.001 *** | 0.23 | <0.001 *** |
| SBP (mmHg) | 0.18 | <0.001 *** | 0.12 | 0.03 |
| DBP (mmHg) | 0.06 | 0.22 | 0.06 | 0.26 |
| FPG (mg/dL) | 0.12 | 0.02 * | 0.15 | 0.004 |
| HDL-C (mg/dL) | −0.20 | <0.001 *** | −0.16 | 0.002 |
| LDL-C (mg/dL) | 0.17 | <0.001 *** | 0.10 | 0.05 |
| TG (mg/dL) | 0.25 | <0.001 *** | 0.17 | 0.001 |
| eGFR (mL/min/1.73 m$^2$) | −0.06 | 0.24 | −0.03 | 0.53 |
| ACR (mg/g) | 0.16 | 0.001 ** | 0.11 | 0.03 * |

Abbreviations: SBP, systolic blood pressure; DBP, diastolic blood pressure; BMI, body mass index; FPG, fasting plasma glucose; HDL-C, high-density lipoprotein cholesterol; hs-CRP, high-sensitivity C-reactive protein; LDL-C, low-density lipoprotein cholesterol; TG, triglyceride; eGFR, estimated glomerular filtration rate; ACR, albumin to creatinine ratio; * $p < 0.05$; ** $p < 0.01$; *** $p < 0.001$.

### 3.3. Associations between Tertiles of hs-CRP and RI

The odds ratio (OR) of RI significantly increased in the high tertile using the low tertile as a reference. This finding was significant, with an OR of 2.25 in model 1 (unadjusted), an OR of 2.22 in model 2 (adjusted for age and sex), and an OR of 2.16 in model 3 (adjusted for age, sex, smoking, BMI, SBP, LDL, FPG, Chinese herb use, and NSAID use). Across increasing hs-CRP tertiles, the trend test of increasing RI was also significant in all three models (Table 3).

Table 3. Associations between tertiles of hs-CRP and renal impairment.

| Tertiles of hs-CRP | Model 1 | | | Model 2 | | | Model 3 | | |
|---|---|---|---|---|---|---|---|---|---|
| | OR | (95% CI) | p-Value | OR | (95% CI) | p-Value | OR | (95% CI) | p-Value |
| | | | Tertiles of hs-CRP | | | | | | |
| Low | 1 | - | - | 1 | - | - | 1 | - | - |
| Middle | 1.49 | (0.77–2.91) | 0.24 | 1.52 | (0.78–2.98) | 0.22 | 1.42 | (0.70–2.90) | 0.33 |
| High | 2.25 | (1.19–4.26) | 0.01 * | 2.22 | (1.17–4.23) | 0.02 * | 2.16 | (1.07–4.93) | 0.03 * |
| p-Value for trend | | | 0.01 * | | | 0.02 * | | | 0.03 * |

Model 1: Unadjusted. Model 2: Multiple logistic regression adjusted for age and sex. Model 3: Multiple logistic regression adjusted for factors in model 2 plus smoking, BMI, SBP, LDL, FPG, Chinese herb use, and NSAID use. Abbreviations: hs-CRP, high-sensitivity C-reactive protein; RI, renal impairment; SBP, systolic blood pressure; BMI, body mass index; FPG, fasting plasma glucose; LDL-C, low-density lipoprotein cholesterol; OR, odds ratio; CI, confidence interval; * $p < 0.05$.

Figure 3 demonstrates the receiver operating characteristic curves for hs-CRP to predict RI in the total (Figure 3a), middle-aged (Figure 3b), and elderly (Figure 3c) groups. Table 4 summarizes the areas under the receiver operating characteristic curve (AUCs), sensitivities, and specificities according to the optimized cutoff points of hs-CRP for predicting RI in these three groups. Based on a cutoff point of 1.61 mg/dL, hs-CRP accurately predicted RI in the total group (AUC = 0.60; $p$ = 0.01; sensitivity = 0.56; specificity = 0.66). Although the predictive value of hs-CRP (cutoff point = 2.03 mg/dL) in the elderly group was promising (AUC = 0.62; $p$ = 0.03; sensitivity = 0.46; specificity = 0.82), its predive value (cutoff point = 1.61 mg/dL) was not significant in the middle-aged group (AUC = 0.59; $p$ = 0.09; sensitivity = 0.58; specificity = 0.63).

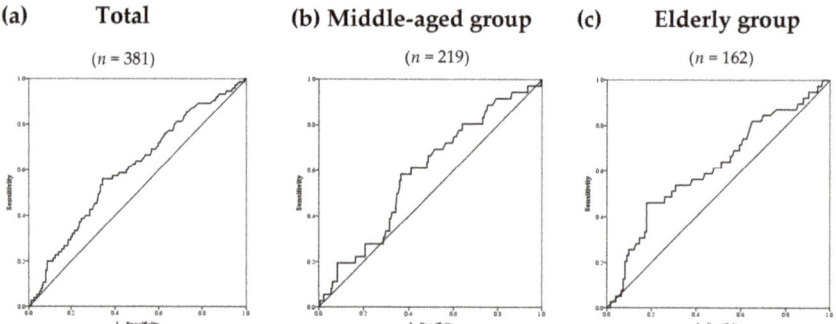

Figure 3. The receiver operating characteristic curves for high-sensitivity C-reactive protein as a predictor of renal impairment in the total group (a), middle-aged group (b), and elderly group (c).

Table 4. Predictive values of hs-CRP for renal impairment in the total, middle-aged, and elderly groups.

| Variables | AUC (95% CI) | p-Value | Cutoff Point | Sensitivity | Specificity |
|---|---|---|---|---|---|
| Total study population ($n$ = 381) | | | | | |
| hs-CRP | 0.60 (0.53–0.67) | 0.01 * | 1.61 mg/dL | 0.56 | 0.66 |
| Middle-aged group (<65 years, $n$ = 219) | | | | | |
| hs-CRP | 0.59 (0.49–0.69) | 0.09 | 1.61 mg/dL | 0.58 | 0.63 |
| Elderly group (≥65 years, $n$ = 162) | | | | | |
| hs-CRP | 0.62 (0.51–0.72) | 0.03 * | 2.03 mg/dL | 0.46 | 0.82 |

Abbreviations: hs-CRP, high-sensitivity C-reactive protein; AUC, area under the receiver operating characteristic curve; * $p < 0.05$.

## 4. Discussion

In our study, hs-CRP was positively associated with conventional cardiometabolic risk factors including BMI, WC, SBP, FPG, LDL, and TGs were negatively associated with HDL. Furthermore, when we divided subjects into tertiles based on hs-CRP levels, the aforementioned variables were significantly different across each group. These findings are compatible with previous reports showing that the level of hs-CRP is highly related to risk factors of cardiovascular diseases (CVD) [10–12].

The results of this study validate our hypothesis; the prevalence of subclinical RI increased across the tertiles of hs-CRP from low to high, and the trend remained significant even after adjusting for many traditional risk factors. Obesity, hypertension, dyslipidemia, and diabetes are well-recognized, major risk factors for kidney damage [13,14]. Diabetic nephropathy is the leading cause of renal failure in many developed countries. However, our study further shows that even after adjusting for conventional risk factors, Chinese herb use, and NSAID use, hs-CRP was independently related to subclinical RI. Notably, hs-CRP was more strongly related to elevated ACR than decreased eGFR and predicted subclinical RI in the elderly population more effectively than in the middle-aged population.

To address the relationship between hs-CRP and subclinical RI, we discuss it from three distinct viewpoints: (1) the biology of hs-CRP as a biomarker of inflammation; (2) the role of chronic inflammation in RI; and (3) the possibility of using hs-CRP in risk stratification for RI. The outcome in this study was RI; however, since CKD is the expected complication when RI lasts over time, we mention both terms frequently as appropriate in the following discussion.

*4.1. Biology of hs-CRP as a Biomarker of Inflammation*

CRP, a member of the pentraxin family, is a ring-shaped protein found in blood plasma that is mainly secreted and released by hepatocytes. CRP is measured as hs-CRP in low-level inflammatory conditions. The production of hs-CRP is triggered by several cytokines, such as interleukin-6 (IL-6). IL-6 is released from activated leukocytes in response to infection or trauma and from vascular smooth muscle cells in response to atherosclerosis [12,15].

hs-CRP is a circulating reactant associated with a wide range of acute and chronic inflammatory conditions. When there is an acute stimulus such as viral or bacterial infection, the level of hs-CRP can increase as much as 100 to 500 mg/L within 4 to 6 h, doubling every 8 h, and can increase up to 10,000-fold in severe cases. The increase in hs-CRP levels tends to be proportional to the intensity of inflammation. hs-CRP levels decrease quickly with a short half-life of approximately 4 to 7 h when inflammation subsides. The above characteristics make hs-CRP a particularly useful clinical biomarker to reflect the presence and degree of inflammation [15,16]. hs-CRP concentrations between 2 and 10 mg/L are considered to indicate metabolic inflammation, which has been postulated as an important pathway linked to atherosclerosis and subsequent CVD. Abundant studies have reported a positive association between hs-CRP level and cardiometabolic risk factors [10,11].

*4.2. Role of Chronic Inflammation in Subclinical RI*

Under normal conditions, inflammation is a protective physiological response to harmful stimuli. However, in conditions such as chronic RI, when inflammation becomes persistent and deregulated, it becomes maladaptive and debilitating [17]. The role of systemic inflammation in chronic RI has been prodigiously investigated, especially in the context of ESRD [18]. Systemic inflammation is considered to be not only a risk factor for mortality but also a catalyst for other complications, and is related to a premature aging phenotype. The pathophysiological mechanisms underlying this process are complicated and intricate, such as premature aging of the immune system, defective regulation of inflammatory processes, abnormalities in mineral metabolism, and gut dysbiosis [19].

The other factor that inflammation and RI are both linked to is atherosclerosis. The concept of inflammation being central to the initiation and progression of atherosclerotic changes is now mature, originating from observations in the 1800s. Atherosclerosis is now considered an inflammatory disease characterized by the progressive accumulation of lipids in the vessel wall [20,21]. Atherosclerosis leads to CVDs such as coronary artery disease, stroke, and peripheral vascular disease [22]. RI, as a common comorbidity among patients with CVD, has been postulated as both a predisposing factor and a consequence of atherosclerosis. RI accelerates atherosclerosis via the augmentation of inflammation, perturbation of lipid metabolism, and other mechanisms [19], which in turn can contribute to the progression of renal decline [13,23].

*4.3. Possibility of Using hs-CRP in Risk Stratification for RI*

Patients with CKD have a considerably higher incidence of CVD events and premature death. A substantial volume of research has focused on finding biomarkers for better risk stratification in this population. hs-CRP is one of the earliest and most frequently used biomarkers. The positive association between hs-CRP level and CVD events, as well as overall morality in CKD patients, is evident [24–26], although some still debate its clinical application [27]. Some other parameters have also been suggested to serve this purpose, such as microalbuminuria, natriuretic peptides, troponins, adiponectin, leptin, phosphorus, parathyroid hormone, vitamin D, fibroblast growth factor 23, and matrix metalloproteinases [27,28].

While the literature extensively addresses hs-CRP for the prediction of outcomes of late-stage CKD patients, there is still limited research on the associations between hs-CRP and mild or early RI. A few studies have reported an inverse association between the hs-CRP level and GFR [29,30]. A recent study has also reported a link between hs-CRP elevation and urinary alpha-1 microglobulin (A1MG), an early sign of renal damage, in type II diabetes patients [31]. Our study provided evidence of the linkage of systemic inflammation and subclinical RI in seemingly healthy middle-aged and elderly community populations. This finding can help clinicians identify patients in need of more aggressive and focused preventive measures to improve future outcomes. Concerning the high prevalence of metabolic syndrome, as well as the high availability and easy interpretation of hs-CRP, this finding has practical clinical application.

The advantages of this study included a clear design, a sufficient sample size, a comprehensive inclusion of relevant confounders, and a well-performed data analysis. The novelty of this study was, from a community approach, to report different cutoff values of hs-CRP among the middle-aged and elderly cohorts to better predict subclinical renal impairment in these two specific age groups. However, the participants in our study were recruited from a few communities in northern Taiwan, and the characteristics of this cohort might differ from those of the general population. A possible selection bias and the single Han ethnicity of the subjects might limit the generalizability of this research. Also, RI was defined using a single urine and blood measurement, based on which the duration and nature of RI were not easy to clarify. Additionally, the study was cross-sectional and thus not able to examine causal relationships. A prospective case–control study is warranted to externally verify our present findings.

## 5. Conclusions

hs-CRP is significantly and independently associated with subclinical RI. Careful evaluation and early intervention should be considered in the middle-aged and elderly population with systemic inflammation and other comorbidities. Future studies with a prospective design will be of interest.

**Author Contributions:** Conceptualization, W.-C.L. and J.-Y.C.; methodology, J.-Y.C.; software, J.-Y.C.; validation, J.-Y.C.; formal analysis, J.-Y.C.; investigation, H.-H.C. and J.-Y.C.; resources, R.-H.L. and J.-Y.C.; data curation, H.-H.C. and J.-Y.C.; writing—original draft preparation, H.-H.C.; writing—review and editing, H.H.C.; visualization, J.-Y.C.; supervision, R.-H.L. and J.-Y.C.; project administration, W.-C.Y., Y.-A.L., and J.-Y.C.; funding acquisition, H.-H.C. and J.-Y.C. All authors have read and agreed to the published version of the manuscript.

**Funding:** This work was supported by Chang Gung Memorial Hospital, grant numbers CORPG3C0171, 3C0172, 3G0021, 3G0022, 3G0023, CZRPG3C0053 (J.Y.C.); CMRPG3F0491, 3F0492, 1H0061, and 1H0062 (H.H.C.).

**Conflicts of Interest:** The authors declare no conflicts of interest.

## References

1. Mazidi, M.; Toth, P.P.; Banach, M. C-reactive Protein is associated with prevalence of the metabolic syndrome, hypertension, and diabetes mellitus in US adults. *Angiology* **2017**, *69*, 438–442. [CrossRef] [PubMed]
2. Abu-Farha, M.; Behbehani, K.; Elkum, N. Comprehensive analysis of circulating adipokines and hsCRP association with cardiovascular disease risk factors and metabolic syndrome in Arabs. *Cardiovasc. Diabetol.* **2014**, *13*, 76. [CrossRef] [PubMed]

3. Thomas, G.; Sehgal, A.R.; Kashyap, S.R.; Srinivas, T.R.; Kirwan, J.P.; Navaneethan, S.D. Metabolic syndrome and kidney disease: A systematic review and meta-analysis. *Clin. J. Am. Soc. Nephrol.* **2011**, *6*, 2364–2373. [CrossRef]
4. Levin, A.; Tonelli, M.; Bonventre, J.; Coresh, J.; Donner, J.-A.; Fogo, A.B.; Fox, C.S.; Gansevoort, R.T.; Heerspink, H.J.L.; Jardine, M.J.; et al. Global kidney health 2017 and beyond: A roadmap for closing gaps in care, research, and policy. *Lancet* **2017**, *390*, 1888–1917. [CrossRef]
5. Banerjee, D.; Recio-Mayoral, A.; Chitalia, N.; Kaski, J.C. insulin resistance, inflammation, and vascular disease in nondiabetic predialysis chronic kidney disease patients. *Clin. Cardiol.* **2011**, *34*, 360–365. [CrossRef]
6. Lin, L.; Peng, K.; Du, R.; Huang, X.; Lu, J.; Xu, Y.; Xu, M.; Chen, Y.; Bi, Y.; Wang, W. Metabolically healthy obesity and incident chronic kidney disease: The role of systemic inflammation in a prospective study. *Obesity* **2017**, *25*, 634–641. [CrossRef]
7. Schei, J.; Stefansson, V.; Eriksen, B.O.; Jenssen, T.G.; Solbu, M.D.; Wilsgaard, T.; Melsom, T. Association of TNF receptor 2 and CRP with GFR decline in the general nondiabetic population. *Clin. J. Am. Soc. Nephrol.* **2017**, *12*, 624–634. [CrossRef] [PubMed]
8. Schei, J.; Stefansson, V.T.; Mathisen, U.D.; Eriksen, B.O.; Solbu, M.D.; Jenssen, T.G.; Melsom, T. Residual associations of inflammatory markers with eGFR after accounting for measured GFR in a community-based cohort without CKD. *Clin. J. Am. Soc. Nephrol.* **2015**, *11*, 280–286. [CrossRef] [PubMed]
9. Duffy, J.R.; Salerno, M. New blood test to measure heart attack risk: C-reactive protein. *J. Cardiovasc. Nurs.* **2004**, *19*, 425–429. [CrossRef]
10. Sigdel, M.; Kumar, A.; Gyawali, P.; Shrestha, R.; Tuladhar, E.T.; Jha, B. Association of high sensitivity C-reactive protein with the components of metabolic syndrome in diabetic and non-diabetic individuals. *J. Clin. Diagn. Res.* **2014**, *8*, CC11–CC13. [CrossRef]
11. Hotamisligil, G.S. Inflammation and metabolic disorders. *Nature* **2006**, *444*, 860–867. [CrossRef] [PubMed]
12. Yousuf, O.; Mohanty, B.D.; Martin, S.S.; Joshi, P.H.; Blaha, M.J.; Nasir, K.; Blumenthal, R.S.; Budoff, M.J. High-sensitivity C-reactive protein and cardiovascular disease. *J. Am. Coll. Cardiol.* **2013**, *62*, 397–408. [CrossRef] [PubMed]
13. Schiffrin, E.L.; Lipman, M.L.; Mann, J.F. Chronic kidney disease. *Circulation* **2007**, *116*, 85–97. [CrossRef]
14. Zammit, A.; Katz, M.J.; Derby, C.; Bitzer, M.; Lipton, R.B. Chronic kidney disease in non-diabetic older adults: Associated roles of the metabolic syndrome, inflammation, and insulin resistance. *PLoS ONE* **2015**, *10*, e0139369. [CrossRef]
15. Thompson, D.; Pepys, M.B.; Wood, S.P. The physiological structure of human C-reactive protein and its complex with phosphocholine. *Structure* **1999**, *7*, 169–177. [CrossRef]
16. Bray, C.; Bell, L.N.; Liang, H.; Haykal, R.; Kaiksow, F.; Mazza, J.J.; Yale, S.H. Erythrocyte sedimentation rate and C-reactive protein measurements and their relevance in clinical medicine. *WMJ Off. Publ. State Med. Soc. Wis.* **2016**, *115*, 317–321.
17. Scrivo, R.; Vasile, M.; Bartosiewicz, I.; Valesini, G. Inflammation as "common soil" of the multifactorial diseases. *Autoimmun. Rev.* **2011**, *10*, 369–374. [CrossRef]
18. Cobo, G.; Lindholm, B.; Stenvinkel, P. Chronic inflammation in end-stage renal disease and dialysis. Nephrology, dialysis, transplantation. *Off. Publ. Eur. Dial. Transpl. Assoc. Eur. Ren. Assoc.* **2018**, *33*, iii35–iii40.
19. Kooman, J.P.; Dekker, M.J.; Usvyat, L.; Kotanko, P.; Van Der Sande, F.M.; Schalkwijk, C.G.; Shiels, P.; Stenvinkel, P. Inflammation and premature aging in advanced chronic kidney disease. *Am. J. Physiol. Physiol.* **2017**, *313*, F938–F950. [CrossRef]
20. Storey, R.H.; Vilahur, G.; Badimon, L. Update on lipids, inflammation and atherothrombosis. *Thromb. Haemost.* **2011**, *105*, S34–S42. [CrossRef]
21. Wong, B.W.; Meredith, A.; Lin, D.; McManus, B.M. The Biological role of inflammation in atherosclerosis. *Can. J. Cardiol.* **2012**, *28*, 631–641. [CrossRef]
22. Gisterå, A.; Hansson, G.K. The immunology of atherosclerosis. *Nat. Rev. Nephrol.* **2017**, *13*, 368–380. [CrossRef] [PubMed]
23. Jara, A.; Mezzano, S. Vascular damage in chronic kidney disease. *Rev. Med. Chile* **2008**, *136*, 1476–1484. [PubMed]
24. Chen, T.; Hassan, H.I.C.; Qian, P.; Vu, M.; Makris, A. High-sensitivity troponin T and C-reactive protein have different prognostic values in hemo and peritoneal dialysis populations: A cohort study. *J. Am. Heart Assoc.* **2018**, *7*, e007876. [CrossRef] [PubMed]

25. Hsu, H.-J.; Yen, C.-H.; Hsu, K.-H.; Wu, I.-W.; Lee, C.-C.; Sun, C.-Y.; Chou, C.-C.; Chen, C.-Y.; Yang, S.-Y.; Tsai, C.-J.; et al. chronic kidney disease stage is a modulator on the association between high-sensitivity C-reactive protein and coronary vasospastic angina. *Sci. World J.* **2014**, *2014*, 1–9. [CrossRef] [PubMed]
26. Dai, L.; Golembiewska, E.; Lindholm, B.; Stenvinkel, P. End-stage renal disease, inflammation and cardiovascular outcomes. *Contrib. Nephrol.* **2017**, *191*, 32–43. [CrossRef]
27. D'marco, L.; Bellasi, A.; Raggi, P. Cardiovascular biomarkers in chronic kidney disease: State of current research and clinical applicability. *Dis. Mark.* **2015**, *2015*, 1–16. [CrossRef]
28. Provenzano, M.; Andreucci, M.; Garofalo, C.; Faga, T.; Ashour, M.; Ielapi, N.; Grande, R.; Sapienza, P.; De Franciscis, S.; Mastroroberto, P.; et al. The association of matrix metalloproteinases with chronic kidney disease and peripheral vascular disease: A light at the end of the tunnel? *Biomolecules* **2020**, *10*, 154. [CrossRef]
29. Amin, H.K.; El-Sayed, M.-I.K.; Leheta, O.F. Homocysteine as a predictive biomarker in early diagnosis of renal failure susceptibility and prognostic diagnosis for end stages renal disease. *Ren. Fail.* **2016**, *38*, 1–9. [CrossRef]
30. Adejumo, O.A.; Okaka, E.I.; Okwuonu, C.G.; Iyawe, I.O.; Odujoko, O.O. Serum C-reactive protein levels in pre-dialysis chronic kidney disease patientsin southern Nigeria. *Ghana Med. J.* **2016**, *50*, 31–38. [CrossRef]
31. Wan, X.; Zhang, L.; Gu, H.; Wang, S.; Liu, X. The Association of serum hsCRP and urinary Alpha1-microglobulin in patients with type 2 diabetes mellitus. *BioMed Res. Int.* **2019**, *2019*, 6364390. [CrossRef] [PubMed]

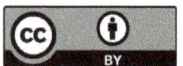

© 2020 by the authors. Licensee MDPI, Basel, Switzerland. This article is an open access article distributed under the terms and conditions of the Creative Commons Attribution (CC BY) license (http://creativecommons.org/licenses/by/4.0/).

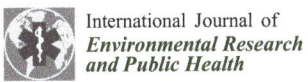

*Article*

# Food Insecurity Is Associated with Depression among a Vulnerable Workforce: Early Care and Education Workers

Ivory H. Loh [1,*], Vanessa M. Oddo [2,3] and Jennifer Otten [1,4]

1. Nutritional Sciences Program, University of Washington School of Public Health, 305 Raitt Hall, P.O. Box 353410, Seattle, WA 98195, USA; jotten@uw.edu
2. Department of Health Services, University of Washington School of Public Health, 1959 NE Pacific St., P.O. Box 357660, Seattle, WA 98195, USA; voddo@uw.edu
3. Department of Kinesiology and Nutrition, University of Illinois Chicago, 1919 West Taylor St., MC 517, Chicago, IL 60612, USA
4. Department of Environmental and Occupational Health Sciences, University of Washington School of Public Health, 1959 NE Pacific St., P.O. Box 353410, Seattle, WA 98195, USA
\* Correspondence: ivoryloh@uw.edu

**Abstract:** *Objective:* We aimed to explore the association between food insecurity and depression among early care and education (ECE) workers, a vulnerable population often working in precarious conditions. *Design:* We utilized cross-sectional data from a study exploring the effects of wage on ECE centers. Participants were enrolled between August 2017 and December 2018. Food insecurity was measured using the validated six-item U.S. Household Food Security Survey Module and participants were categorized as food secure (score = 0–1), low food security (score = 2–4), and very low food security (score = 5–6). Depression (defined as a score ≥ 16) was measured using the 20-item Center for Epidemiologic Studies Depression Scale-Revised. We employed a logistic regression model to examine the relationship between food insecurity and depression. All models controlled for marital status, nativity, race/ethnicity, number of children in the household, job title, weekly hours of work, education, income, and study site. *Setting:* Participants were from Seattle (40%) and South King County (26%), Washington, and Austin, Texas (34%). *Participants:* Participants included 313 ECE workers from 49 ECE centers. *Results:* A majority of participants were female, non-Hispanic White, born in the U.S., and did not have children. Compared to being food secure, very low and low food insecurities were associated with a 4.95 (95% confidence interval (CI): 2.29, 10.67) and 2.69 (95% CI: 1.29, 5.63) higher odds of depression, respectively. *Conclusions:* Policies and center-level interventions that address both food insecurity and depression may be warranted, in order to protect and improve the health of this valuable, yet vulnerable, segment of the U.S. workforce.

**Keywords:** food insecurity; depression; mental health; early care and education; childcare

## 1. Introduction

In 2019, 10.5% of U.S. households (13.7 million households) experienced low or very low food security, defined as households that lack stable access to sufficient food [1]. Of U.S. households with children, 6.5% (2.4 million households) were food insecure in 2019, with very low food secure households reporting that children experienced hunger, skipped a meal, or did not eat for an entire day due to inability to purchase food [1]. Food insecurity is associated with greater depressive symptoms among both the general U.S. population [2–4] and a more vulnerable population: female welfare recipients [5]. Furthermore, food insecurity may contribute to children's self-perceived psychological distress [6]. Prior studies also find high prevalence rates of both food insecurity and depression among the early care and education (ECE) workforce [7–9], a vulnerable population who typically earns low wages, works long hours, and lacks fringe benefits [7,8]. ECE settings include sites in which children younger than age six are cared for by a caregiver other than their parents or primary caregivers and include both center-based (e.g., childcare centers, preschools) and home-based care arrangements (e.g., nanny or babysitting in the child's home) [8,10]. Despite the high prevalence rates of both food insecurity and depression, and the precarious work conditions faced by ECE workers in the U.S., studies have yet to explore the relationship between food insecurity and depression among this population [7].

Several prior studies have examined the relationship between food insecurity and adverse mental health outcomes [11–15], and most report that food insecurity is associated with a higher prevalence of depressive symptoms in the U.S. [2–5,11,16–18]. In particular, a 2019 meta-analysis (N = 57 cross-sectional studies) [12] reported that the odds of depression were 174% higher among those who were food insecure (compared to food secure). Similarly, a longitudinal study reported a dose–response relationship between food insecurity and depressive symptoms and poor mental health, among women at risk of or living with HIV, i.e., women experiencing more severe food insecurity had higher odds of probable depression when compared with food secure women [18]. At the same time, longitudinal analyses suggest that the relationship could be bidirectional, meaning that food insecurity is both associated with depressive symptoms and depressive symptoms are associated with food insecurity [11]. For example, a 2016 analysis using data from the Early Childhood Longitudinal Study—Birth Cohort reported that severe maternal depression was associated with a higher probability of child (79%) and household (69%) food insecurity [4].

There are several mechanisms through which food insecurity might directly be related to mental health. First, food insecurity may act as a stressor, as individuals are plagued with a constant anxiety about household food supply and worried about meeting practical needs [11,15]. Chronic stress has been found to induce physiological changes, including hyper-activation of the hypothalamic-pituitary-adrenal (HPA) axis and increased cortisol levels, that predispose individuals to depression [19]. In addition, the way in which an individual interprets their food insecurity status relative to the psychosocial environment and their social positioning may evoke shame, as well as trigger stress and adverse physiological responses [2]. Food insecurity may also be related to poor mental health by limiting one's ability to consume a nutritious diet [2,20], provide self-care, and/or adhere to medical recommendations [11,15]. Poor self-management of chronic mental and physical health conditions may also increase an individual's health care costs, which, in turn, can lead to additional financial strain, continued food insecurity, and limited access to health care.

Food insecurity may also indirectly harm mental health through participation in food assistance programs. The Supplemental Nutrition Assistance Program (SNAP) is the largest federal food and nutrition assistance program that supports low-income Americans [14]. Although SNAP participation is associated with a significant reduction in both prevalence and severity of food insecurity [14], participation in food assistance programs and the stigma associated with receiving food assistance have been linked to adversely affect mental health [3,5].

The ECE workforce is predominantly female and a particularly vulnerable, yet very important, segment of the U.S. workforce [7,21]. ECE jobs are often precarious or lower quality, characterized by low wages, high stress, long hours, lack of fringe benefits, and short tenure [7,21]. Compared to national averages or women of similar demographics, this workforce has been found to have unhealthier diets, lower rates of physical activity, fewer hours of sleep, and higher rates of depression and diabetes [7,8]. Moreover, this population has a high prevalence of both food insecurity and depression [7–9]. A study in North Carolina found that 36% of ECE workers reported clinically depressive symptoms—about five times the national rate of depression for Americans [7]. Similarly, a 2017 Arkansas workforce study reported that 33% of their sample of ECE teachers were at risk for depression, and 40% reported being food insecure [9]. A 2020 scoping review on the health status of the U.S. ECE workforce and health-promoting interventions targeting this population further validated that this workforce experiences significant mental health challenges, including stress and depression, and has a heightened chronic disease risk due to suboptimal health behaviors, regardless of ECE setting (e.g., federally funded Head Start Programs for low-income households vs. for-profit or non-profit childcare centers) and job title [22].

When examining the ECE workforce beyond the U.S., research shows that workplace stress is common among workers in other countries [22]. ECE workers in other countries, such as Singapore, also experience low pay, high turnover rate, and poor prestige [23]. The policy context for ECE varies by country. The policies, systems, regulations, practices, and culture of ECE within each country, therefore, significantly shape the health and quality of the workforce [24]. For example, the U.S. has a national recommendation on the maximum number of children per staff member based on the age of child, such as 4:1 for children up to 1 year old and 10:1 for children 2 to 5 years old, with regulations enforced by individual states [24]. The Russian Federation, on the other hand, bases its staff-to-child ratio on the available floor space of the ECE center rather than age of child. Nonetheless, there is a growing recognition among governments worldwide on the importance of investing in quality early education through the development of an effective and accessible ECE system with a well-trained and sustainable workforce [24].

The primary objective of this analysis was to explore the association between food insecurity and depression among ECE workers, as prior studies have yet to investigate this association among this high-risk population. Given the prior literature that focuses on female welfare recipients and households with children, we hypothesized that food insecurity will be associated with higher odds of depression among this vulnerable segment of the U.S. workforce. The secondary objective of this analysis was to investigate the extent to which the relationship between food insecurity and depression varied by wages and participation in food assistance programs. A better understanding of this relationship is needed to inform interventions and policies that are designed to improve the health and well-being of the ECE workforce, which may benefit the workers themselves, as well as the children whom they care for [25,26].

## 2. Methods

The cross-sectional data presented in this paper were collected as part of baseline data collection from a 2017–2020 prospective study titled "Exploring the Effects of Wage on the Culture of Health in Early Childhood Education Centers," which explores the effects of wage on early care and education centers in Seattle and South King County, Washington, and Austin, Texas [8,27].

### 2.1. Participants, Recruitment, and Data Collection

The study population and study recruitment are described in detail elsewhere [8]. Briefly, between August 2017 and December 2018, ECE centers that served children ages 0–6 were recruited in comparable urban areas, specifically Seattle, South King County, and Austin. Seattle and South King County share similar key cost-of-living measures, including food costs and housing-cost burden [28]. Austin, TX, was also chosen as an additional comparison site to Seattle, WA, due to its similarity in cost of living, demographic characteristics, and the ECE context (Supplemental Table S1). Forty-nine (15–19%) of ECE centers that were contacted in Seattle (N = 16), South King County (N = 16), and Austin (N = 17) were enrolled. In-person worker recruitment meetings were then conducted by study staff at each enrolled ECE center. Inclusion criteria included the following: being an adult worker ($\geq$18 years old); being employed part-time or full-time in one of the 49 ECE centers, in a position that cared for children; and being able to read and speak English. All eligible workers were invited to participate in the study. Of 504 workers who initially expressed interest in participating, 366 enrolled in the study and completed the baseline questionnaire. Of these 366 participants, 313 workers had complete case information. Participants were compensated with a $30 gift card upon completion of the baseline survey.

The baseline survey was offered online or on paper. All interested participants (n = 504) were e-mailed a link to the online survey or mailed a paper copy of baseline surveys based on their preference. Data were collected on sociodemographic characteristics (e.g., age, race/ethnicity, education, marital status, household and individual annual income, food assistance participation), employment characteristics (e.g., job title, average paid hours of work per week), and workers' health (e.g., self-reported depressive symptoms and food security).

The Institutional Review Board at the University of Washington approved all study protocols.

### 2.1.1. Key Exposure Variable

Our primary exposure was food insecurity, which was measured using the validated six-item U.S. Household Food Security Survey Module developed by the National Center for Health Statistics [29]. This module queries individuals about their household food situation with questions about how often in the last 12 months the participant and/or adults in his/her household ran out of food and did not have money to buy more and how often they could not afford to eat balanced meals [29]. Participants were also asked questions (yes/no) about whether they and/or adults in their household reduced the size of meals or skipped meals due to lack of money for food in the last 12 months. Affirmative answers to these questions were summed to form a household raw score (range = 0–6). Using established guidelines [29], participants were categorized into three categories: normal to high food security (score = 0 to 1), low food security (score = 2 to 4), and very low food security (score = 5 to 6). Participants categorized in the normal to high food security group are referred to as "food secure" throughout this manuscript.

### 2.1.2. Key Outcome Variable

Our primary outcome was depression, which was measured using the validated 20-item Center for Epidemiologic Studies Depression Scale-Revised (CESD-R) [30,31]. Respondents answered questions about how often they experience nine different groups of depressive symptoms: sadness, loss of interest, appetite, sleep, thinking/concentration, guilt, tired, movement, and suicidal ideation. Each item was scored as follows: 0 ("not at all or less than one day"), 1 ("1–2 days"), 2 ("3–4 days"), and 3 ("5–7 days, or nearly every day for 2 weeks"). The overall CESD-R score is a sum of the responses to the 20 questions and ranges from 0–60 [30]. For the purposes of this analysis and using previously established cutoffs from the CESD-R, participants were coded into binary categories: clinically significant depression (score $\geq$ 16) and not depressed (score < 16) [30].

### 2.1.3. Effect Measure Modifiers and Confounders

Based on prior literature [3,5,17,32], we hypothesized that the effect of food insecurity and depression may vary by wages and food assistance program participation. Food assistance participation was defined as self-reported participation in at least one food assistance program, which included Supplemental Nutrition Assistance Program (SNAP), the Special Supplemental Nutrition Program for Women, Infants, and Children (WIC), farmers market WIC program, food bank, and reduced-price or free school program. Participants receiving any food assistance were categorized together due to small sample sizes for each individual food assistance program.

Workers' wages were collected as a continuous variable. Wage was dichotomized based on the median value for each study site (i.e., <median versus $\geq$median). The hourly wage median at each study site was $17.35 in Seattle, $14.08 in South King County, and $14.82 in Austin.

A directed acyclic graph (DAG) was used to identify potential confounders, which were defined as variables associated with the exposure and outcome that are not along the causal pathway [33]. Existing literature was used to support assumptions made about the role of each variable and the completeness of our DAG. From our DAG, a minimally sufficient set of confounders was identified and included as covariates in our primary model. Confounders included age (continuous), marital status (never married, now married, other), birth country (U.S. versus other), race/ethnicity (Non-Hispanic Black/African American, Non-Hispanic White, Other, Hispanic), number of children in the household (0, 1, ≥2 children), job title (center director, lead teacher or instructor, teacher or instructor, assistant teacher or instructor, other), average paid hours of work per week (continuous), highest level of education (≤high school/GED, some college/associates/ECE certificate, ≥bachelor's degree), total household income (>$25,000, $25,000–$49,999, ≥$50,000, don't know), and an indicator variable for study site (Seattle, South King County, Austin).

*2.2. Statistical Analysis*

We employed a logistic regression model to examine the relationship between food insecurity and depression, and controlled for the aforementioned covariates.

Two sensitivity analyses were performed for the primary model. First, sex was included as an additional covariate in the model, because 94% of our sample was female. Second, annual household income was replaced with annual individual income, as a covariate. Our primary model assumed that household income more strongly influences food insecurity and depression versus individual income.

Finally, in two separate models, an interaction term was used to assess whether food assistance participation (food assistance (yes/no) × food insecurity) and wage (median wage (below/at or above) × food insecurity) modified the association between food insecurity and depression.

All statistical analyses were conducted in STATA 13 (StataCorp., College Station, TX, USA).

## 3. Results

Our primary model included 313 ECE workers, with complete case information, from 49 ECE centers in Seattle, WA (n = 126, 40%), South King County, WA (n = 81, 26%), and Austin, TX (n = 106, 34%). Fifty-three participants, who lacked complete case information, were excluded from this analysis. Compared to participants with complete data, those excluded were more likely to be foreign-born, Hispanic, not have any children in the household, and had lower educational attainment.

Demographic characteristics of our analytic sample by food security status are presented in Table 1 (additional details presented in Supplemental Table S2). The majority of participants was female (94%), non-Hispanic White (56%), born in the U.S. (86%), and did not have children (63%). Compared with workers who reported being food secure, workers who reported low and very low food security, on average, had lower household incomes. A greater proportion of these workers also reported never having been married, having two or more child dependents, having less than a bachelor's degree, earning wages below the site median, and participating in food assistance programs. Workers who reported that they were food secure were generally older. Of the total sample (N = 313), 72 (23%) participants were participating in food assistance programs, with 37 (12%) participants or members of their households receiving SNAP benefits.

When examining the association between depression and food insecurity, we see that mean CESD-R depression raw scores increased with higher levels of food insecurity (Figure 1). In our primary model, after controlling for covariates, very low and low food insecurities, compared to being food secure, were associated with a 4.95 (95% Confidence Interval (CI): 2.29, 10.67) and 2.69 (95% CI: 1.29, 5.63) higher odds of depression, respectively (Table 2). In the sensitivity analyses, the magnitude, direction, and statistical significance were similar when we controlled for sex (low food security Odds Ratio (OR) = 2.75; 95% CI: 1.32, 5.79, very low food security OR = 5.00; 95% CI: 2.31, 10.83) and when we controlled for household versus individual annual income (low food security OR = 3.06; 95% CI: 1.49, 6.27; very low food security OR = 5.49; 95% CI: 2.63, 11.46) (Table 3).

Table 1. Characteristics of the study cohort of 313 early care and education (ECE) providers, by food security status, 2017.

| Demographic Factor * | Food Secure (n = 185) | Low Food Security (n = 64) | Very Low Food Security (n = 64) |
|---|---|---|---|
| Age, mean (SD) | 39.5 (13) | 35.5 (13) | 33.3 (12) |
| Females, n (%) | 171 (93%) | 59 (92%) | 61 (97%) |
| U.S. Born, n (%) | 155 (84%) | 55 (86%) | 58 (91%) |
| Study Site, n (%) | | | |
| Seattle, WA | 81 (44%) | 26 (41%) | 19 (30%) |
| South King County, WA | 50 (27%) | 16 (25%) | 15 (23%) |
| Austin, TX | 54 (29%) | 22 (34%) | 30 (47%) |
| Race/Ethnicity, n (%) | | | |
| Non-Hispanic White | 118 (64%) | 30 (47%) | 27 (42%) |
| Non-Hispanic Black/African-American | 17 (9%) | 10 (16%) | 14 (22%) |
| Non-Hispanic, Other | 27 (15%) | 3 (5%) | 6 (9%) |
| Hispanic | 23 (12%) | 21 (33%) | 17 (27%) |
| No Children (<18) in Household, n (%) | 125 (68%) | 32 (50%) | 40 (63%) |
| Highest Level of Education, n (%) | | | |
| ≤High School or GED | 17 (9%) | 18 (28%) | 16 (25%) |
| Some college, Associate's degree, ECE certificate | 65 (35%) | 23 (36%) | 32 (50%) |
| Bachelor's degree or higher | 103 (56%) | 23 (36%) | 16 (25%) |
| ECE Job Title, n (%) | | | |
| Center Director | 20 (11%) | 3 (5%) | 3 (5%) |
| Lead Teacher or Instructor | 55 (30%) | 24 (38%) | 28 (44%) |
| Teacher or Instructor | 50 (27%) | 14 (22%) | 14 (22%) |
| Assistant Teacher or Instructor | 41 (22%) | 12 (19%) | 13 (20%) |
| Other | 19 (10%) | 11 (17%) | 6 (9%) |
| Average Paid Hours of Work Per Week, mean (SD) | 37.7 (8) | 37.2 (7) | 36.5 (8) |
| Individual Annual Income ($), median (25th–75th percentile) | 31,340 (25,480–37,502) | 25,935 (17,160–31,221) | 26,000 (15,600–30,000) |
| Household income, n (%) | | | |
| Below $25,000 | 22 (12%) | 20 (31%) | 20 (31%) |
| $25,000–$49,999 | 55 (30%) | 20 (31%) | 28 (43%) |
| $50,000 or more | 96 (52%) | 18 (28%) | 15 (23%) |
| Don't know | 12 (7%) | 6 (9%) | 1 (2%) |
| Hourly Wage in Comparison to Median Site Wage, n (%) | | | |
| Below median | 73 (41%) | 34 (55%) | 41 (66%) |
| Depression CESD-R Score [†], mean (SD) | 11.8 (8) | 18.7 (12) | 23.1 (12) |
| Non-clinical Depression [‡], n (%) | 138 (75%) | 31 (48%) | 21 (33%) |
| USDA Food Security 6-item Raw Score [§], mean (SD) | 0.2 (0.4) | 2.8 (0.8) | 5.6 (0.5) |
| Participates in Food Assistance Program [◊], n (%) | 32 (17%) | 20 (31%) | 20 (31%) |

* Percentages provided for each demographic factor reflect proportions of participants in each food security subgroup (i.e., for each demographic factor, percentages within the same column sum to 100%). [†] The Center for Epidemiologic Studies Depression Scale-Revised (CESD-R) scores are based on responses to 20 questions and range from 0 to 60, with higher scores indicating more depressive symptoms [30]. [‡] Categorical depression was based on the CESD-R scores from 0–60 and categorized accordingly: (1) Non-clinical Depression (score = 0–16) and (2) Clinical Depression, including Major, Probable, Possible, and Sub-threshold Depression (score ≥ 16), based on previously established cutoffs [30]. [§] The United States Department of Agriculture (USDA) Food Security six-item Raw Scores ranged from 0 to 6, with a higher score being indicative of more severe food insecurity. Food security was categorized accordingly: (1) Normal to High Food Security (score = 0 to 1), (2) Low Food Security (score = 2–4), and (3) Very Low Security (score = 5–6) [29]. [◊] Out of a total of 313 samples, 37 (12%) participants or members of their households received Supplemental Nutrition Assistance Program (SNAP) benefits, 22 (7%) received Women, Infants and Children (WIC) program benefits, four (1%) received farmers market nutrition program for WIC, 13 (4%) received benefits from food bank or pantry, 24 (8%) received benefits from free or reduced school breakfast or lunch for kids, and one (0.3%) received benefits from another program.

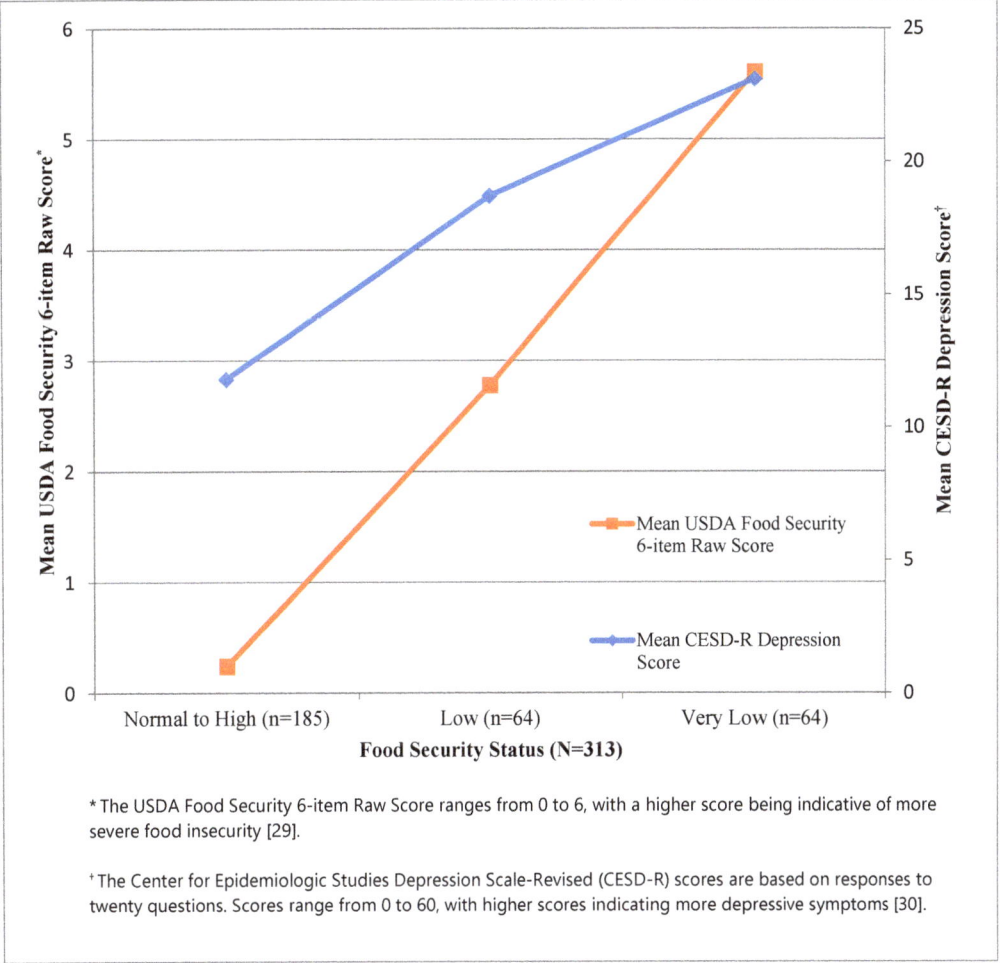

* The USDA Food Security 6-item Raw Score ranges from 0 to 6, with a higher score being indicative of more severe food insecurity [29].

† The Center for Epidemiologic Studies Depression Scale-Revised (CESD-R) scores are based on responses to twenty questions. Scores range from 0 to 60, with higher scores indicating more depressive symptoms [30].

**Figure 1.** Mean USDA food security and CESD-R depression raw scores by food security status among 313 early care and education providers.

**Table 2.** Primary model with logistic regression estimates (odds ratios) for the association between food insecurity and depression among a cohort of 313 early care and education (ECE) providers in Washington and Texas *.

| Food Security Status | Odds Ratio | 95% Confidence Interval | $p$-Value |
|---|---|---|---|
| Low Food Security (N = 64) | 2.69 | (1.29, 5.63) | 0.011 |
| Very Low Food Security (N = 64) | 4.95 | (2.29, 10.67) | 0.000 |

* Presented values were estimated using logistic regression models for the association between food insecurity and depression after controlling for age, marital status, birth country, race/ethnicity, number of children in the household, job title, average paid hours of work per week, highest level of education, total household income, and an indicator variable for study site. The reference group is participants who are food secure (N = 185).

Table 3. Sensitivity analyses with logistic regression estimates (odds ratio) for the association between food insecurity and depression among a cohort of 313 early care and education (ECE) providers in Washington and Texas *.

| Food Security Status | Odds Ratio | 95% Confidence Interval | p-Value |
|---|---|---|---|
| Sensitivity Analysis 1: Primary Model + Sex (N = 311) [†] | | | |
| Low Food Security (n = 64) | 2.75 | (1.32, 5.79) | 0.009 |
| Very Low Food Security (n = 63) | 5.00 | (2.31, 10.83) | 0.000 |
| Sensitivity Analysis 2: Primary Model, replacing Annual Household Income with Annual Individual Income (N = 299) [‡] | | | |
| Low Food Security (n = 61) | 3.06 | (1.49, 6.27) | 0.002 |
| Very Low Food Security (n = 62) | 5.49 | (2.63, 11.46) | 0.000 |

* Presented values were estimated using logistic regression models for the association between food insecurity and depression. The primary model controls for age, marital status, birth country, race/ethnicity, number of children in the household, job title, average paid hours of work per week, highest level of education, total household income, and an indicator variable for study site. [†] The reference group is participants who are food secure (n = 184). [‡] The reference group is participants who are food secure (n = 176).

Finally, our study found that the association between food insecurity and depression did not vary by participation in a food assistance program ($p = 0.71$) or median site wage ($p = 0.41$). Table 4 presents estimates, stratified by food assistance program participation and wage status.

Table 4. Logistic regression estimates (odds ratios) for the association between food insecurity and depression among a cohort of early care and education (ECE) providers in Washington and Texas, stratified by food assistance program participation and wage *.

| Food Security Status | Food Assistance Program Participation (N = 313) [†] | | Individual Wage (N = 303) [†] | |
|---|---|---|---|---|
| | Yes (n = 72) | No (n = 241) | Below Site Median (n = 146) [‡] | At or Above Site Median (n = 155) |
| Low Food Security | 2.58 (0.41, 16.35) | 2.73 (1.17, 6.38) | 1.62 (0.52, 5.04) | 4.11 (1.28, 13.24) |
| Very Low Food Security | 6.77 (1.02, 44.80) | 6.11 (2.48, 15.02) | 6.67 (2.19, 20.38) | 5.18 (1.32, 20.32) |
| Global p value | 0.71 | | 0.41 | |

* Presented values were estimated using logistic regression models for the association between food insecurity and depression after controlling for age, marital status, birth country, race/ethnicity, number of children in the household, job title, average paid hours of work per week, highest level of education, total household income, and an indicator variable for study site. [†] The reference group is participants who are food secure. [‡] Individuals with a job title of center director who earned below median site wage (n = 1) were not included in this model.

## 4. Discussion

To our knowledge, this is the first study to investigate the association between food insecurity and depression among ECE workers. Prevalence rates for food insecurity and depression in our sample were 41% and 39%, respectively, which are higher than national prevalence rates of food insecurity among American households (10.5%) [1] and of depression among U.S. females (9%) [34]. However, the prevalence rates in our sample were comparable to rates noted in recent studies with ECE samples and nursing home employees, a comparable low-wage worker population [7,9,25,32].

The association between food insecurity and depression noted in our ECE sample is consistent with that of several previous studies that look at this association within vulnerable populations and predominantly female samples [4,5,18,35]. In a recent cross-sectional analysis of the National Health and Nutrition Examination Survey (2011–2014), authors report a dose–response relationship between food insecurity and depressive symptoms among diabetic adults with an odds ratio of similar magnitude to those noted in our study [35]. A second cross-sectional analysis of low-income, diabetic participants, in King County, WA, also found that being food insecure (versus secure) was associated with almost 3-times higher odds of depression, similar to our finding for food insecure adults [36]. Results from the Women's Employment Study similarly reported that household food insufficiency was associated with depression among low-income female welfare recipients [5]. Moreover, using longitudinal data, Tuthill et al. [18] found that women with very low food security had five times the odds of depression, compared to food secure women [18].

Regarding our secondary study objective, we did not find that food assistance participation modified the association between food insecurity and depression. These findings differ from that of some studies, which reported that the association between food insecurity and depression varied by food assistance program participation [2,3,17,37]. Some nationally representative data suggest that the association between food insecurity and emotional distress or depression was higher among SNAP participants compared to SNAP-eligible nonparticipants [2,3]. Heflin and Ziliak's [2] longitudinal analysis also noted that the magnitude of the association between food insufficiency (i.e., food insecurity with hunger) and emotional distress was larger when participants were initially transitioning onto SNAP, possibly due to the increased stigma and participants' inexperience in navigating the system. Similarly, Leung et al. concluded that the odds of depression, in relation to food insecurity, were higher for most SNAP participants versus SNAP-eligible nonparticipants [3]. Unlike these studies, which focused on only SNAP participation, our study examined the heterogeneity in the association by food program participation in any food assistance program, because we were not powered to solely examine SNAP participation. Only 72 sample participants received benefits from any food assistance program, and only 12% of sample participants or household members (n = 34) were enrolled in SNAP, which was much smaller than that of previous studies [2,3]. This may have been attributable to differences in SNAP eligibility requirements, as our study focused on ECE workers in only two states, rather than a nationally representative sample; our sample also mostly consisted of working, able-bodied adults without dependents (ABAWD), who must abide by specific work requirements (e.g., averaging 80 work hours/month) in order to receive SNAP benefits and are only eligible for SNAP benefits for three months in a three-year period [38,39]. Additional barriers to participation may have also played a role. In focus groups conducted with our ECE providers (N = 15), participants mentioned several barriers to participation, including stigma, individual resistance to ask for help, limited time, and having a household income that was slightly over the eligibility threshold. This is consistent with prior literature [40,41], which emphasizes the administrative hurdles associated with both applying and maintaining eligibility for SNAP, as well as the program's inability to account for short-term income volatility among SNAP-eligible participants. In addition to differences in sampling, the absence of effect modification noted in our study may also be due to the fact that food assistance participation could be acting as a mediator, rather than an effect modifier, of the relationship between food insecurity and mental health.

Surprisingly, our study also did not find that individual-level wage modified the association between food insecurity and depression. Household financial income is consistently found to be the strongest predictor of food insecurity risk [14], and the association between financial instability and poor mental health is well documented [13,18,32]. We hypothesized that participants with the lowest wage would have a larger magnitude of effect between food insecurity and depression. One possible explanation for our findings may have to do with the narrow range of income represented in this sample. Our overall sample size was also relatively small and, therefore, we may have been insufficiently powered to detect heterogeneity in the association. Another possible explanation for our findings may be related to whether the respondent was the primary wage earner in the household and, thus, subject to higher levels of stress due to financial strain. For example, a study examining low-wage nursing home workers, which is also a highly vulnerable workforce, found that the association of depression with household financial strain and food insufficiency varied by primary wage earner status [32]. Among primary wage earner participants, the odds of depressive symptoms were found to be 3.6 times higher in relation to food insufficiency (vs. food security), whereas food insufficiency was not associated with depressive symptoms, among non-primary wage earners [32]. Our survey did not include a measure that would allow for identification of primary wage earner status.

Overall, this study suggests the need for policies and interventions that address both mental health and food insecurity in this valuable yet vulnerable workforce. Although our study focused on the ECE workforce in the U.S., the issue of low wages in this employment sector may not be unique to this country, and the availability and generosity of food assistance benefits may differ. A well-nourished and healthy ECE workforce is needed in all countries to optimize the growth and development of the next generation [24]. More children than ever are enrolled in ECE programs, and these children spend a significant amount of developmental time and may receive most of their daily nutrition in this setting [42,43]. In order to provide high-quality care and education to the children they serve, ECE workers need support in their work environments; one possible approach to help optimize their working conditions and health is through population-level strategies [25,26].

Potential policy-level strategies in the U.S. could include incorporating ECE workers as recipients of the federally reimbursed nutritious meals and snacks already served on-site to children via the Child and Adult Care Food Program or adopting legislation or provisions that improve financial security for ECE workers (e.g., tax credits, raised minimum wage [44]). Centers could also provide workers with resources and connections to nutrition education and food assistance programs, as misunderstandings and uncertainty around eligibility for food stamp benefits are fairly common, and population-specific outreach and education around food assistance participation eligibility may encourage participation [45].

Centers can also look for opportunities to create on-site programs or create synergies with existing local programs (e.g., home preparation meal kits, weekly produce markets, or food pantries). For example, Hungry Harvest partners with various public schools in Baltimore City to provide reduced-cost, recovered produce to staff, students, and families in low-income neighborhoods [46]. In Seattle and South King County, the Good Food Bags program provides a weekly subscription to subsidized, fresh produce to lower-income families through preschools, community centers, and other community partner organizations [47]. On-site programs established through a community effort [48] are not only more accessible but may also reduce the stigma associated with food assistance [45] and thereby encourage use of these resources. Finally, potential centers could include routine staff training on mental health and emotional well-being, coping skills, and stress management.

There are several limitations of this analysis. First, a cross-sectional analysis precludes our ability to infer a causal relationship between food insecurity and depression. Second, our study also included a relatively small sample of predominantly female, non-Hispanic white, and low-wage ECE workers in two states in the U.S., which limits generalizability. Third, we did not collect data on the total number of children or adults *outside of the home* who may rely upon the incomes of the ECE workers in our sample. However, an additional sensitivity controlling for the total number of people in the household produced results similar in magnitude, direction, and statistical significance to our primary specification where we only controlled for the total number of children (Supplemental Table S3). Finally, our study findings, like most survey research, are limited by selection bias. Participants who were interested and willing to complete our baseline survey may differ from non-respondents, which could bias our study results. Nonetheless, key strengths of this study include the use of validated measures and a rigorous assessment of the relationship between food insecurity and depression among a sample of ECE workers.

## 5. Conclusions

This study found that food insecurity is associated with depression among a sample of ECE workers. Considering the high prevalence rates of food insecurity and depression within this population, policies and center-level interventions that address both food insecurity and depression may be warranted in order to protect and improve the health of this valuable, yet vulnerable, workforce. A healthy ECE workforce is vital to the delivery of quality childcare.

**Supplementary Materials:** The following are available online at https://www.mdpi.com/1660-4601/18/1/170/s1. Table S1: Comparison of Seattle, WA, and Austin, TX, by cost of living, demographic, and childcare center employee wages. Table S2: Additional characteristics of a cohort of 313 early care and education (ECE) providers in Washington and Texas participating in baseline data collection of a prospective study exploring the effects of wage on ECE provider health, by food security status, 2017. Table S3: Sensitivity analyses with logistic regression estimates (odds ratio) for the association between food insecurity and depression among a cohort of 313 early care and education (ECE) providers in Washington and Texas.

**Author Contributions:** Conceptualization, J.O. and I.H.L.; methodology, J.O.; formal analysis, I.H.L. and V.M.O.; investigation, J.O. and I.H.L.; resources, J.O.; writing—original draft preparation, I.H.L.; writing—review and editing, I.H.L., J.O. and V.M.O.; visualization, I.H.L.; supervision, J.O.; project administration, J.O.; funding acquisition, J.O. All authors have read and agreed to the published version of the manuscript.

**Funding:** This research was primarily funded by the Robert Wood Johnson Foundation Evidence for Action, No. 74458. Additional support was provided by the National Center for Advancing Translational Sciences of the National Institutes of Health, No. UL1 TR002319, as well as the Center for Studies in Demography and Ecology at the University of Washington, No. P2C HD042828. Ivory H. Loh was supported by the University of Washington Nutritional Sciences Program through the Top Scholar Award.

**Institutional Review Board Statement:** This study was conducted according to the guidelines of the Declaration of Helsinki, and approved by the Institutional Review Board of the University of Washington (STUDY00002664, 7/27/2017-7/26/2020).

**Informed Consent Statement:** Informed consent was obtained from all subjects involved in the study.

**Data Availability Statement:** The data presented in this study are available on request from the corresponding author. The data are not publicly available due to privacy reasons.

**Acknowledgments:** The authors thank the individuals and early care and education centers who generously dedicated their time to participate in this study. They also thank Bert Stover, the statistician of the research team.

**Conflicts of Interest:** The authors declare no conflict of interest. The funders had no role in the design of the study; in the collection, analyses, or interpretation of data; in the writing of the manuscript, or in the decision to publish the results.

# References

1. Coleman-Jensen, A.; Rabbitt, M.P.; Gregory, C.A.; Singh, A. Household Food Security in the United States in 2019. Economic Research Service, 2020. Available online: https://www.ers.usda.gov/publications/pub-details/?pubid=99281 (accessed on 27 December 2020).
2. Heflin, C.M.; Ziliak, J.P. Food Insufficiency, Food Stamp Participation, and Mental Health. *Soc. Sci. Q.* **2008**, *89*, 706–727. [CrossRef]
3. Leung, C.W.; Epel, E.S.; Willett, W.C.; Rimm, E.B.; Laraia, B.A. Household Food Insecurity Is Positively Associated with Depression among Low-Income Supplemental Nutrition Assistance Program Participants and Income-Eligible Nonparticipants. *J. Nutr.* **2015**, *145*, 622–627. [CrossRef] [PubMed]
4. Noonan, K.; Corman, H.; Reichman, N.E. Effects of maternal depression on family food insecurity. *Econ. Hum. Biol.* **2016**, *22*, 201–215. [CrossRef] [PubMed]
5. Heflin, C.M.; Siefert, K.; Williams, D.R. Food insufficiency and women's mental health: Findings from a 3-year panel of welfare recipients. *Soc. Sci. Med.* **2005**, *61*, 1971–1982. [CrossRef]
6. Leung, C.W.; Stewart, A.L.; Portela-Parra, E.T.; Adler, N.E.; Laraia, B.A.; Epel, E.S. Understanding the Psychological Distress of Food Insecurity: A Qualitative Study of Children's Experiences and Related Coping Strategies. *J. Acad. Nutr. Diet.* **2020**, *120*, 395–403. [CrossRef]
7. Linnan, L.; Arandia, G.; Bateman, L.A.; Vaughn, A.; Smith, N.; Ward, D. The Health and Working Conditions of Women Employed in Child Care. *Int. J. Environ. Res. Public Health* **2017**, *14*, 283. [CrossRef]
8. Otten, J.J.; Bradford, V.A.; Stover, B.; Hill, H.D.; Osborne, C.; Getts, K.; Seixas, N. The Culture of Health in Early Care and Education: Workers' Wages, Health, and Job Characteristics. *Health Aff. (Proj. Hope)* **2019**, *38*, 709–720. [CrossRef]

9. McKelvey, L.; Forsman, A.; Morrison-Ward, J. Arkansas Workforce Study: Instructional Staff in Child Care & Early Childhood Education, 2017. Good to Great. 2017. Available online: https://familymedicine.uams.edu/wp-content/uploads/sites/57/2018/04/Staff-Workforce-Study-Report_FINAL.pdf (accessed on 27 December 2020).
10. Morrissey, T. The Effects of Early Care and Education on Children's Health. Health Affairs. 2019. Available online: https://www.healthaffairs.org/do/10.1377/hpb20190325.519221/full/ (accessed on 27 December 2020).
11. Maynard, M.; Andrade, L.; Packull-McCormick, S.; Perlman, C.M.; Leos-Toro, C.; Kirkpatrick, S.I. Food Insecurity and Mental Health among Females in High-Income Countries. *Int. J. Environ. Res. Public Health* **2018**, *15*, 1424. [CrossRef]
12. Arenas, D.J.; Thomas, A.; Wang, J.; DeLisser, H.M. A Systematic Review and Meta-analysis of Depression, Anxiety, and Sleep Disorders in US Adults with Food Insecurity. *J. Gen. Intern. Med.* **2019**, 1–9. [CrossRef]
13. Jessiman-Perreault, G.; McIntyre, L. The household food insecurity gradient and potential reductions in adverse population mental health outcomes in Canadian adults. *Ssm-Popul. Health* **2017**, *3*, 464–472. [CrossRef]
14. Loopstra, R. Interventions to address household food insecurity in high-income countries. *Proc. Nutr. Soc.* **2018**, *77*, 270–281. [CrossRef] [PubMed]
15. Gundersen, C.; Ziliak, J.P. Food Insecurity and Health Outcomes. *Health Aff. (Proj. Hope)* **2015**, *34*, 1830–1839. [CrossRef] [PubMed]
16. Brostow, D.; Gunzburger, E.; Abbate, L.; Brenner, L.; Thomas, K. Mental Illness, Not Weight Status, Predicts Increased Odds of Food Insecurity in the Health and Retirement Study (OR02-06-19). *Curr. Dev. Nutr.* **2019**, *3*. [CrossRef]
17. Kim, K.; Frongillo, E.A. Participation in Food Assistance Programs Modifies the Relation of Food Insecurity with Weight and Depression in Elders. *J. Nutr.* **2007**, *137*, 1005–1010. [CrossRef]
18. Tuthill, E.L.; Sheira, L.A.; Palar, K.; Frongillo, E.A.; Wilson, T.E.; Adedimeji, A.; Merenstein, D.; Cohen, M.H.; Wentz, E.L.; Adimora, A.A.; et al. Persistent Food Insecurity Is Associated with Adverse Mental Health among Women Living with or at Risk of HIV in the United States. *J. Nutr.* **2019**, *149*, 240–248. [CrossRef]
19. Dean, J.; Keshavan, M. The neurobiology of depression: An integrated view. *Asian J. Psychiatry* **2017**, *27*, 101–111. [CrossRef]
20. Rao, T.S.S.; Asha, M.R.; Ramesh, B.N.; Rao, K.S.J. Understanding nutrition, depression and mental illnesses. *Indian J. Psychiatry* **2008**, *50*, 77–82.
21. Whitebook, M.; McLean, C.; Austin, L.J.E.; Edwards, B. Early Childhood Workforce Index 2018. In *Center for the Study of Child Care Employment*; University of California: Berkeley, CA, USA, 2018.
22. Lessard, L.M.; Wilkins, K.; Rose-Malm, J.; Mazzocchi, M.C. The health status of the early care and education workforce in the USA: A scoping review of the evidence and current practice. *Public Health Rev.* **2020**, *41*, 2. [CrossRef]
23. Mongeau, L. Time to Change How We Think about Early Education, International Study Finds. Available online: https://hechingerreport.org/time-to-change-how-we-think-about-early-education-international-study-finds/ (accessed on 4 December 2020).
24. Bertram, T.; Pascal, C. *Early Childhood Policies and Systems in Eight Countries: Findings from IEA's Early Childhood Education Study*; Springer Open: Cham, Switzerland, 2016.
25. Whitaker, R.C.; Becker, B.D.; Herman, A.N.; Gooze, R.A. The Physical and Mental Health of Head Start Staff: The Pennsylvania Head Start Staff Wellness Survey, 2012. *Prev. Chronic Dis.* **2013**, *10*, E181. [CrossRef]
26. Cumming, T. Early Childhood Educators' Well-Being: An Updated Review of the Literature. *Early Child. Educ. J.* **2017**, *45*, 583–593. [CrossRef]
27. Loh, I.H.; Oddo, V.M.; Otten, J. Food Insecurity Is Associated with Depression among a Vulnerable Workforce: Early Care and Education Workers. *Curr. Dev. Nutr.* **2020**, *4*, 228. [CrossRef]
28. King County Council. King County Technical Appendix B to the 2012 Comprehensive Plan: Housing. 2016. Available online: https://www.kingcounty.gov/~{}/media/Council/documents/CompPlan/2016/2016-0155/AppendixBHousing.ashx?la=en (accessed on 27 December 2020).
29. Department of Agriculture, Economic Research Service. U.S. Household Food Security Survey Module: Six-Item Short Form. Available online: https://www.ers.usda.gov/media/8282/short2012.pdf (accessed on 4 December 2020).
30. Eaton, W.W.; Smith, C.; Ybarra, M.; Muntaner, C.; Tien, A. *Center for Epidemiological Depression Scale: Review and Revision (CESD and CESD-R)*; Maruish, M.E., Ed.; The Use of Psychological Testing for Treatment Planning and Outcomes Assessment; Lawrence Erlbaum Associates: Mahwah, NJ, USA, 2004; pp. 363–377.
31. Van Dam, N.T.; Earleywine, M. Validation of the Center for Epidemiologic Studies Depression Scale—Revised (CESD-R): Pragmatic depression assessment in the general population. *Psychiatry Res.* **2011**, *186*, 128–132. [CrossRef] [PubMed]
32. Okechukwu, C.A.; El Ayadi, A.M.; Tamers, S.L.; Sabbath, E.L.; Berkman, L. Household Food Insufficiency, Financial Strain, Work–Family Spillover, and Depressive Symptoms in the Working Class: The Work, Family, and Health Network Study. *Am. J. Public Health* **2012**, *102*, 126–133. [CrossRef] [PubMed]
33. Glymour, M.M. *16. Using Causal Diagrams to Understand Common Problems in Social Epidemiology*; Methods in Social Epidemiology: San Francisco, CA, USA, 2006; pp. 393–428. Available online: http://publicifsv.sund.ku.dk/~{}nk/epiF14/Glymour_DAGs.pdf (accessed on 27 December 2020).
34. National Institute of Mental Health Major Depression. Available online: https://www.nimh.nih.gov/health/statistics/major-depression.shtml (accessed on 27 December 2020).
35. Montgomery, M.J.; Lu, D.J.; Ratliff, M.S.; Mezuk, D.B. Food Insecurity and Depression among Adults with Diabetes: Results from the National Health and Nutrition Examination Survey (NHANES). *Diabetes Educ.* **2017**, *43*, 260. [CrossRef] [PubMed]

36. Silverman, J.; Krieger, J.; Kiefer, M.; Hebert, P.; Robinson, J.; Nelson, K. The Relationship between Food Insecurity and Depression, Diabetes Distress and Medication Adherence among Low-Income Patients with Poorly-Controlled Diabetes. *J. Gen. Intern. Med.* **2015**, *30*, 1476–1480. [CrossRef] [PubMed]
37. Oddo, V.M.; Mabli, J. Association of Participation in the Supplemental Nutrition Assistance Program and Psychological Distress. *Am. J. Public Health* **2015**, *105*, e30–e35. [CrossRef] [PubMed]
38. Texas Health and Human Services SNAP Food Benefits. Available online: https://hhs.texas.gov/services/food/snap-food-benefits (accessed on 27 December 2020).
39. Washington State Legislature WAC 388-444-0030. Available online: https://app.leg.wa.gov/WAC/default.aspx?cite=388-444-0030 (accessed on 27 December 2020).
40. Keith-Jennings, B.; Llobrera, J.; Dean, S. Links of the Supplemental Nutrition Assistance Program with Food Insecurity, Poverty, and Health: Evidence and Potential. *Am. J. Public Health (1971)* **2019**, *109*, 1636–1640. [CrossRef]
41. Gaines-Turner, T.; Simmons, J.C.; Chilton, M. Recommendations From SNAP Participants to Improve Wages and End Stigma. *Am. J. Public Health (1971)* **2019**, *109*, 1664–1667. [CrossRef]
42. Alberdi, G.; McNamara, A.; Lindsay, K.; Scully, H.; Horan, M.; Gibney, E.; McAuliffe, F. The association between childcare and risk of childhood overweight and obesity in children aged 5 years and under: A systematic review. *Eur. J. Pediatr.* **2016**, *175*, 1277–1294. [CrossRef]
43. Kaphingst, K.M.; Story, M. Child care as an untapped setting for obesity prevention: State child care licensing regulations related to nutrition, physical activity, and media use for preschool-aged children in the United States. *Prev. Chronic Dis.* **2009**, *6*, A11.
44. Economic Opportunity Institute Washington State Career and Wage Ladder Evaluation. Available online: http://www.opportunityinstitute.org/research/post/washington-state-career-and-wage-ladder-evaluation/ (accessed on 27 December 2020).
45. Bartlett, S.; Burstein, N.; Hamilton, W.; Kling, R. *Food Stamp Program Access STUDY Final Report*; E-FAN; Economic Research Service: Washington, DC, USA, 2004; Volume 3-013-3.
46. Hungry Harvest about Produce in a SNAP. Available online: https://www.produceinasnap.com/our-roots (accessed on 23 November 2019).
47. Good Food Bags. Available online: http://www.tilthalliance.org/about/good-food-bags (accessed on 23 November 2019).
48. Snelling, A.; Maroto, M.; Jacknowitz, A.; Waxman, E. Key Factors for School-Based Food Pantries: Perspectives from Food Bank and School Pantry Personnel. *J. Hunger Environ. Nutr.* **2014**, *9*, 350–361. [CrossRef]

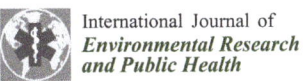

*Article*

# Factors Influencing the Preventive Practice of International Students in South Korea against COVID-19 during the Pandemic

Gun Ja Jang [1], Ginam Jang [2] and Sangjin Ko [3,*]

1. Department of Nursing, Daegu University, Daegu 42400, Korea; kjjang14@daegu.ac.kr
2. School of International Studies, Yeungnam University, Gyeongsan 38541, Korea; jjggnn@hanmail.net
3. Department of Nursing, University of Ulsan, Ulsan 44610, Korea
* Correspondence: sangjinko@ulsan.ac.kr; Tel.: +82-52-259-1298

**Abstract:** As the novel coronavirus disease (COVID-19) spreads worldwide, quarantine guidelines are being constantly updating to prevent the transmission of this virus. Regardless of which country international students live in, they might receive limited crucial quarantine guidelines from that country's government. The purpose of this study was to identify factors influencing the preventive practice of international students in South Korea during the COVID-19 pandemic. This was a cross-sectional descriptive study. Data were collected from international students in three universities from July 10 to July 31 in 2020. A total of 261 international students participated in the survey, using an online questionnaire. Data were analyzed by independent t-test, one-way ANOVA, Pearson correlation coefficients, and multiple regression analysis. Preventive practice during the COVID-19 pandemic was affected by duration of stay in Korea ($\beta = -0.21$, $p < 0.001$), attitudes ($\beta = 0.22$, $p = 0.001$), and trust in Korea's quarantine system ($\beta = 0.33$, $p < 0.001$). This study showed that attitudes and trust in the quarantine system could affect personal preventive practice during the outbreak of a highly contagious disease such as COVID-19.

**Keywords:** coronavirus; infection control; quarantine; students

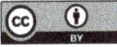

## 1. Introduction

The novel coronavirus disease 2019 (COVID-19), also called severe acute respiratory syndrome coronavirus 2 (SARS-CoV-2), is the cause of an ongoing worldwide pandemic [1]. Its main symptoms include fever, cough, sore throat, and many other respiratory symptoms. It was first reported in those with pneumonia of unknown cause in Wuhan, China, in December 2019 [1]. In Korea, the first COVID-19 patient was a 35-year-old Chinese woman who arrived from Wuhan on 19 January 2020 [2]. Despite the imposition of Wuhan's entry restrictions on 4 February, the number of confirmed COVID-19 cases in Korea sharply increased, starting with the 31st identified patient in Daegu city, a city with 2.5 million residents [3]. The number of patients reached 7755 in Korea on 12 March 2020, with the country ranking second globally. As COVID-19 can spread very rapidly in a specific cluster (Christchurch), 87.3% of all confirmed South Korean cases occurred only in Daegu and the adjacent Gyeongbuk province, as of 17 March 2020 [3,4].

It is essential to know and adhere to proper prevention guidelines for infection control. During the emergence of an unknown novel virus, the guidelines from the World Health Organization (WHO) [5], Centers for Disease Control and Prevention (CDC) [6], and Korea Disease Control and Prevention Agency (KDCA) [7] continue to be updated and revised. However, sometimes, the information provided in these guidelines is confusing or conflicting [8]. Therefore, it is difficult for most international students living in Daegu and Gyeongbuk to keep track of the continually changing guidelines announced by Korea's government or to find relevant information. Mostly, many international students often obtain COVID-19 related information through social media [9], so they need to be managed to avoid exposure to misinformation, particularly during the COVID-19 pandemic. Most of them are non-English speakers and may have difficulty understanding the official announcements provided in Korean and English. For a highly contagious disease such as COVID-19, individuals' prevention practices are of the utmost importance in preventing infectious diseases, and it is necessary to investigate the preventive practices of international students, who are often overlooked, during quarantine.

According to the Knowledge–Attitude–Practice (KAP) model, knowledge allows individuals to change their attitudes, and finally, to change their practices [10]. Each person's compliance with preventive guidelines is mostly affected by their KAP toward COVID-19 under KAP theory [11]. In previous studies about infectious diseases, including Middle East respiratory syndrome (MERS) [12] and severe acute respiratory syndrome (SARS) [13], the knowledge and attitudes were found to be correlating variables with preventive practice. A few KAP studies on COVID-19 reported similar findings, and most of them were conducted on native college or university students majoring in nursing or medicine [14–16], which may be not be generalizable to international students. Moreover, very few studies have explored the relationship between trust in a quarantine system and preventive practice. Therefore, the aim of this study was, for international students who are likely to be marginalized by the national quarantine system, to investigate the relationship between KAP towards COVID-19 and influencing factors of preventive practice.

## 2. Methods

### 2.1. Study Design

This study utilized a cross-sectional descriptive study design. It was conducted in two steps. First, a pilot study was conducted to test the feasibility and reliability of the measuring instruments. In particular, whether international students could entirely understand a questionnaire written in Korean was assessed. After completing the pilot study, the primary survey was conducted to identify factors influencing international students' preventive practice during the COVID-19 pandemic. The questionnaire developed by researchers consisted of demographic characteristics, knowledge, attitudes, trust in Korea's quarantine system, and preventive practice related to the COVID-19 pandemic.

### 2.2. Participants

Participants were conveniently sampled, and they were voluntarily recruited through a recruitment announcement from three (Y, D, another D) universities located in Daegu and Gyeongbuk, Korea. These universities are private universities with 68, 91, and 37 departments, respectively, and Korean language education centers. Around 2900 international students are registered in the three universities, which are the leading universities in terms of the number of international students enrolled [17]. The number of eligible participants was 1200 based on the inclusion and exclusion criteria. Among them, 300 international students participated in the online survey, and 43 were excluded due to unresponsive items. Finally, data from 256 international students were used for statistical analysis. Inclusion criteria were as follows: (1) those who registered in a university or a language school of a university and took online or offline lectures; (2) those who had a level 3 in the Test of Proficiency in Korean (TOPIK) [18] that allowed international students to be accepted by a Korean university for studying as a minimal requirement; (3) those who had been living in South Korea for more than six months and voluntarily participated in the online survey. Exclusion criteria were as follows: (1) age of younger than 20 years or more than 30 years; and (2) those who had a regular job as foreign workers, although they were studying in a university.

## 2.3. Measures

### 2.3.1. Knowledge about COVID-19 Pandemic

The researchers developed a COVID-19 pandemic knowledge scale based on the CDC's guidelines [6] and the questions used to survey MERS-related knowledge among Korean nursing students [19]. This scale consisted of 10 items. Its content validity index (CVI) was rated by three nursing professors using a 4-point Likert scale (1 = not relevant, 4 = very relevant). In the pilot study, ten foreign students were asked to respond to some words in vague terms ("droplet infection" and "olfactory paralysis"). Subcategories were onset (1 item), symptoms (4 items), transmission (3 items), and prevention (2 items). A correct answer was given 1 point, and an incorrect answer or "do not know" response was given 0 points, with a higher score indicating a higher level of knowledge. The final CVI of the scale was 0.88. Its reliability (Kuder–Richardson 20) was 0.73.

### 2.3.2. Attitudes toward the COVID-19 Pandemic

The researchers developed five items relating to attitudes toward the COVID-19 pandemic by referring to previous studies [20,21]. Each item was rated on a 5-point Likert scale from "Not at all" (1 point) to "Absolutely yes" (5 points), with a higher score indicating that the participant was more likely to feel that that the COVID-19 pandemic was a severe health issue. Ambiguous words and phrases were revised through a pilot study. Cronbach's $\alpha$ of the scale in the primary study was 0.72.

### 2.3.3. Trust in Korea's Quarantine System during the COVID-19 Pandemic

The researchers developed three items relating to trust in Korea's quarantine system during the COVID-19 pandemic. Each item was rated on a 5-point Likert scale (1 = "Not at all" to 5 = "Absolutely yes"). Regarding the reliability of the scale, Cronbach's $\alpha$ in the primary study was 0.86.

### 2.3.4. Preventive Practice during the COVID-19 Pandemic

Preventive behaviors during the COVID-19 pandemic are related to the respondents' practice behaviors to prevent the transmission of the disease during the previous two weeks. The scale, based on CDC guidelines [6] and developed by the researchers, consisted of ten items. Three nursing professors tested the scale, and its CVI was 0.89. Each item could be rated on a 4-point Likert scale (0 = "Not performed" or "Not applicable" to 3 = "Performed all the time"), with a higher score meaning greater performance of the preventive practice. The reliability (Cronbach's $\alpha$) of the scale was 0.86 in the primary study.

## 2.4. Data Collection

Before developing scales for this study, the researchers completed an online course entitled COVID-19 Contact Tracing, authorized by Johns Hopkins University, to guarantee researchers' expertise regarding COVID-19. This study was approved by the Institutional Review Board (IRB) of U University in Korea (No. 1040968-A-2020-009).

A pilot study was conducted from 3 July to 7 July 2020, to correct these scales. The primary study was conducted from 10 July to 31 July 2020. International students were notified and encouraged to participate in the study through a voice recording or an announcement via the three universities' Learning Management Systems. If they intended to participate in the study, they could follow a link to access the survey. The first page of the online survey included the consent to participate in the research, and all subjects proceeded to the survey after agreeing to participate in the research.

## 2.5. Data Analysis

Data of 256 participants were analyzed using SPSS/WIN 25.0 software. General characteristics and knowledge about COVID-19 were expressed as mean, standard deviation, frequencies, and percentages. Differences in preventive practice according to general characteristics were analyzed using t-test, ANOVA, and post-hoc Scheffe test. Attitudes, trust in Korea's quarantine system, and preventive practice during COVID-19 were presented as mean, standard deviation, and minimum–maximum values. Correlation between study variables was analyzed using Pearson's correlation test. Factors influencing COVID-19 preventive practice were identified by hierarchical multiple linear regression analysis.

## 3. Results

*3.1. Preventive Practice According to General Characteristics*

Participants' average age was 22.90 years, and there were slightly more males (50.8%) than females (49.2%). There were more undergraduate students (56.3%) than language school students (43.8%) in the affiliation. Regarding their duration of stay in Korea, durations of 1 to 2 years were the most common (49.6%), and a duration of more than three years (9.8%) represented the lowest proportion. As for nationality, Vietnamese (43.0%) represented a higher proportion than Uzbekistani (27.0%), Chinese (18.8%), and other nationalities (11.3%). Other countries included Japan, the Philippines, and Malaysia.

There were significant differences in preventive practice by gender (t = 4.19, $p < 0.001$), affiliation (t = 5.47, $p < 0.001$), and duration of stay in Korea (F = 8.93, $p < 0.001$). As a result of the post-hoc comparison test, students who stayed for 1 to 2 years practiced significantly lower preventive behaviors than those who stayed for more than two years (Table 1).

Table 1. Preventive practice according to general characteristics (N = 256).

| Variables | Categories | Mean ± SD or n (%) | Preventive Practice | | |
|---|---|---|---|---|---|
| | | | Mean ± SD | t or F | p (post-hoc) |
| Age (yrs) | | 22.90 ± 2.41 | | | |
| Gender | Male | 130 (50.8) | 2.66 ± 0.44 | 4.19 | <0.001 |
| | Female | 126 (49.2) | 2.42 ± 0.46 | | |
| Affiliation | Undergraduate | 144 (56.3) | 2.68 ± 0.37 | 5.47 | <0.001 |
| | Language school | 112 (43.8) | 2.36 ± 0.51 | | |
| Stay duration in Korea (yrs) | Less than 1 | 56 (21.9) | 2.58 ± 0.43 | 8.93 | <0.001 (a < b,c) |
| | 1-2 [a] | 127 (49.6) | 2.41 ± 0.49 | | |
| | 2-3 [b] | 48 (18.8) | 2.71 ± 0.38 | | |
| | More than 3 [c] | 25 (9.8) | 2.79 ± 0.30 | | |
| Nationality | Vietnam | 110 (43.0) | | | |
| | Uzbekistan | 69 (27.0) | | | |
| | China | 48 (18.8) | | | |
| | Others | 29 (11.3) | | | |

*3.2. Knowledge about COVID-19*

The total correct rate was 85.5% for knowledge about COVID-19 among international students in South Korea. The item with the highest correct answer rate (99.2%) was about prevalent symptoms such as fever, cough, and a sore throat in the symptoms category. However, students most lacked information on the two-week quarantine period in the transmission category (57.0%) (Table 2).

Table 2. Knowledge about COVID-19 (N = 256).

| Items | Answer | Category | Correct n (%) |
|---|---|---|---|
| 1. COVID-19 is a respiratory infectious disease caused by coronavirus (SARS-CoV-2) | True | Onset | 247 (96.5) |
| 2. COVID-19 is transmitted by close contact with the infected person | True | Symptoms | 249 (97.3) |
| 3. Fever, cough, a sore throat, muscle pains, and shortness of breath are possible symptoms of COVID-19 | True | Symptoms | 254 (99.2) |
| 4. Nausea, diarrhea, taste, and olfactory dysfunction are possible non-specific symptoms of COVID-19 | True | Symptoms | 203 (79.3) |
| 5. It requires people who have recently had close contact with someone with COVID-19 to go into quarantine for 1 week | False | Transmission | 146 (57.0) |
| 6. COVID-19 vaccine is available in markets | False[1] | Prevention | 159 (62.1) |
| 7. Using face masks can help in the prevention of disease transmission | True | Transmission | 252 (98.4) |
| 8. COVID-19 could be fatal only for the elderly | False | Transmission | 201 (78.5) |
| 9. You could have been infected and spread COVID-19 to others even if you do not have symptoms | True | Symptoms | 232 (90.6) |
| 10. If soap and water are not readily available, use a hand sanitizer that contains at least 60% of alcohol | True | Prevention | 237 (92.6) |
| Total | | | 85.5% |

[1] It was scored false because there was no vaccine during the data collection period in June 2020.

### 3.3. Attitudes, Trust in Korea's Quarantine System, and Preventive Practice for COVID-19

The mean score of participants' attitudes toward COVID-19 was 4.40 out of 5. The highest scoring item (4.41) was about social distancing, and the lowest scoring item (3.04) was about recognition of the dangers of COVID-19.

The mean score of participants' trust in Korea's quarantine system was 4.13 out of 5. They were satisfied with the order of the healthcare system (score of 4.26), government quarantine system (score of 4.10), and local government quarantine system (score of 4.01).

The mean score of their preventive practice was 2.54 out of 3. The highest score was 2.82 for the item about wearing a face mask in public, and the lowest score was 2.29 for the item of avoiding touching one's own face with unwashed hands (Table 3).

Table 3. Attitudes, trust in Korea's quarantine system, and preventive practice related to COVID-19 (N = 256).

| Variables | Mean ± SD | Min-Max |
|---|---|---|
| **Attitudes** | 4.40 ± 0.57 | 3–5 |
| 1. Do you have confidence that we can win the battle against the COVID-19 virus? | 4.31 ± 0.97 | 1–5 |
| 2. Do you have confidence that you can prevent COVID-19 infection by following the precautions well? | 4.39 ± 0.75 | 2–5 |
| 3. Do you carefully read and follow the instructions on COVID-19 from the (provincial) government and university? | 4.40 ± 0.83 | 1–5 |
| 4. COVID-19 is a very dangerous contagious disease | 3.04 ± 1.49 | 1–5 |
| 5. The activities in my daily life needs to be limited to prevent COVID-19 | 4.41 ± 0.79 | 2–5 |
| **Trust in Korea's quarantine system** | 4.13 ± 0.81 | 2–5 |
| 1. In general, are you satisfied with how the government handles the COVID-19 outbreak? | 4.10 ± 0.95 | 1–5 |
| 2. In general, are you satisfied with how your provincial government handles the COVID-19 outbreak? | 4.04 ± 0.97 | 1–5 |
| 3. In general, are you satisfied with healthcare system in South Korea? | 4.26 ± 0.82 | 2–5 |

Table 3. Cont.

| Variables | Mean ± SD | Min-Max |
|---|---|---|
| **Preventive practice (During past 2 weeks)** | 2.54 ± 0.47 | 1–3 |
| 1. Have washed my hands often with soap and water for at least 20 seconds | 2.49 ± 0.70 | 0–3 |
| 2. Have avoided touching my eyes, nose, and mouth with unwashed hands | 2.29 ± 0.89 | 0–3 |
| 3. Have avoided close contact with people who are sick, even inside my home | 2.41 ± 0.84 | 0–3 |
| 4. Have stayed out of crowded places and avoided mass gatherings | 2.50 ± 0.73 | 0–3 |
| 5. Have worn a face mask when I have to go out in public | 2.82 ± 0.44 | 1–3 |
| 6. Have covered my mouth and nose with a tissue when I coughed or sneezed or used the inside of my elbow, if I did not have a mask on in a private setting | 2.59 ± 0.70 | 0–3 |
| 7. Have thrown used tissues in the trash, and immediately washed my hands after coughing or sneezing | 2.60 ± 0.64 | 1–3 |
| 8. Have cleaned and disinfected frequently touched surfaces on daily basis | 2.42 ± 0.74 | 0–3 |
| 9. Have been alert for related symptoms | 2.69 ± 0.53 | 0–3 |
| 10. Have taken temperature if symptoms were shown | 2.61 ± 0.65 | 0–3 |

### 3.4. Correlations among Variables

Knowledge, attitude, and trust in Korea's quarantine system were positively correlated with each other. Preventive practice for COVID-19 showed significantly positive correlations with knowledge ($r = 0.29$, $p < 0.001$), attitudes ($r = 0.46$, $p < 0.001$), and trust in Korea's quarantine system ($r = 0.48$, $p < 0.001$) (Table 4).

Table 4. Correlations among variables ($N = 256$).

| Variables | Attitudes | Trust in Korea's Quarantine System | Preventive Practice |
|---|---|---|---|
| Knowledge | 0.44 (<0.001) | 0.36 (<0.001) | 0.29 (<0.001) |
| Attitudes |  | 0.46 (<0.001) | 0.46 (<0.001) |
| Trust in Korea's quarantine system |  |  | 0.48 (<0.001) |

### 3.5. Factors Influencing Preventive Practice against COVID-19

A hierarchical multiple linear regression was conducted to analyze factors influencing preventive practice. The Durbin-Watson statistic showed an approximate value of 2, indicating no problem assuming the independence of residuals. The variance expansion index was all less than 10, indicating that there was no multicollinearity problem. In model 1, regression analysis was performed by gender, affiliation, and Stay duration in Korea, significant variables among general characteristics, as dummy variables. Regression equation was significant ($F = 22.15$, $p < 0.001$) and the explained power was 14%. Gender ($\beta = 0.19$, $p = 0.001$) and stay duration in Korea ($\beta = -0.30$, $p < 0.001$) were significant variables. In model 2, preventive practice against COVID-19 was affected by the stay duration in Korea ($\beta = -0.21$, $p < 0.001$), attitudes ($\beta = 0.22$, $p = 0.001$), and trust in Korea's quarantine system ($\beta = 0.33$, $p < 0.001$). Final regression equation was significant ($F = 26.58$, $p < 0.001$) and the explained power was 33% (Table 5).

Table 5. Factors influencing preventive practice against COVID-19 (N = 256).

| Variables | B | SE | beta | t | p |
|---|---|---|---|---|---|
| Model 1 | | | | | |
| Constant | 2.57 | 0.05 | | 52.79 | <0.001 |
| Gender (Ref. male) | 0.18 | 0.06 | 0.19 | 3.28 | 0.001 |
| Stay duration in Korea (Ref. 1 to 2 years) | −0.28 | 0.06 | −0.30 | −5.01 | <0.001 |
| | $R^2 = 0.15$, adj.$R^2 = 0.14$, F = 22.15, $p < 0.001$ | | | | |
| Model 2 | | | | | |
| Constant | 0.94 | 0.23 | | 4.14 | <0.001 |
| Gender (Ref. male) | 0.03 | 0.05 | 0.03 | 0.54 | 0.593 |
| Stay duration in Korea (Ref. 1 to 2 years) | −0.20 | 0.05 | −0.21 | −3.94 | <0.001 |
| Knowledge | 0.12 | 0.22 | 0.03 | 0.56 | 0.579 |
| Attitudes | 0.18 | 0.05 | 0.22 | 3.49 | 0.001 |
| Trust in Korea's quarantine system | 0.19 | 0.04 | 0.33 | 5.46 | <0.001 |
| | $R^2 = 0.35$, adj.$R^2 = 0.33$, F = 26.58, $p < 0.001$ | | | | |

## 4. Discussion

The highly infectious nature of COVID-19 is causing dramatic changes in the lifestyles of millions of people worldwide. In particular, in South Korea, the spread of COVID-19 resulted in a dramatic increase in the number of confirmed cases per day, reaching 741 in Daegu only ten days after discovering the 31st patient in Daegu on 18 February 2020 [3,4]. At that time, Daegu and Gyeongbuk had to fight a novel epidemic without being prepared. Above all, international students, mostly from non-English-speaking countries, had difficulty obtaining information from a daily updated national policy for novel infectious diseases. Therefore, this study was performed to identify influencing factors associated with preventive practice during the COVID-19 pandemic for international students who might have been marginalized during information transmission. There have been very few studies on preventive practice during COVID-19 among international students, to our knowledge.

According to the KAP model, knowledge, attitudes, and practice are inter-related [9,10], and previous studies have found that knowledge is the most crucial factor in preventive behavior regarding novel influenza A [22]. However, the result of the final hierarchical regression analysis in this study found that participants' attitudes, but not their knowledge about COVID-19, affected their preventative practice, although they also showed significant positive relationships [23–25].

Knowledge about COVID-19 was moderate (85.5%), and four out of 10 items showed a correct answer rate of less than 80%. This study's knowledge level was lower than that of 300 international students in Hubei province in China, which showed only two out of 13 items were correctly answered, at a rate of less than 80% [11]. It also was lower than that of 93.2%, measured in 474 nursing students in the study of Sun et al. [26], and 90%, measured in 6910 residents in China [20]. Of course, a direct comparison might be difficult due to differences in the instruments used and the different populations.

These results indicate that it is difficult for international students to obtain accurate, newly updated information and national policy. In particular, students lacked information on the two-week quarantine period (57.0%) and the absence of a COVID-19 vaccine (as of June 2020) (62.1%). However, results showed a very high correct answer rate in regard to wearing a face mask to prevent COVID-19 (98.4%), and in regard to preventive practice during the previous two weeks, wearing a face mask in public achieved the highest score. This result was higher than that of 58.2%, measured in the Iranian population, who responded that they always wear a mask [27]. Because COVID-19 is transmitted via droplets [6], personal preventive equipment (PPE), especially face masks, can play a critical role in controlling COVID-19 [28]. This is thought to be because KDCA actively encouraged and promoted the wearing of face masks [7]. Regarding the attitudes, subjects agreed that disease prevention would be possible if they complied with quarantine regulations, including social distancing. Moreover, their trust in Korea's quarantine system was high (score of 4.13). In March, the Korean government attempted to prevent the spread of COVID-19 by introducing a 5-day rotation system for mask distribution so that people can purchase disposable face masks each week, by sending text messages about safety guidance, such as wearing a mask, social distancing, and hand washing, and by briefing residents on the situation twice a day on television [29]. It was believed that such an active response from the government improved international students' trust in the quarantine system. Direct comparison is difficult because there is no previous study on the correlation between preventive practice and the quarantine system. However, people with low trust in the healthcare system are associated with low adherence to human immunodeficiency virus (HIV) care and poorer health outcomes [30]. Therefore, having trust in quarantine systems and demonstrating compliance with guidelines might be more important than having a high level of knowledge regarding factors affecting preventative practice.

## 5. Conclusions

In this study, international students residing in Daegu and Gyeongbuk, with the highest number of confirmed COVID-19 cases in Korea, were investigated for factors affecting preventive practice regarding COVID-19. Results indicate that having the right attitudes and trust in the public quarantine system are more important in maintaining individual preventive actions than having the right knowledge about infectious diseases in a pandemic situation.

This study has some limitations. First, many participants in this study were Asian and from the southeast or northeast regions, so the findings were limited and cannot be generalized to all international students from all continents. However, to ensure the samples' representativeness, we sought to secure the number of samples according to international students' national distribution. Second, participants in this study were limited to international students enrolled in three universities, so international students who left Korea before the COVID-19 pandemic and were in their home countries were omitted. This was because they were international students who did not experience Korea's quarantine system and prevention guidelines in the context of the COVID-19 pandemic and did not match this study's purpose. Despite some limitations, this study was meaningful in that it sought ways to promote the preventive practices of international students living in regions where the number of confirmed cases was increasing and the fear of residents was high.

**Author Contributions:** Conceptualization, G.J.J. and S.K.; methodology, G.J.J. and G.J. and S.K.; investigation, G.J.J. and G.J.; data curation, S.K.; writing—original draft preparation, G.J.J. and S.K.; writing—review and editing, G.J.J. and S.K.; funding acquisition, G.J.J. All authors have read and agreed to the published version of the manuscript.

**Funding:** This research was funded by Daegu University, grant number 20160037.

**Institutional Review Board Statement:** The study was conducted according to the guidelines of the Declaration of Helsinki and approved by the Institutional Review Board of University of Ulsan (No.1040968-A-2020-009).

**Informed Consent Statement:** Informed consent was obtained from all subjects involved in the study.

**Conflicts of Interest:** The authors declare no conflict of interest.

## References

1. Sharma, A.; Tiwari, S.; Deb, M.K.; Marty, J.L. Severe acute respiratory syndrome coronavirus-2 (SARS-CoV-2): A global pandemic and treatment strategies. *Int. J. Antimicrob. Agents* **2020**, *56*, 106054. [CrossRef]
2. Choi, J.Y. COVID-19 in South Korea. *Postgrad. Med. J.* **2020**, *96*, 399–402. [CrossRef] [PubMed]
3. Shim, E.; Tariq, A.; Choi, W.; Lee, Y.; Chowell, G. Transmission potential and severity of COVID-19 in South Korea. *Int. J. Infect. Dis.* **2020**, *93*, 339–344. [CrossRef]

4. COVID-19 National Emergency Response Center; Epidemiology and Case Management Team; Korea Centers for Disease Control and Prevention. Coronavirus disease-19: The first 7755 cases in the republic of Korea. *Osong. Public Health Res. Perspect.* **2020**, *11*, 85–90. [CrossRef]
5. World Health Organization. Coronavirus (COVID-19) Outbreak. Available online: https://www.who.int/westernpacific/emergencies/covid-19 (accessed on 15 February 2021).
6. Centers for Disease Control and Prevention. Guidance Documents. Available online: https://www.cdc.gov/coronavirus/2019-ncov/communication/guidance-list.html?Sort=Date%3A%3Adesc (accessed on 22 May 2020).
7. Korea Disease Control and Prevention Agency. Guidelines. Available online: http://www.kdca.go.kr/board/board.es?mid=a20507020000&bid=0019 (accessed on 15 February 2021).
8. Perz, C.A.; Lang, B.A.; Harrington, R. Validation of the fear of COVID-19 scale in a US college sample. *Int. J. Ment. Health Addict.* **2020**, *25*, 1–11. [CrossRef] [PubMed]
9. Wu, X.L.; Munthali, G.N.C. Knowledge, attitudes, and preventive practices (KAPs) towards COVID-19 among international students in China. *Dovepress* **2021**, *14*, 507–518. [CrossRef]
10. Monde, M.D. The KAP Survey Model (Knowledge, Attitudes, and Practices). Available online: https://www.springnutrition.org/publications/tool-summaries/kap-survey-model-knowledge-attitudes-and-practices (accessed on 20 December 2020).
11. Ajilore, K.; Atakiti, I.; Onyenankey, K. College students' knowledge, attitudes, and adherence to public service announcements on Ebola in Nigeria: Suggestions for improving future Ebola prevention education programmes. *Health Educ. J.* **2017**, *76*, 648–660. [CrossRef]
12. Choi, J.S.; Kim, J.S. Factors influencing preventive behavior against Middle East Respiratory Syndrome-Coronavirus among nursing students in South Korea. *Nurse Educ. Today* **2016**, *40*, 168–172. [CrossRef]
13. Ejeh, F.E.; Saidu, A.S.; Owoicho, S.; Maurice, N.A.; Jauro, S.; Madukaji, L.; Okon, K.O. Knowledge, attitude, and practice among healthcare workers towards COVID-19 outbreak in Nigeria. *Heliyon* **2020**, *6*, e05557. [CrossRef] [PubMed]
14. Taghrir, M.H.; Borazjani, R.; Shiraly, R. COVID-19 and Iranian medical students; a survey on their related-knowledge, preventive behaviors and risk perception. *Arch. Iran. Med.* **2020**, *23*, 249–254. [CrossRef] [PubMed]
15. Albaqawi, H.M.; Alquwez, N.; Balay-odao, E.; Bajet, J.B.; Alabdulaziz, H.; Alsolami, F.; Tumala, R.B.; Alsharari, A.F.; Tork, H.M.M.; Felemban, E.M. Nursing students' perceptions, knowledge, and preventive behaviors toward COVID-19: A multi-university study. *Front. Public Health* **2020**, *8*. [CrossRef]
16. Kim, H.R.; Choi, E.Y.; Park, S.Y.; Kim, E.A. Factors influencing preventive behavior against coronavirus disease 2019 (COVID-19) among medically inclined college students. *J. Korean Acad. Fundam. Nurs.* **2020**, *27*, 428–437. [CrossRef]
17. Higher Education in Korea. Student. Available online: https://www.academyinfo.go.kr/index.do?lang=en (accessed on 16 February 2021).
18. Test of Proficiency in Korean. TOPIK Test Information. Available online: https://www.topik.go.kr/usr/lang/index.do?home_seq=221&lang=en (accessed on 16 February 2021).
19. Kim, J.S.; Choi, J.S. Middle East respiratory syndrome-related knowledge, preventive behaviours and risk perception among nursing students during outbreak. *J. Clin. Nurs.* **2016**, *25*, 2542–2549. [CrossRef]
20. Huynh, G.; Nguyen, T.N.H.; Tran, V.K.; Vo, K.N.; Vo, V.T.; Pham, L.A. Knowledge and attitude toward COVID-19 among healthcare workers at District 2 Hospital, Ho Chi Minh City. *Asian Pac. J. Trop Med.* **2020**, *13*. [CrossRef]
21. Zhong, B.L.; Luo, W.; Li, H.M.; Zhang, Q.Q.; Liu, X.G.; Li, W.T.; Li, Y. Knowledge, attitudes, and practices towards COVID-19 among Chinese residents during the rapid rise period of the COVID-19 outbreak: A quick online cross-sectional survey. *Int. J. Biol. Sci.* **2020**, *16*, 1745–1752. [CrossRef]
22. Choi, J.S.; Yang, N.Y. Perceived knowledge, attitude, and compliance with preventive behavior on influenza A (H1N1) by university students. *J. Korean Acad. Adult Nurs.* **2010**, *22*, 250–259. (In Korean)
23. Ferdous, M.Z.; Islam, M.S.; Sikder, M.T.; Mosaddek, A.S.M.; Zegarra-Valdivia, J.A.; Gozal, D. Knowledge, attitude, and practice regarding COVID-19 outbreak in Bangladesh: An online-based cross-sectional study. *PLoS ONE* **2020**, *15*, e0239254. [CrossRef]
24. Papagiannis, D.; Malli, F.; Raptis, D.G.; Papathanasiou, I.V.; Fradelos, E.C.; Daniil, Z.; Rachiotis, G.; Gourgoulianis, K.I. Assessment of knowledge, attitudes, and practices towards new coronavirus (SARS-CoV-2) of health care professionals in Greece before the outbreak period. *Int. J. Environ. Res. Public Health* **2020**, *17*, 4925. [CrossRef]
25. Akalu, Y.; Ayelign, B.; Molla, M.D. Knowledge, attitude and practice towards COVID-19 among chronic disease patients at Addis Zemen Hospital, Northwest Ethiopia. *Infect. Drug Resist.* **2020**, *13*, 1949–1960. [CrossRef]
26. Sun, Y.; Wang, D.; Han, Z.; Gao, J.; Zhu, S.; Zhang, H. Disease prevention knowledge, anxiety, and professional identity during COVID-19 pandemic in nursing Students in Zhengzhou, China. *J. Korean Acad. Nurs.* **2020**, *50*, 533. [CrossRef]
27. Firouzbakht, M.; Omidvar, S.; Firouzbakht, S.; Asadi-Amoli, A. COVID-19 preventive behaviors and influencing factors in the Iranian population; a web-based survey. *BMC Public Health* **2021**, *21*, 143. [CrossRef] [PubMed]
28. Chu, D.K.; Akl, E.A.; Duda, S.; Solo, K.; Yaacoub, S.; Schünemann, H.J. COVID-19 Systematic Urgent Review Group Effort (SURGE) study authors. Physical distancing, face masks, and eye protection to prevent person-to-person transmission of SARS-CoV-2 and COVID-19: A systematic review and meta-analysis. *Lancet* **2020**, *395*, 1973–1987. [CrossRef]

29. Kang, J.; Jang, Y.Y.; Kim, J.; Han, S.H.; Lee, K.R.; Kim, M.; Eom, J.S. South Korea's responses to stop the COVID-19 pandemic. *Am. J. Infect. Control* **2020**, *48*, 1080–1086. [CrossRef] [PubMed]
30. Graham, J.L.; Shahani, L.; Grimes, R.M.; Hartman, C.; Giordano, T.P. The influence of trust in physicians and trust in the healthcare system on linkage, retention, and adherence to HIV care. *AIDS Patient Care STDS* **2015**, *29*, 661–667. [CrossRef]

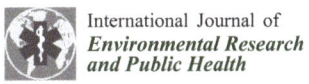

International Journal of
*Environmental Research and Public Health*

*Article*

# Determinants of Perceived Accessibility of Maternity Leave and Childcare Leave in South Korea

Eun Jung Kim [1], Won Ju Hwang [2] and Mi Jeong Kim [1,*]

[1] School of Architecture, Hanyang University, Seoul 04763, Korea; ejkim82@hanyang.ac.kr
[2] College of Nursing Science, Kyung Hee University, Seoul 02447, Korea; hwangwj@khu.ac.kr
* Correspondence: mijeongkim@hanyang.ac.kr; Tel.: +82-2-2220-1249

**Abstract:** This study examined the determinants of perceived accessibility of maternity leave and childcare leave in South Korea. Although maternity leave and childcare leave are mandated in Korea, many employees are hesitant to use the policies. The purpose of this study was to empirically examine why some women are more likely than others to perceive the policies as inaccessible and to identify what those women's characteristics are. The results revealed that nonregular workers were significantly less likely than regular workers with secure contracts to perceive the policies as accessible even though they were eligible for them. In addition, workers who worked in the private sector, did not belong to a labor union, worked in small firms, or worked long hours were significantly less likely to perceive the policies as accessible than those who worked in the public sector, belonged to a labor union, worked in large firms, or worked short hours. Further, workers with low salaries were significantly less likely than workers with high salaries to perceive the policies as accessible. The study underscores that accessibility of leave policies in Korea is significantly correlated with women's employment status and wage level in the labor market.

**Keywords:** childcare leave; determinants; maternity leave; perceived accessibility; South Korea

**Citation:** Kim, E.J.; Hwang, W.J.; Kim, M.J. Determinants of Perceived Accessibility of Maternity Leave and Childcare Leave in South Korea. *IJERPH* **2021**, *18*, 10286. https://doi.org/10.3390/ijerph181910286

**Academic Editor:** Paul B. Tchounwou

**Received:** 12 August 2021
**Accepted:** 27 September 2021
**Published:** 29 September 2021

**Publisher's Note:** MDPI stays neutral with regard to jurisdictional claims in published maps and institutional affiliations.

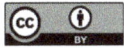

**Copyright:** © 2021 by the authors. Licensee MDPI, Basel, Switzerland. This article is an open access article distributed under the terms and conditions of the Creative Commons Attribution (CC BY) license (https://creativecommons.org/licenses/by/4.0/).

## 1. Introduction

In 2020, the total fertility rate in South Korea (hereafter referred to as Korea) was 0.84, the lowest in the world [1]. Difficulties balancing work and family responsibilities have been associated with women's reluctance to have children in Korea [2]. According to a 2009 Organisation for Economic Co-operation and Development (OECD) report, while married Korean working women spent on average 3 h per day on unpaid domestic work, men spent on average 30 min per day [3]. The Confucian patriarchal culture has placed many burdens on Korean working women, who are still considered responsible for the majority of household tasks [4]. In an effort to increase fertility among working women and promote work–family balance, the Korean government has actively expanded maternity leave and childcare leave since the 2000s [4]. However, despite the government's effort, the fertility rate has constantly dropped in Korea, and the actual use of maternity leave and childcare leave by working women still remains relatively low [4]. According to a 2012 national report, 24% of Korean employed women who gave birth used maternity leave, and 35% used childcare leave [5].

Although maternity leave and childcare leave are mandated by the government, many Korean companies disapprove of employees taking advantage of the policies. Hence, a considerable number of Korean employees perceive maternity leave and childcare leave as inaccessible because they fear negative reprisals (i.e., being demoted to unfavorable positions, being passed over for promotions, and being laid off after their contract ends). In a 2008 report by the Korean Women's Development Institute (KWDI), 56% and 59% of wage-earning working women reported that their companies did not provide or allow maternity leave and childcare leave, respectively [6].

Despite the low use of maternity and childcare leave in Korea, until now, to our knowledge, no study has empirically examined the reasons why some women in Korea are less likely than others to perceive maternity leave and childcare leave as accessible and to identify what those women's characteristics are on a national scale. Kim examined 1000 working Korean mothers with preschool children from five metropolitan areas in 2011–2012 and found that intent to use family policy was influenced by work-oriented attitude, household financial status, informal (i.e., family members and neighbors) support, work sector (i.e., private sector vs public sector), and awareness and familiarity with family policies [7]. However, Kim's findings cannot be generalizable because the study only relies on five metropolitan areas. In Korea, significant differences exist between people dwelling in metropolitan areas and rural areas (i.e., income, age, and social infrastructures). For example, income is important because it is directly related to affordability of leaves. In 2012, the annual average household income for rural residents was substantially lower than for residents dwelling in metropolitan areas (USD 30,000 vs USD 54,000 [7]. Additionally, rural areas have fewer social infrastructures such as childcare centers to help working parents with childcare and other domestic responsibilities. Hence, the goal of the present study was to address this gap in the literature. Using the 2007–2012 Korean Longitudinal Survey of Women and Families (KLoWF), the present study examined on a national scale the factors associated with working women's perceived accessibility of maternity leave and childcare leave in Korea. Findings from this study will help policymakers to develop policies that better facilitate working women's access to maternity leave and childcare leave in Korea.

## 2. Maternity Leave and Childcare Leave in Korea

In Korea, both maternity leave and childcare leave are mandated under the Act on Equal Employment and Support for Work-Family Balance. To be eligible for maternity leave and childcare leave in Korea, workers must have been employed at their workplaces and enrolled in the National Employment Insurance program for more than 180 days. In Korea, all companies—except for (1) unincorporated businesses with four or fewer full-time employed workers in agricultural, forestry, fishing, or hunting industries; (2) small construction companies with a yearly total construction cost of less than KRW 20 million (approximately USD 17,300); and (3) self-employed businesses—are mandated to provide the National Employment Insurance to their employees. Hence, except for the few above-mentioned cases, the majority of wage-earning Korean workers should be automatically eligible for maternity leave and childcare leave if they have worked at the workplace for more than 180 days. The penalty for the company refusing to provide maternity or childcare leave is KRW 5,000,000 (USD 4500) per case, but it only applies when reported by a refused employee. Over the years, the Korean government has expanded maternity leave and childcare leave to promote work–family balance and fertility.

*2.1. Maternity Leave*

Maternity leave was originally introduced in 1953 as a paid 60-day leave policy but was extended in 2001 to 90 days in Korea. Currently, in Korea, maternity leave can be used prior to birth for up to 45 days. Working Korean women are eligible to receive full replacement wages for the first 60 days of their leave from employers and partial or full-wage replacement from the National Employment Insurance program for the remaining 30 days up to a maximum of KWR 2,000,000 (USD 1750).

*2.2. Childcare Leave*

Childcare leave was first introduced in 1987 as unpaid one-year leave for mothers with children under one year old. In 2008, this policy was revised to provide paid leave at a flat rate of KRW 500,000 (USD 450) per month and was expanded to include both mothers and fathers with children under three years old. In 2010, the leave was further expanded to include children under six years old. In 2011, the flat rate was revised from KRW 500,000 (USD 450) per month to a wage replacement equivalent to 40% of the receiver's monthly salary within a range of KRW 500,000–1,000,000 (USD 450–900). In 2014, it was revised to include children under eight years old (or until they enter the second year of primary education). In 2018, the wage replacement rate was revised to 80% of their monthly salary within a range of KRW 700,000–1,500,000 (USD 600–1300) for the first 3 months of their leave, and 40% of their salary within a range of KRW 500,000–1,000,000 (USD 450–900) for the remaining 9 months. Additionally, from 2018, to promote mothers' return to work, only a partial 75% of the benefit is provided during the leave period and the remaining 25% of the benefit is paid as a lump sum 6 months after mothers return to work.

Employees who are unable to take full-time one-year absence may use reduced working hours as an alternative to childcare leave. To be eligible for such leave, employees must work for a minimum of 15 h per week and a maximum of 35 h per week and may use the leave for up to a maximum of 2 years in one or two blocks before the child's eighth birthday.

*2.3. Low Uptake of Maternity Leave and Childcare Leave*

In comparison with other OECD countries, the overall length of statutory maternity and childcare leave support in Korea is quite extensive. Mothers in Korea can take up to 65 weeks of paid leave in total, which is longer than the OECD average of 55 weeks [8]. However, as mentioned above, the uptake rate of maternity leave and childcare leave remains low in Korea. For children born in 2017, only about 23% of mothers used maternity leave benefits, and 11% of them worked in the civil public sector or teaching professions [9]. Regarding childcare leave, for children born in 2018, only about 30% of parents claimed the benefit, and 53% of them were government officials or teachers (in schools or universities). Compared with other OECD countries, this uptake is relatively low. For example, in Germany in 2016, approximately 94 mothers and 35 fathers claimed childcare leave for every 100 births [9].

## 3. Literature Review of Determinants of Maternity Leave and Childcare Leave Accessibility

A possible reason for the low usage of maternity leave and childcare leave is that employees believe that access to such provisions is restricted [10]. The literature explains this as a gap between "policy and practice" [11–13]. Employees might not report that leave policies are accessible to them even if they are available at their workplaces for several reasons. First, companies may offer certain benefits only to specific groups of employees (i.e., uneven coverage within a workplace). Second, employees may not be aware of the benefits to which they are entitled. Lastly, employees may feel that these policies are inaccessible because of various barriers, such as financial constraints, impracticalities, and fear of reprisals [10].

However, in Korea, since maternity leave and childcare leave are statutory, companies do not have the discretion to choose to whom to provide provisions. In addition, because maternity leave and childcare leave have been implemented since 1953 and 1987, respectively, it is unlikely that employees' reason for not using the policies is the lack of awareness of the programs in Korea. Dulk and Peper argued that employees must have a sense of entitlement for them to access and use the policies and contended that social atmosphere and institutional features pose as barriers or enablers to employees' sense of entitlement to policies [14]. Since there is a lack of studies on policy accessibility and its determinants in Korea, the present study used studies from Western countries (e.g., the Netherlands, United Kingdom, and United States) [10,14,15] to understand the mechanisms behind why some women are less likely than others to perceive the leave policies as accessible. We believe it would be interesting to examine whether in Korea the results would be different. Compared with Western countries, Korea has a strong collectivist workplace culture, which places "team/group" above "individual" [16]. On the other hand, in Western cultures, there is more focus on the individual and that collective goods are to serve individual rights, not vice versa. Hence, personal and family time is a priority; however, in Korea, priority is often given to work [16]. Such differences may yield different results.

### 3.1. Public Sector Employees

Dulk and Peper's arguments are corroborated by findings from Budd and Mumford's examination of the relationship between institutional context (i.e., norms, regulations, and social expectations) and employees' perceived access to policies in the United Kingdom [10,14]. They posited that some employees are more sensitive to institutional pressure than other employees, based on their visibility and influence in society, and found that public sector employees were more likely to feel entitled to maternity and childcare leave and to perceive the policies as accessible because they were more visible to the public and sensitive to government policies. Hence, in this study, we hypothesized that:

**Hypothesis 1 (H1)**: *Women working in the public sector are more likely to perceive maternity leave and childcare leave as accessible in Korea.*

### 3.2. Labor Union Members

Budd and Mumford also discovered that more than those who did not belong to labor unions, employees who belonged to labor unions were more likely to perceive leave policies as accessible because they had stronger collective bargaining power to negotiate benefits and, having been educated through union letters and workshops, had greater awareness of maternity leave and childcare leave, and thus felt a stronger sense of entitlement to these policies [10]. In Korea, although a majority of the people are aware of the existence of the policies, some employees may not be aware that they are also eligible for the policies. Hence, those who belong to labor unions are more likely to be aware of their entitlements and have greater bargaining power to fight against employers who refuse to provide maternity leave or childcare leave. Hence, in this study, we hypothesized that:

**Hypothesis 2 (H2)**: *Working women belonging to labor unions are more likely to perceive maternity leave and childcare leave as accessible in Korea.*

### 3.3. Nonregular Temporary Workers

Budd and Mumford also discovered that regular employees were more likely than nonregular workers to perceive leave policies as accessible because they had greater job security [10]. In Korea, nonregular workers are often deprived of their right to apply for maternity and childcare leave because of the workplace culture and regulations that forbid them from taking the leave or simply do not acknowledge their rights. Although in Korea, the law stipulates that employees are automatically eligible for maternity leave and childcare leave, regardless of their contract status, as long as they are employed for more than 6 months at their workplaces. However, nonregular workers may not know this or feel they cannot use the policies. According to a survey conducted by the KWDI in 2009, about half of nonregular workers did not apply for maternity leave, and about a third of those who did not apply reported that they did not apply because their workplace regulations forbade them from taking leave, which is not only discriminatory but also illegal [17]. However, nonregular workers dared not challenge the companies' regulations for fear of losing their work contract in the subsequent year. Hence, we hypothesized that:

**Hypothesis 3 (H3)**: *Women who are regular workers are more likely to perceive maternity leave and childcare leave as accessible in Korea.*

### 3.4. Company Size

It has also been reported that smaller firms are more likely than big companies in Korea to have work regulations that forbid workers from using leave [18]. This is possibly because the first two months of maternity leave are paid for by the employer, and smaller firms may have less financial capability to support such costs. In addition, it was reported that a significant share of women in Korea prefer not to take the leave in order to avoid penalizing their coworkers, because companies often do not fill temporary vacancies [19]. Smaller firms are less likely than bigger companies to have the human and financial resources to fill the vacancies when employees take leave; therefore, they are more likely to have workplace cultures or internal regulations that hinder employees from using maternity and childcare leave. Hence, we hypothesized that:

**Hypothesis 4 (H4)**: *Women who work in small companies are less likely to perceive maternity leave and childcare leave as accessible in Korea.*

### 3.5. Gendered-Discriminatory Workplace and Long Working Hours

The internal culture of the organization is argued to also influence the extent to which employees feel entitled to leave policies [14]. There is mounting evidence that workplace culture substantially affects workers' perceived access to and use of maternity and childcare leave [20]. Fried discovered that in workplaces where the workforce composition was a "gendered pyramid, with the greatest number of women at the bottom and increasingly fewer women as one moves up to the top", long working hours were valued, the workplaces were often permeated by a male-defined culture (i.e., competition, aggression, and singular focus on career, usually at the expense of family), and employees tended to perceive leave polices as less accessible [15] (p. 40). In Korea, work culture is marked by long working hours (46.8 h per week, compared with the OECD average of 42 h; OECD 2019) and strong work ethics, primarily dominated by male managers [4]. According to a survey conducted by Job Korea in 2010, more than half of the 1623 female workers interviewed reported that it was difficult to use maternity and childcare leave because of the pressure from their workplaces [21], and according to a survey conducted by Samsung Economic Research Institute, 42% of female respondents reported that they feared receiving low evaluations during or after they returned from maternity and childcare leave [22]. Hence, in this study, we hypothesized that:

**Hypothesis 5a (H5a)**: *Women who work in a gender-discriminatory workplace culture are less likely to perceive maternity leave and childcare leave as accessible in Korea.*

**Hypothesis 5b (H5b)**: *Women who work long hours are less likely to perceive maternity leave and childcare leave as accessible in Korea.*

### 3.6. Managerial Positions

Lastly, Fried also discovered that neither men nor women at the upper levels used leave policy, and middle-level managers used it sparingly in the United States [15]. The largest cohort of leave-takers comprised female non-managers. In addition, according to the 2010 Korean Women Manager Panel, only 36% of managers applied for childcare leave, and among those who did not apply, one-fourth responded that they could not apply for the leave because, according to their workplace culture, it is customary not to apply [23]. In a similar line of reasoning, the present study expected women workers with high salaries to be less likely to perceive maternity leave and childcare leave as accessible than workers with lower salaries because they have greater work responsibilities and higher peer pressure. In this study, because of data limitations, salary was used as a proxy variable to measure career-level position. The literature indicates that there is a significant positive correlation between salary and career [24]. Moreover, considering that only a partial rate of the salary is paid during the leave period, for employees with higher salaries, the opportunity cost of leaving work to take care of children will be higher, and hence, they may be less inclined to take maternity and childcare leave than employees' with lower salaries. Hence, we hypothesized that:

**Hypothesis 6 (H6)**: *Women with higher wages are less likely to perceive maternity leave and childcare leave as accessible in Korea.*

## 4. Methodology

### 4.1. Data

The KLoWF was used for this study. The KLoWF uses a multi-stage, stratified clustered design and surveys 9997 women aged 19 to 64 who live in 9068 households across the nation. The survey was first conducted in 2007 and subsequently in 2008, 2010, and 2012. The KLoWF is an unbalanced panel survey and refreshment samples were added to supplement for attrition. To treat for possible attrition biases, the present study used post-stratification survey weights provided by the KLoWF. Post-stratification weights adjust attrition by assuming that dropouts occur randomly within weighting classes defined by observed variables that are associated with dropouts [25].

### 4.2. Analytical Sample

In this study, to ensure that our analytical sample was eligible for maternity and childcare leave, our analytical sample included married, wage-earning, full-time working women of childbearing age (16–49) and those who had worked at their workplaces for more than 6 months, excluding those who were self-employed and worked in agricultural, forestry, fishing, or hunting industries with fewer than four full-time employees. We were unable to exclude those working in small construction companies with a yearly total construction cost of less than KRW 20 million because of data limitations: however, we posit that this number would have been minimal because the percentage of women working in construction is very small in Korea.

Based on these criteria, a total sample of 4559 observations (wave 2007 = 1174, wave 2008 = 1154, wave 2010 = 1118, wave 2012 = 1113) was examined. To treat for possible biases due to repeated measures, random effects modeling was used in this study, which is further explained in Section 4.4.

### 4.3. Measures

#### 4.3.1. Outcome Variables

The outcome variables for this study were working women's perceived access (whether employees could actually use the policies if they wished) to maternity leave and childcare leave. Accessibility was measured as a binary response (yes or no).

#### 4.3.2. Predictor Variables

Employment status (regular or nonregular worker), work sector (public or private), and belonging to a labor union (yes or no) were measured as dichotomous variables. Company size was measured as a categorical variable (1 = below 5 employees, 2 = 5–9 employees, 3 = 10–29 employees, 4 = 30–99 employees, 5 = more than 100). Average work hours per day and logged monthly salary were measured as a continuous variable. Gender-discriminatory workplace culture was measured using the following six items: (1) "If candidates have similar qualifications for appointment, men are preferred to women"; (2) "Even with identical or similar careers, male workers are promoted faster than female counterparts"; (3) "Even in identical or similar positions, male workers receive higher wages and bonuses than female workers"; (4) "Duties are fixed or customarily divided between men and women"; (5) "Even with similar duties, men have more opportunities to receive education and training than women"; and (6) "In case of restructuring, female workers are more likely to be forced to quit". The KLoWF reports the six items using a 4-point Likert scale (1: nondiscriminatory to 4: discriminatory), and in this study, the items were summed and averaged to measure gender-discriminatory workplace culture.

#### 4.3.3. Control Variables

A range of demographic variables was controlled in this study. Participants' age, average hours spent on unpaid household chores, and logged yearly household income were measured as continuous variables and controlled. Number of children was measured as a categorical variable (0 = none, 1 = one child, 2 = two children, 3 = three or more children). Education attainment was measured as a 4-point ordinal scale (1 = middle school degree or below, 2 = high school degree, 3 = two-year community college degree, 4 = four-year bachelor's degree or master's or higher). We have summarized the variables in Table 1.

Table 1. Summary of the variables.

| | Variables | Measures |
|---|---|---|
| Outcome | Perceive maternity leave as accessible | No (=0)/Yes (=1) |
| | Perceive childcare leave as accessible | No (=0)/Yes (=1) |
| Predictor | Employed in public sector | Private (=0)/Public (=1) |
| | Labor union member | No (=0)/Yes (=1) |
| | Regular worker | Nonregular (=0)/Regular (=1) |
| | Company size | Below 5 (=1)/5–9 (=2)/10–29 (=3)/30–99 (=4)/ more than 100 (=5) |
| | Gender-discriminatory workplace | Six-item Likert scale (1–4) |
| | Working hours | Average daily working hour (continuous) |
| | Monthly wage | Logged after-tax wage KRW 10,000 (continuous) |
| Control | Age | Age (continuous) |
| | Household chores | Average hours spent on household chores (continuous) |
| | Number of children | 0 (=0)/1 (=1)/2 (=2)/3 or more (=3) |
| | Household income | Logged yearly after-tax household income (continuous) |
| | Education | (1 = middle school degree or below, 2 = high school degree, 3 = two-year community college degree, 4 = four-year bachelor's degree or master's or higher) |

### 4.4. Modeling

Since the KLoWF is a longitudinal panel survey, a pooled ordinary least squares (OLS) regression model with year dummies may yield biased results because of potential omitted variables (i.e., unobserved heterogeneity), such as social and cultural attitudes. Considering that leave policies are closely related to contextual influences such as social and cultural attitudes toward working women, it is important to control for such variables [26].

Both a fixed effects model and random effects model can account for unobserved heterogeneity [27]. The purpose of both fixed and random effects estimators is to consider treatment effects whilst controlling for unobserved individual-specific effects. In the model below, this is represented by $\alpha_i$

$$Y_{it} = \beta X_{it} + \alpha_i + e_{it},$$

where,

- $Y_{it}$ is the dependent variable (i = individual, t = time);
- $X_{it}$ is the independent variable;
- $\beta$ is the coefficient;
- $\alpha_i$ is the individual-specific intercept;
- $e_{it}$ is the error term.

In a fixed effects modeling, unobserved heterogeneity is accounted for by allowing each individual to have its own intercept ($\alpha_i$). In fixed effects modeling, each individual is assigned a specific intercept value (hence, the name fixed effects), and by doing so, we eliminate all individual-specific effects, including both observable and unobservable individual-level factors and focus solely on the impact of variables that vary over time. A disadvantage, however, is that time-invariant variables cannot be estimated. Since individual-level intercepts are essentially separate independent variables in a fixed effects model, we assume that the intercepts are correlated with the independent variables.

In a random effects model, individual-specific effects, including unobservable factors, are captured by the composite error terms ($\alpha_i + e_{it}$), which assumes that individual intercepts ($\alpha_i$) are randomly distributed (hence, the name random effects), unlike in the fixed effects model, which assigns fixed specific values. In order to capture individual heterogeneity, random effects modeling estimates error variances specific to cross-sectional units [27]. Since in the random effects model, the variation across individuals is random, we assume that the intercepts are uncorrelated with the independent variables. Hence, in a random effects model, a one-unit increase in independent variable "X" may have two meanings: (1) differences between individuals when there is a unit difference in "X" between them (i.e., between effect) and (2) differences within an individual when "X" increases by one (i.e., within effect). The random effects model estimates that the two effects are the same [25].

Since this study was interested in estimating the overall effect of determinants of perceived accessibility of maternity and childcare leave between and within individuals, the random effects model was selected. Hausman specification tests were conducted to test whether fixed effects or random effects modeling was a better model fit, and the results confirmed the appropriateness of using random effects modeling over fixed effects modeling. Here, we used a random effects logistic model since our dependent variables were binary variables.

Further, we controlled for possible sample selection bias (i.e., bias due to a flaw in the sample selection process, where a subset of the data is systematically excluded due to a particular attribute [26]) by using STATA 16 extended regression model (ERM) analysis (see Appendix A Table A1). Since in our study perceived accessibility of maternity leave and childcare leave was only observed among working women, there was the possibility that working women may have had attributes that were significantly different and non-random from women not participating in the labor market. That is, women who were less likely to perceive maternity leave and childcare leave as accessible may have been less likely to join the labor market from the start (i.e., selection bias). However, the ERM results showed that no significant sample selection bias existed in our model; hence, in this study, we used the more parsimonious random effects logistic model as our final model.

In addition, if we were to run a pooled ordinary least squares regression model with year dummies, the results may have been biased because of autocorrelation due to repeated measures (i.e., correlation between residuals at a given wave and the ones for the previous one) [26]. To control for the possible existence of autocorrelation, we used cluster-robust standard errors in all the models [26].

## 5. Results

Table 2 presents the accessibility rates by time. The results show that approximately 26% and 21% of working women reported that they felt they could use maternity leave and childcare leave, respectively, if they wished to. Over the years, despite the government's efforts, a lower percentage of people have perceived the leave policies as accessible.

**Table 2.** Maternity leave and childcare leave accessibility time.

|  | Wave 2007 | Wave 2008 | Wave 2010 | Wave 2012 | Overall |
| --- | --- | --- | --- | --- | --- |
| Maternity leave | 32.2% | 26.3% | 23.1% | 21.5% | 25.8% |
| Childcare leave | 28.4.% | 23.3% | 19.7% | 13.9% | 21.4% |

Table 3 presents the unadjusted bivariate results between policy accessibility and the predictors and covariates. First, with regard to maternity leave, while 60% of regular workers perceived maternity leave as accessible, less than 5% of nonregular workers perceived maternity leave as accessible ($p < 0.001$). Likewise, while the majority (72%) of workers who belonged to labor unions perceived maternity leave as accessible, only 18% of workers who did not belong to labor unions perceived maternity leave as accessible ($p < 0.001$). In addition, women who worked in the public sector (61%) were approximately 3 times more likely to perceive maternity leave as accessible than those who worked in the private sector (23%; $p < 0.001$). Moreover, workers who worked in larger companies were also significantly more likely to perceive maternity leave as accessible ($p < 0.001$), and those who worked longer hours were more likely to perceive maternity leave as accessible

($p < 0.001$). Workers who worked in more gender-discriminatory workplaces were more likely to perceive maternity leave as accessible, but this was not statistically significant. Lastly, working women whose salary was higher were significantly likely to perceive maternity leave as accessible ($p < 0.001$).

Table 3. Bivariate analyses ($N = 4559$).

| Frequency (%) | Maternity Leave | | | Childcare Leave | | |
|---|---|---|---|---|---|---|
| | Not Accessible | Accessible | $x^2$ ($df$) | Not Accessible | Accessible | $x^2$ ($df$) |
| **Employment type** | | | | | | |
| Regular worker | 49.10% | 50.90% | 1129.7 (1) *** | 58.90% | 41.10% | 904.4 (1) *** |
| Nonregular worker | 95.20% | 4.80% | | 97.20% | 2.80% | |
| **Labor union** | | | | | | |
| No | 81.80% | 18.20% | 902.8 (1) *** | 87.10% | 12.90% | 921.8 (1) *** |
| Yes | 28.30% | 71.70% | | 37.30% | 62.80% | |
| **Work sector** | | | | | | |
| Private | 77.00% | 23.10% | 421.9 (1) *** | 84.00% | 16.00% | 548.5 (1) *** |
| Public | 38.80% | 61.20% | | 43.00% | 57.00% | |
| **Company size** | | | | | | |
| 5 below | 94.90% | 5.10% | | 97.40% | 2.60% | |
| 5–9 | 85.90% | 14.10% | 837.2 (4) *** | 91.50% | 8.50% | 752.1 (4) *** |
| 10–29 | 74.50% | 25.50% | | 80.90% | 19.10% | |
| 30–99 | 52.40% | 47.60% | | 58.30% | 41.70% | |
| 100 or more | 42.20% | 57.80% | | 53.80% | 46.20% | |
| **Education attainment** | | | | | | |
| Middle school or below | 98.50% | 1.50% | | 98.60% | 1.40% | |
| High school | 87.60% | 12.40% | 765.1 (3) *** | 91.40% | 8.60% | 736.4 (3) *** |
| 2-year community collage | 64.8.% | 35.20% | | 79.10% | 20.90% | |
| 4-year college or above | 47.30% | 52.70% | | 53.60% | 46.40% | |
| **Number of children** | | | | | | |
| 0 | 62.30% | 38.70% | | 71.80% | 28.20% | |
| 1 | 56.10% | 43.90% | 164.6 (3) *** | 65.60% | 34.40% | 111.9 (3) *** |
| 2 | 75.60% | 24.40% | | 80.60% | 19.40% | |
| 3 or more | 82.90% | 17.10% | | 87.00% | 13.00% | |
| **Mean** [1] | Not Accessible | Accessible | $t$-Test ($df$) | Not Accessible | Accessible | $t$-Test ($df$) |
| Gender-discriminatory workplace culture [2] | 2.9 (0.1) | 3.1 (2.9 × $10^{-2}$) | −2.0 (7914) * | 2.8 (0.1) | 3.1 (2.8 × $10^{-2}$) | −3.7 (7914) *** |
| Average daily working hours | 6.8 (0.5) | 7.2 (0.5) | −3.5 (7868) *** | 6.8 (0.1) | 7.1 (0.1) | −1.7 (7681) |
| Monthly salary (KRW 10,000) | 111.3 (1.5) | 239.6 (3.5) | −58.3 (7814) *** | 116.5 (1.6) | 255.3 (3.8) | −56.6 (7629) *** |
| Age | 40.6 (0.2) | 36.4 (0.2) | 27.8 (7914) *** | 40.2 (0.2) | 37.6 (0.3) | 23.1 (7727) *** |
| Average daily unpaid housework minutes | 196.1 (10.2) | 242.1 (10.8) | −11.2 (6166) *** | 201.0 (3.7) | 234.3 (8.6) | −8.6 (6069) *** |
| Yearly household income (KRW 10,000) | 4197.1 (240.5) | 6207.5 (115.2) | −29.5 (7781) *** | 4291.2 (57.4) | 6419.9 (120.6) | −27.9 (7596) *** |

Note: Values are weighted; [1] standard errors in parentheses; [2] Likert scale 1: nondiscriminatory to 4: discriminatory; * $p < 0.05$, *** $p < 0.001$.

Second, with regard to childcare leave, similarly, regular workers (42%) were significantly ($p < 0.001$) more likely to perceive the policy as accessible than nonregular workers (3%). Likewise, those who belonged to labor unions (63%) were significantly ($p < 0.001$) more likely to perceive childcare leave as accessible than those who did not belong to labor unions (13%). Working women who worked in the public sector (84%) were approximately 2 times more likely to perceive childcare leave as accessible than those in the private sector (43%). In addition, those working in larger companies were significantly more likely to perceive childcare leave as accessible ($p < 0.001$). The results show that those who work in gender-discriminatory workplaces were significantly more likely to perceive childcare leave as accessible ($p < 0.001$), while those who worked longer hours were also more likely to perceive childcare leave as accessible, but this was not statistically significant. Lastly, working women whose salary was higher were significantly likely to perceive childcare leave as accessible ($p < 0.001$).

Table 4 presents the random effects logistic model results after controlling for other model covariates. First, regarding maternity leave, the results indicate that the odds of public sector workers perceiving maternity leave as accessible were 2.87 times higher than for private sector workers ($p < 0.001$). Likewise, those who were labor union members were 2.58 times more likely to perceive maternity leave as accessible than non-labor union members ($p < 0.001$). The odds of regular workers perceiving maternity leave as accessible were 12.25 times higher than nonregular workers ($p < 0.001$). In addition, those working in larger companies were significantly more likely to perceive maternity leave as accessible ($p < 0.001$), and long working hours were reported to significantly decrease the odds of perceiving maternity leave as accessible ($p < 0.01$). The odds of perceiving maternity leave as accessible increased by 8.19 times with every additional 1% increase in monthly salary ($p < 0.001$). However, gender-discriminatory workplaces did not have significant associations with working women's perception of maternity leave accessibility.

**Table 4.** Multivariate logistic random effects model for determinants of leave accessibility.

|  | Maternity Leave OR (95% CI) | Childcare Leave OR (95% CI) |
|---|---|---|
| Public sector | 2.87 (1.91, 4.32) *** | 3.72 (2.39, 5.78) *** |
| Labor union | 2.58 (1.79, 3.72) *** | 2.57 (1.80, 3.68) *** |
| Regular worker | 12.25 (7.85, 19.11) *** | 13.39 (8.11, 22.11) *** |
| Company size (ref: below 5) |  |  |
| 5–9 employees | 2.28 (1.33, 3.91) ** | 2.20 (1.16, 4.17) * |
| 10–29 employees | 4.58 (2.65, 7.91) *** | 4.95 (2.69, 9.11) *** |
| 30–99 employees | 6.30 (3.63, 10.93) *** | 6.63 (3.60, 12.21) *** |
| 100 or more employees | 19.11 (10.50, 34.77) *** | 14.30 (7.50, 27.23) *** |
| Gender-discriminatory workplace culture | 1.25 (0.60, 2.09) | 1.20 (0.53, 2.30) |
| Work hour | 0.92 (0.84, 0.99) ** | 0.83 (0.76, 0.92) *** |
| Logged salary | 8.19 (5.39, 1.01) *** | 7.32 (4.69, 11.44) *** |
| Age | 0.87 (0.84, 0.90) *** | 0.90 (0.87, 0.93) *** |
| Number of children (ref: 0) |  |  |
| 1 | 1.68 (0.89, 3.17) | 1.71 (0.88, 3.32) |
| 2 | 1.29 (0.70. 2.37) | 1.25 (0.66, 2.37) |
| 3 or more | 1.61 (0.78, 3.32) | 1.73 (0.79, 3.79) |
| Unpaid housework hour | 1.00 (0.99, 1.00) | 1.00 (0.99, 1.00) |
| Logged household income | 1.20 (0.99, 1.72) | 1.09 (0.74, 1.58) |
| Education (ref: middle school or below) |  |  |
| High school degree | 6.54 (1.73, 24.64) ** | 2.52 (0.87, 7.27) |
| 2-year community college | 10.29 (2.65, 39.90) ** | 2.75 (0.89, 8.49) |
| 4-year college or higher | 11.58 (2.99, 44.75) *** | 5.50 (1.82, 16.54) ** |
| Constant | $1.03 \times 10^{-6}$ ($3.98 \times 10^{-9}$, $2.64 \times 10^{-5}$) *** | $3.43 \times 10^{-6}$ ($1.32 \times 10^{-7}$, $8.89 \times 10^{-5}$) |
| Sigma_u | 1.25 (Robust SE: 0.16) | 1.37 (Robust SE: 0.16) |
| rho | 0.32 (Robust SE: 0.05) | 0.36 (Robust SE: 0.05) |

* $p < 0.05$, ** $p < 0.01$, *** $p < 0.001$.

Second, regarding childcare leave, results similarly indicate that the odds of public sector workers perceiving childcare leave as accessible were 3.72 times higher than for private sector workers ($p < 0.001$). Likewise, those who were labor union members were 2.57 times more likely to perceive childcare leave as accessible than non-labor union members ($p < 0.001$). The odds of regular workers perceiving childcare leave as accessible were 13.39 times higher than for nonregular workers ($p < 0.001$). Further, those working in larger companies were significantly more likely to perceive childcare leave as accessible ($p < 0.001$), and long working hours were reported to significantly decrease the odds of perceiving childcare leave as accessible ($p < 0.001$). The odds of perceiving childcare leave as accessible increased 7.32 times with every 1% increase in monthly salary ($p < 0.001$).

Gender-discriminatory workplaces did not have significant associations with the perception of childcare leave accessibility.

We summarize the results in comparison with our initial hypotheses in Table 5. Contrary to our hypotheses, gender-discriminatory workplace culture was not significantly associated with working women's perception of access to both maternity leave and childcare leave. Moreover, while we initially hypothesized that those with higher salaries would be less likely to perceive the leave policies as accessible, the results show that, on the contrary, they were more likely to perceive maternity leave and childcare leave as accessible in Korea, which we believe is because in Korea, salary is not only associated with managerial positions but also with company characteristics. Korea's labor market is highly polarized by company size [28]. Even among similar industries, large companies usually provide much higher salaries with better fringe benefits than smaller companies, which has been accelerated since the Asian Economic Crisis of 1997 [29].

**Table 5.** Summary of the results.

| Predictors | Hypotheses | Results |
|---|---|---|
| Public sector | Positively significant | Positively significant |
| Labor union | Positively significant | Positively significant |
| Regular worker | Positively significant | Positively significant |
| Large firm size | Positively significant | Positively significant |
| Gender-discriminatory workplace culture | Negatively significant | Insignificant |
| Long working hour | Negatively significant | Negatively significant |
| High Salary | Negatively significant | Positively significant |

## 6. Discussion

This study examined the determinants of perceived access to maternity leave and childcare leave among Korean wage-earning full-time working women of childbearing age. First, the results show that despite the government's efforts to expand leave policies, the majority of working women perceived the leave policies as inaccessible. On average, only 26% and 21% of the sample reported that they could use maternity leave and childcare leave, respectively, if they wished to. Second, the results indicate that those who worked in the public sector, belonged to labor unions, worked in big companies, were regular workers, and earned high salaries were more likely to perceive maternity leave and childcare leave as accessible, whereas those who worked long hours were less likely to perceive maternity leave and childcare as accessible.

### 6.1. Limitations

Before discussing the study implications, the limitations require consideration. First, the study focused on examining the determinants of maternity leave and childcare leave quantitatively. Further qualitative studies are warranted to understand the complex mechanisms behind working women's perception of maternity leave and childcare leave. Second, the present study examined the determinants of women's perceived accessibility and not the actual usage. Different factors may play a role in women's use of maternity leave and childcare leave. For example, women in higher positions may have greater authority and thus may perceive leave policies as being more accessible; however, they may voluntarily choose to not use these policies because they are more work-oriented. Further studies are needed that compare the determinants of perceived accessibility and actual usage of leave policies. Third, since in this study we did not lag (i.e., create variables that were one period behind in time) our predictor variables, we cannot guarantee a causal relationship. We decided not to lag our predictor variables because we were interested in examining how the respondents' current status was associated with their current perception of maternity leave and childcare leave, as a result, strictly speaking, we examined association instead of causality. Nonetheless, based on Dulk and Peper [14] and other previous studies [10–13,15], we assume that the respondents' current status affected their perceived accessibility of maternity leave and childcare leave. Fourth, due to data limitations, salary was used as a proxy variable to measure career-level position. We acknowledge that salaries differ in particular sectors of the economy, size classes of cities, regions, and occupations. However, we believed it would still be interesting and meaningful to examine salary. Future studies are called for with improved data.

Despite these limitations, the study has notable strengths. The study is the first Korean study to empirically examine the determinants of perceived accessibility of maternity leave and childcare leave using a national sample of working women. Restricted accessibility has been a common recurring issue not only in Korea but also internationally; however, there are very few empirical studies on why some employees are less likely to perceive maternity leave and childcare leave as accessible. This paper contributes to understanding the determinants of working women's perceived access to maternity leave and childcare leave, and informs policymakers of factors that could help improve policy accessibility, and possibly usage.

*6.2. Policy Implications*

Our results have important policy implications. First, in our study, only one in four working women and one in five working women perceived maternity leave and childcare leave as accessible, respectively. A possible reason may be because currently, penalties against employers who violate the requirement to provide leave policies are weak in Korea [30]. For instance, companies that refuse to provide leave to employees are penalized only KRW 5,000,000 (USD 4500) when reported by the refused employee [30]. Hence, the authors believe stricter penalties and heightened enforcement should be implemented for employers who do not follow the law in order to increase accessibility. In addition, it is important to create a workplace culture where employees feel they can use the policies without the fear of reprisal.

Second, among all the predictors, regular work had the most significant association with women's perceptions of the accessibility of maternity leave and childcare leave. Regular workers perceiving maternity leave and childcare leave as accessible was 12 times and 13 times higher than for nonregular workers, respectively. Considering that all the samples analyzed in this study had worked for more than 180 days and were eligible to apply for the policies, this disparity is striking. Although nonregular workers are often involved in the same or similar tasks in the workplace as regular workers in Korea, their terms (i.e., wages) and employment conditions (i.e., exclusion from company benefits) tend to fall below those of regular workers [28]. Nonregular employment contracts became a popular form of contract in Korea during the 1997 Asian Economic Crisis to avoid providing full-time job security and welfare entitlements, which was justified as a necessity to overcome the crisis and to remain economically solvent at the time. However, it remained popular even after the crisis ended [28]. It is likely that nonregular workers, in fear of losing their jobs or contracts in subsequent years, will not request leave policies as frequently as regular workers, whose job security is protected by the Labor Standard Act and Social Security Act. Under these Acts, regular workers cannot be subject to a definite employment termination date unless they reach the mandatory retirement age or have committed substantial misconduct. Although it is illegal to deprive nonregular workers of maternity leave and childcare leave, some companies forbid (both directly and indirectly) nonregular workers from taking leave in their regulations or contracts [31]. In 2016, 40% of total Korean female workers were nonregular workers [32]. As a result, a possible reason for Korea's low policy usage rate may be the high number of female nonregular workers and their inability to access maternity leave and childcare leave, in addition to the government's failure to properly regulate discrimination against nonregular workers in the labor market.

Third, the results show that those who worked in the public sector were 2.9 times and 3.7 times more likely to perceive maternity leave and childcare leave as being accessible, respectively. This is probably because the public sector is more sensitive to government policies, and hence it is a workplace environment that is more accepting of and accommodating to employees using leave policies. Statistics show that in 2017, among mothers who used maternity leave, approximately one-third of them worked in the public sector [9], manifesting that, as hypothesized, in Korea those who work in the public sector are more likely to perceive leave policies as accessible.

Fourth, the results indicate that, in contrast to Western studies and our initial hypothesis, women with higher salaries were significantly more likely to perceive maternity leave and childcare leave as being accessible in Korea. We believe this is because, in Korea, as previously mentioned, higher-earnings are associated not only with managerial positions but also with company characteristics. Korea's labor market is highly polarized between those employed in small companies with low wages and those employed in large companies with high salaries and good fringe benefits [28]. Hence, those earning high salaries are more likely to be employed in large companies. However, the problem lies in the fact that a substantial number of Korean working women are low-wage workers, earning less than two-thirds of the median-salary wage earners [33]. In 2014, 38% of Korean working women were low-wage workers earning less than KRW 6712 (USD 5.84) an hour [31]. Although childcare leave is paid in Korea, it currently only covers a maximum of 40% of a mother's monthly salary, within the range of USD 450–900. Working mothers, especially mothers with low earning capacity, hence are likely not able to take leave or afford a lower income. Thus, in this study, we suggest expanding the benefit amounts to be more generous to increase accessibility and use of maternity leave and childcare leave in Korea.

Lastly, long working hours were negatively associated with working women's perceived accessibility of maternity leave and childcare leave. In 2019, a Korean worker worked on average 1967 h per year, which is 241 h more than the OECD average and the highest among the OECD countries [34]. Korean work culture emphasizes strong a work ethic and long working hours, which makes it difficult to reconcile work and family lives [35]. What we found in this study was that it is important to decrease working hours in order to increase accessibility and usage of maternity leave and childcare leave.

## 7. Conclusions

In summary, the present study is the first to empirically examine the determinants of Korean working women's perceptions of the accessibility of maternity leave and childcare leave in Korea using a national sample. The study discovered that employment status (regular vs nonregular worker), working in the public sector, belonging to a labor union, company size, and salary were the important determinants of perceived accessibility of leave policies in Korea. However, a significant number of Korean working women are nonregular low-wage workers who work in small companies without labor unions. Hence, we suspect this may be one of the reasons for Korea's low leave usage and probably Korea's very low fertility rate. Whilst the period of the so-called "demographic transition" involves a significant decline in fertility linked with economic development, this negative relationship has weakened, and some countries such as France and Sweden have experienced an increase in fertility rates since the late 1990s, while their economies continue to grow [9]. On the other hand, East Asian countries such as Singapore, Korea, and Taiwan experienced a continued drop in their fertility, hovering around 1.0–1.2 children per woman—the lowest low fertility (i.e., total fertility rate at or below 1.3) [36]. Reports show that countries that experienced an increase in their fertility had relatively high work–family balance and gender-equality [9,36]. For example, Sweden offered a comprehensive support system for working parents through a combination of generous leave policies and widely available childcare services. The uptake rate of maternity leave and childcare leave is also high in Sweden [37]. Hence, policymakers interested in increasing fertility rates should therefore consider addressing these issues and try to improve the accessibility and use of maternity leave and childcare leave. Laws that prohibit discrimination against nonregular workers and policies that promote women's status in the labor market should be considered.

**Author Contributions:** Conceptualization, E.J.K., W.J.H. and M.J.K.; methodology, E.J.K.; formal analysis E.J.K.; writing—original draft preparation E.J.K., W.J.H. and M.J.K.; supervision, M.J.K.; funding acquisition, M.J.K. All authors have read and agreed to the published version of the manuscript.

**Funding:** This research was supported by a grant (21AUDP-B127891-05) from the Architecture & Urban Development Research Program, funded by the Ministry of Land, Infrastructure and Transport of the Korean government.

**Institutional Review Board Statement:** Not applicable.

**Informed Consent Statement:** Not applicable.

**Data Availability Statement:** Publicly available datasets were analyzed in this study. The data can be found here: https://klowf.kwdi.re.kr/portal/eng/dataSet/rdssListPage.do?phDivCd=P (accessed on 5 March 2021).

**Conflicts of Interest:** The authors declare no conflict of interest.

# Appendix A

**Table A1.** Extended Regression Model (ERM) probit analysis controlling for selection bias.

| | Maternity Leave Coeff. (Robust SE) | Childcare Leave Coeff. (Robust SE) |
|---|---|---|
| Public sector | 0.48 (0.12) *** | 0.59 (0.10) *** |
| Labor union | 0.49 (0.12) *** | 0.50 (0.09) *** |
| Regular worker | 1.05 (0.19) *** | 1.02 (0.14) *** |
| Company size (ref: below 5) | | |
| 5–9 employees | 0.36 (0.12) ** | 0.32 (0.11) ** |
| 10–29 employees | 0.72 (0.16) *** | 0.70 (0.13) *** |
| 30–99 employees | 0.81 (0.17) *** | 0.78 (0.14) *** |
| 100 or more employees | 1.26 (0.25) *** | 1.09 (0.17) *** |
| Gender-discriminatory workplace culture | 0.25 (0.60) | 0.20 (0.53) |
| Work hour | −0.04 (0.01) * | −0.07 (0.02) *** |
| Logged salary | 0.88 (0.19) *** | 0.82 (0.13) *** |
| Age | −0.04 (0.01) * | −0.03 (0.01) ** |
| Number of children (ref: 0) | | |
| 1 | 0.22 (0.14) | 0.23 (0.13) |
| 2 | 0.09 (0.11) | 0.11 (0.12) |
| 3 or more | 0.17 (0.15) | 0.21 (0.14) |
| Unpaid housework hour | $2.78 \times 10^{-4}$ ($1.73 \times 10^{-4}$) | $-8.19 \times 10^{-5}$ ($1.63 \times 10^{-4}$) |
| Logged household income | 0.88 (0.08) | 0.05 (0.07) |
| Education (ref: middle school or below) | | |
| High school degree | 0.85 (0.28) * | 0.56 (0.22) * |
| 2-year community college | 1.03 (0.30) ** | 0.57 (0.23) * |
| 4-year college or higher | 1.04 (0.30) ** | 0.80 (0.23) ** |
| constant | −7.10 (0.69) *** | −6.52 (0.63) *** |
| **Selected equation** | | |
| Education (ref: middle school or below) | −0.02 (0.04) | −0.01 (0.04) |
| High school degree | 0.01 (0.05) | −0.01 (0.05) |
| 2-year community college | 0.01 (0.04) | 0.01 (0.04) |
| 4-year college or higher | | |
| Age | 0.24 (0.01) *** | 0.25 (0.01) *** |
| Age$^2$ | $-3.09 \times 10^{-3}$ (0.01) *** | $-3.12 \times 10^{-3}$ (0.01) *** |
| Log household income | 0.15 (0.01) *** | 0.15 (0.01) *** |
| Have a preschool child | −0.20 (0.02) *** | −0.20 (0.02) *** |
| Constant | −6.86 (0.30) *** | −6.91 (0.29) *** |
| Corr (perceived accessibility, work) | 0.44 (0.48) | 0.46 (0.28) |

* $p < 0.05$, ** $p < 0.01$, *** $p < 0.001$.

## References

1. Lee, K.M.S. Korea's Fertility Rate Marks Record Low in 2020. *Hankyoreh*, 25 February 2021. Available online: https://english.hani.co.kr/arti/english_edition/e_national/984524.html (accessed on 3 August 2021).
2. Lee, J.; Choi, Y. A path analysis on birthplan of married working women: Focus on the relationships of gender role attitude, work-family reconciliation, marriage satisfaction and birth plan. *Korean J. Soc. Welf. Stud.* **2012**, *43*, 5–30. [CrossRef]
3. Organisation for Economic Co-Operation and Development. Data from National Time Use Surveys. Available online: http://www.oecd.org/gender/data/balancingpaidworkunpaidworkandleisure.htm (accessed on 3 August 2021).
4. Chin, M.; Lee, J.; Lee, S.; Son, S.; Sung, M. Family policy in South Korea: Development, current status, and challenges. *J. Child Fam. Stud.* **2012**, *21*, 53–64. [CrossRef]
5. Korea Institute of Child Care and Education. *Corporate Maternity Leave and Child Care Leave Conditions and Challenges*; Korea Institute of Child Care and Education: Seoul, Korea, 2012.
6. Korean Women's Development Institute. *2008 Korean Longitudinal Survey of Women and Families Annual Report*; Korean Women's Development Institute: Seoul, Korea, 2009.
7. Kim, E. Do working mothers with preschool children recognize and intend to use work-family reconciliation policy? An analysis of the differences between time support policy and service provision policy. *Korean Soc. Public Adm.* **2013**, *24*, 617–642.
8. Organisation for Economic Co-Operation and Development. Parental Leave Systems—OECD. Available online: https://www.oecd.org/els/soc/PF2_1_Parental_leave_systems.pdf (accessed on 3 August 2021).
9. Organisation for Economic Co-Operation and Development. *Rejuvenating Korea: Policies for a Changing Society*; OECD Publishing: Paris, France, 2019. [CrossRef]
10. Budd, W.J.; Mumford, K. Family-Friendly Work Practice in Britain: Availability and Perceived Accessibility. *Hum. Resour. Manag.* **2006**, *45*, 23–42. [CrossRef]
11. Forth, J.; Lissenburgh, S.; Callender, C.; Millward, N. *Family Friendly Working Arrangements in Britain,1996*; Research Report No. 16; Policy Studies Institute, Department for Education and Employment: London, UK, 1997.
12. Haas, L.L.; Hwang, P. Parental leave in Sweden. In *Parental Leave: Progress or Pitfall? Research and Policy Issues in Europe*; Moss, P., Deven, F., Eds.; NIDI/CBGS Publications: Brussels, Belgium, 1999; pp. 45–68.
13. Rostgaard, T.; Christoffersen, M.N.; Weise, H. Parental leave in Denmark. In *Parental Leave: Progress or Pitfall? Research and Policy Issues in Europe*; Moss, P., Deven, F., Eds.; NIDI/CBGS Publications: Brussel, Belgium, 1999; pp. 25–44.
14. Dulk, L.D.; Peper, B. Working parents' use of work–life policy. *Sociologia* **2007**, *53*, 51–70.
15. Fried, M. *Taking Time: Parental Leave Policy and Corporate Culture*; Temple University Press: Philadephia, PA, USA, 1998.
16. Bu, N.; MacKeen, C.A. Work and family expectations of the future managers and professionals of Canada and China. *J. Manag. Psychol.* **2000**, *15*, 771–790. [CrossRef]
17. Kim, Y.O.; Chun, K.T. The current status of non-regular worker's utilization of maternity leave and return to workforce. *Labor Rev.* **2007**, *12*, 48–63.
18. Korean Women's Development Institute. *The Analysis of Current Implementation Status of Maternal Protection System and Research Highlight of Improvement Study*; Research Report; Korean Women's Development Institute: Seoul, Korea, 2004.
19. Kim, E.J.; Hong, S.A.; Min, H.; Sung, K. *A Study on the Measures to Ensure Effective Income Security for Parental Leave*; Korea Women's Development Institute: Seoul, Korea, 2016.
20. Thompson, C.A.; Beauvais, L.L.; Lyness, K.S. When work-family benefits are not enough: The influence of work-family culture on benefit utilization, organizational attachment, and work-family conflict. *J. Vocat. Behav.* **1999**, *54*, 392–415. [CrossRef]
21. Kim, Y.M. Re-examination of the exclusion from social insurance coverage of non-standard employment in Korea. *Soc. Welf. Policy* **2010**, *37*, 155–179.
22. Samsung Economic Research Institute. *Report on the Current Condition of Korean Working Moms*; CEO Information: Seoul, Korea, 2010.
23. Korean Women's Development Institute. *Korean Women Manager Panel*; Ministry of Gender Equality and Family, Women's Resources Development Division: Seoul, Korea, 2010.
24. Vasilios, D.K. Job level changes and wage growth. *Int. J. Manpow.* **2009**, *30*, 269–284.
25. Henderson, M.; Hillygus, D.; Tompson, T. "Sour grapes" or rational voting? Voter decision making among thwarted primary voters in 2008. *Public Opin. Q.* **2010**, *74*, 499–529. [CrossRef]
26. Woodridge, J. *Introductory Econometrics: A Modern Approach*, 4th ed.; South-Western Publication: Mason, OH, USA, 2008.
27. Park, H.M. *Practical Guides to Panel Data Modeling: A Step-by-Step Analysis Using Stata*; Tutorial Working Paper; Graduate School of International Relations, International University of Japan: Niigata, Japan, 2011.
28. Chun, J.J. *The Struggles of Irregularly-Employed Workers in South Korea, 1999–2012*; Working Paper; UCLA Institute for Research on Labor and Employment: Los Angeles, CA, USA, 2013.
29. Organisation for Economic Co-Operation and Development. *Towards Better Social and Employment Security in Korea, Connecting People with Job*; OECD Publishing: Paris, France, 2018. [CrossRef]
30. Chin, M.; Lee, J.; Lee, S.; Son, S.; Sung, M. Family policy in South Korea: Development, implementation and evaluation. In *Handbook of Family Policies across the Globe*; Robila, M., Ed.; Springer: Flushing, NY, USA, 2014; pp. 205–318.
31. Baek, S.Y. Maternity and Childcare Leave and the Struggle for Equal Rights in Korean Labor Market. Master's Thesis, KDI School of Public Policy and Management, Yeongi-gun, Korea, November 2011.

32. National Statistics Office of Korea. *Women Labor Force Participation*; National Statistics Office of Korea: Sejong, Korea. Available online: http://www.index.go.kr/potal/main/EachDtlPageDetail.do?idx_cd=1497 (accessed on 15 September 2021).
33. Organisation for Economic Co-Operation and Development. *Wage Levels (Indicator)*, 18th ed.; OECD: Paris, France, 2017. [CrossRef]
34. Kim, Y.S. Korea Has 2nd Longest Working Hours in OECD. *The Korean Herald*, 9 March 2021. Available online: http://www.koreaherald.com/view.php?ud=20210309000162 (accessed on 26 September 2021).
35. Kim, E.; Parish, S.L. Family-supportive workplace policies and South Korean mothers' perceived work-family conflict: Accessibility matters. *Asian Popul. Stud.* **2020**, *16*, 167–182. [CrossRef]
36. Basten, S.; Sobotaka, T.; Zeman, K. Future fertility in low fertility countries. In *World Population and Human Capital Century*; Lutz, W., Butz, W., KC, S., Eds.; Oxford Scholarship: Oxford, UK, 2007; pp. 39–146.
37. Organisation for Economic Co-Operation and Development. *OECD Parents' Use of Childbirth-Related Leave*; OECD: Paris, France, 2019. Available online: https://www.oecd.org/els/family/PF2-2-Use-childbirth-leave.pdf (accessed on 26 September 2021).

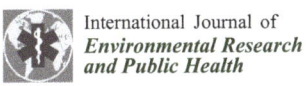

*Article*

# Factors Affecting the Initial Engagement of Older Adults in the Use of Interactive Technology

Lina Lee * and Mary Lou Maher

Department of Software and Information Systems, University of North Carolina at Charlotte, Charlotte, NC 28223, USA; m.maher@uncc.edu
* Correspondence: llee52@uncc.edu

**Abstract:** Smart environments and the use of interactive technology has the potential to improve the quality of life for the senior community as well as to support the connections among the senior community and the world outside their community. In addition to the increasing number of studies in the field of aging and technologies, research is needed to understand the practical issues of user focus, adoption, and engagement for older adults to accept interactive technologies in their lives. In this study, we use two commercial technological interventions (uDraw and GrandPad) to understand technology-related perceptions and behaviors of older adults. We present five case studies that emerge from empirical observations of initial engagement with technology through research methods such as focus group discussions, in-depth interviews, observations, and diary studies. The contributions of this study are identification of the key factors that influence the initial engagement with interactive technology for older adults.

**Keywords:** engagement; older adults; technology; empirical studies

## 1. Introduction

World demographics have shifted in the last twenty years by the drop in the birth rates and an upward shift in life expectancy [1]. As a result, there is a significant rise in the number of older people. Along with this rise in the number of older people, recent years have shown a large rise in the use of technology in all aspects of daily life. Many researchers believe that the application of technology to the aging process can help people "age well" and stay active [2,3]. Various technological inventions have been developed for older adults to facilitate independence when performing essential activities as well as to stay connected with family members and friends [4,5]. Technological literacy is increasingly required to live for the senior community [6] because older adults will be expected to use interactive technologies in their living environments, regardless of their willingness or not to engage with technology [7]. In particular, the COVID 19 pandemic has triggered an urgent need to address societal changes of an aging population due to social isolation and the need for health care [8,9]. This results in an increased demand for the design and adoption of interactive technologies to assure the health of older adults.

This paper has a focus on the need to build an in-depth understanding of older adults' perception and preferences towards technology. Despite the increasing amount of studies in the field of aging and technologies [10,11], not enough research has been done to understand the practical issues of engagement in accepting interactive technologies by older adults. Many studies tend to focus on evaluating the feasibility or usability of technology [12–15]. Recent research about aging and technology tends to underestimate the initial barrier to use technology faced by older adults.

In this study, we address this need by asking the overarching research question: What are the key factors that engage the older population in the use of technology to adapt and live well in the digitized world? We study a senior community and their responses to the use of specific interactive technologies to understand technology-related perceptions

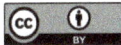

and behaviors of older adults. The goal of this study is to identify the key factors that influence the engagement of older adults in the adoption of interactive technology. To achieve this, we took a more holistic approach, engaging with over 50 people, including multiple stakeholders over six months: program director and staff members in the senior community center, social workers, and volunteers for the activities that provided in the senior center, family members, relatives, or religious group.

Our methodology is a qualitative ethnographic study in which the researcher directly observes and evaluates older adults' technological behavior in the research context [16]. We use data accumulated over six months through research methods such as focus group discussions, in-depth interviews, observations, and a diary study using two commercial products (uDraw (https://en.wikipedia.org/wiki/UDraw_GameTablet (accessed on 14 November 2010))) and GrandPad (https://www.grandpad.net/) (accessed on 1 May 2018). We conduct an inductive thematic analysis on the multiple sources of data [17]. From our analysis, five case studies have emerged that categorically describe the variety of attitudes towards interactive technologies: (1) active towards technology, (2) passive towards technology, (3) social use of technology, (4) diverse use of technology, and (5) family oriented use of technology. Based on these cases, we present new engagement factors that emerge from our empirical observations of older adults and their response to interactive technology.

## 2. Background

In this section, we show that the focus of research on the use of technology by older adults tends to be about the limitations of this population and the impact of the limitations on the design and usability of the technology. In contrast, our study has a focus on the attitudes, perceptions, and engagement of older adults with technology. We also review the methodologies for research on interactive technologies for older adults and recognize a need for ethnographic methods that can provide more in-depth studies of individuals in situ rather than methods that generalize across large numbers of participants in laboratory settings.

### 2.1. Current Research Focus for Older Adults' Use of Technology

Many studies have been conducted to understand the challenges and barriers that older adults face and the factors that affect their adapting to new technologies and their continued use. However, there is a relatively little research exploring older adults' initial and long-term engagement with interactive technology.

In order to design appropriate interactive technology for older adults, understanding aging limitations are important [18–20]. When people start aging, their physical and cognitive abilities tend to reduce slowly and gradually end, which in turn forces them to start developing negative attitudes towards interactive technologies [21]. Older adults may have doubts that technological innovations are real and become nervous since they are not confident in their ability to manage and practically adopt these innovations [22]. The mistrust of technology may escalate to technophobia, which makes older adults less likely to try out new technology [23–25]. Peek et al. [22] explain that technophobia is normal for people who did not grow up in environments that are populated by digital systems and changing mindset does not happen quickly. To support older adults, service providers, researchers, designers, developers, and policymakers have long been working together to better understand how older adults can achieve optimal health and wellbeing with the benefit of technology [26].

Other studies have focused on factors that affect adoption of technology by older adults and its continued usage. Many scholars show a lower level of innovative technology adoption by older adults [27–30]. To make interactive technologies more acceptable, the notions of usability [31,32], independence, convenience [33,34], devices to support physical activity [35,36], technology training and education [37,38], the role of caregiver [39,40], innovation (focus on developing new features) [41–43], affordability [44,45] and potential or continued benefit [28,29] have been explored by many scholars over the past decades. These studies focus on technologies that are usable or adoptable and suitable for continued use, but they typically do not focus on providing pleasurable and positive experiences to encourage initial and long-term engagement.

Older adults' engagement and enthusiasm are key elements in determining the success in their use of interactive technology. By reviewing the literature, we learn that despite the barrier to adoption being the most difficult stage, there is a lack of research for understanding older adults' initial engagement. Due to age-related factors, older people often have difficulty overcoming the initial barrier to use interactive technology [46,47]. The significant problem in the use of technology by older adults is that even though a broad and advanced range of tools and platforms for older adults are being developed, the number of older adults who actively utilize the technology remain few. Therefore, our research explores the complex phenomena of human values to understand the essential behavioral characteristics and identify the key factors that influence the initial engagement of older adults with technology.

### 2.2. Current Research Challenges for Older Adults

There are methodological and design challenges in studying older adults [48], including recruitment, informed consent, reliable responses, communication with older adults, and providing appropriate instruction about research. Older adults may fear that refusing to participate in a study. The number of participants may affect the quality and validity of the finding of the study [49]. According to Birkland [48], many researchers conduct user studies with older adults that rely on self-report methods. Empirical studies that use a mixed-method design are rare. The main problem of short-term surveys or interviews is that these rely on users' recollection and self-interpretations. Older adults tend to provide responses to researchers that are more positive or more frequent than in reality. Results show that older adults often assess the technology as positive, however, they fail to show clear evidence that older adults will adopt new emerging technology into their lives [50,51]. Many studies heavily focus on testing the usability by older adults with a lab study over a short period of time [52–54].

The vast majority of the research use age as the sampling criteria [48]. In many studies, older adults are often considered as a homogeneous group in technology research studies regardless of their characteristics, abilities, or technology experiences [55,56]. However, older adults are heterogeneous, and it is difficult to generalize the characteristics of technology use due to various factors such as physical, psychological, emotional, social, and economic situations of older adults [57]. This research explores the behavioral characteristics of older adults when asked to initiate the engagement of new technology rather than to evaluate the usability of new technology. Instead of focusing on a specific target demographic who need to supplement their physical ability, we focus on broad engagement themes as a starting point in studying older adults' engagement towards technology. This study conducts an ethnographic study to understand the complex phenomena surrounding older adults which enable researchers and designers to predict and provide the processes to develop engaging technologies for older adults [13].

### 3. Methodology for Studying the Factors That Affect Older Adults' Initial Engagement with Technology

The methodology for this study includes choosing the technology interventions and using a mixed methods approach that includes ethnographic observational data. We explain the reason for choosing commercial products for the intervention. Then, we describe the mixed methods studies specific to our research goal of identifying the factors that increase older adults' initial interest and their subsequent engagement with interactive technology.

### 3.1. Technological Intervention

Initially, we conducted a pilot study with five senior residents living in a retirement community to learn about the factors that may stimulate their interest in the use of technology [58,59]. The main topic of the discussion was about activities that interest older adults and how to spend leisure time. We found that many older adults enjoy being creative, playing games, and being social. With the results, we decided to focus on two user experiences using interactive technology: (1) social creative expression in public space, and (2) emotional attachment in a private setting.

When selecting the interactive technology for the longitudinal study reported in this paper, we chose two commercial products as the context in which we observed and collected data so that we could reduce the issues related to poor usability that occur in technologies developed by research students. The uDraw Game Tablet is an embodied interactive technology that facilitates creative social expression by allowing users to create free form drawings, artwork, and games. GrandPad is a communication technology that enables older adults to easily communicate with their loved ones. In the context of a longitudinal study, older adults may lose interest quickly if they experience difficulty in understanding how to use the system. We wanted to avoid disinterest due to using a prototype system that might have unexpected usability issues or is an unstable implementation. If the purpose of this study was to propose a new practical solution to older adults with a specific problem through technology, the user-related study would have been carried out using technology designed on our own. However, since this research is not intended to evaluate the feasibility of technology or focus on technological solutions but to observe cases in which older adults are engaged when experiencing technology, commercial products were used.

*3.2. Mixed Methods Studies*

Our methodology includes participant observation, augmented by a range of other approaches: the use of focus groups, semi-structured interviews, participant diaries. Our findings are based on interacting with older adults in the context of previous research and the accumulated experience of the researcher.

3.2.1. uDraw Study of Initial Engagement in a Community Center
Observation (with Facilitator)

Participant observation is a central data collection method in the uDraw study. We collected data at a shared community room at a senior residence. The researcher visited the site for three hours each visit, three times a week, over three months. We recorded the activities, participant attitudes or behaviors, and noted relevant details. To observe senior residents effectively, we operated a help desk to engage in participant observation to gain insight into the culture of the community of older adults. Significant time and effort were given to open-ended conversations with residents. We offered training in the uDraw system and provided personal help for older adults to learn mobile apps, web search, and other appliances that tailor to their interests. Although there were about 40 residents in the community we observed, we used the data from 19 residents that were most involved in the technology interventions and help desk support activities. Of the 19 residents, 11 experienced the uDraw system with the help of researchers; 8 residents made use of the help desk (7 males and 1 female); 3 out of the 8 visited the help desk repeatedly with the main purpose to learn mobile apps.

Video recorded data is used to observe the natural behavior around the system when a facilitator is not located. The uDraw system was constantly running in a shared community room throughout the three month research period. Residents were free to try and use the uDraw system. Two video recording devices (Google Nest Cam) were located near the screen to capture the study area. One was directed toward the user and the tablet, to record all behaviors occurring when the system was used, while the other was toward the public large display, to record social behaviors around the system. The motion activated cameras would turn on and start recording when they detected motion. This study was approved by the Institutional Review Board (IRB) to collect data from people who walked down the hall or past the interaction area but who had no intention of interacting. We collected video data over 92 days. We segmented this data so we could identify data referring directly to the usability of the uDraw system, referring to content about hobbies or interests of older adults, or referring to technology-related matters. This particular situation was separately extracted, and the issues were noted and discussed. Most residents watched TV while knitting, using a coffee machine, or using a copy machine, with 21 residents showing a repeating pattern. Of the residents, 12 appeared to be interested in activities provided by the community center and in using digital devices provided by volunteers. In the case of the uDraw system we provided, only one person was observed using the uDraw system voluntarily, and the number of times this individual used the uDraw system without the help of a researcher was 9 times.

We conducted in-person semi-structured interviews to understand general attitudes towards interactive technology with regard to 8 factors (positive affect, comfort, feel involved, perceived benefits and usefulness, controllability, help, discoverability and learnability, and persistence) as shown in Table 1. We interviewed 4 residents, and they also participated in the focus group discussions. All interviews were audio recorded and transcribed with the participants' consent. While participant observation gives information on the action and behavior of older adults in the context of interactive technologies, interviews provide us with data on how people directly reflect on their own behavior, circumstances, identities, and events.

**Table 1.** Interview Questions used for qualitative study.

| Interview Questions |
|---|
| Positive Affect: Can you explain how you feel while using feature X? |
| Comfort: Are you comfortable when using feature X? |
| Feel involved: How helpful do you think feature X is for your social interaction? |
| Perceived benefits and usefulness: How much do you think using feature X improves the quality of your life? |
| Control: How easily do you think you can control feature X? |
| Help: How much do you think you need the support to be able to use feature X? |
| Discoverability and Learnability: How easily do you think you understand feature X? |
| Persistency: How frequently do you use feature X? |

The first question asked in the interview: What do you like the best about your cellphone? X in follow up questions is based on individual's responses.

The focus group discussions were conducted every two weeks, a total of five focus group discussions with four residents. We let participants play the uDraw Pictionary game before participating in the focus group discussion. This game is an art-based video game in which players can play on a uDraw Game Tablet. In uDraw Pictionary, the players refer to a particular subject to draw a picture. The teammates are then tasked with the challenge of guessing the words each image is supposed to portray. After one hour of play, we discussed the same 8 factors as the interview prompts used in the pre-interview questions (slightly modified) to gain insights about older adults' engagement in the use of the given system. The focus group was audio recorded and transcribed.

3.2.2. GrandPad Study of Initial Engagement in a Family Setting

The diary study is a central data collection method of the GrandPad study with a total of 3 older adults and family members. In this study, the older adults received one GrandPad tablet for three months. Family members could connect to GrandPad's private family network via iPhone, Android phone, or desktop computer. They could manage the functions for older adults from the convenient companion app. The researcher purchased and created an account on the GrandPad app with a monthly subscription including the convenience of unlimited data. We gathered data from the usage log. The researcher collected usage records every day. Since the fact of recording their usage may affect their behavior; it was not mentioned to the older adults. We also gathered data from diary studies submitted by the family member for each older adult with approval from our institution's IRB. There are a lot of limitations in conducting a diary study with older adults. Older adults feel writing a diary is an extra burden, so the likelihood of a negative impact on the use of a GrandPad device cannot be excluded. For this reason, the diary study was conducted with family members. Using mobile diary studies software, the participant wrote a diary about older adults' GrandPad usage through a smartphone. One or two younger family members who are in the closest relationship with older adults played a role in sending a prompt to encourage older adults to use the GrandPad. The researcher sent journal prompts to family members through text or email at 9 am every day, however younger family members could create their prompts as well. The prompts were created in a way to encourage older adults to actively use the GrandPad App. These prompts were used for seniors to inspire them to be creative, share significant memories, and keep their minds healthy and active.

There was a significant difference in the frequency of GrandPad use of the three families. The first user was given the first GrandPad on 7 November 2019, and used it until 22 January 2020, and 73 diary entries were recorded, and the total usage time was 141 h. The second family started using it on 8 November 2019, but the last recorded date of using the GrandPad was 20 November, with the device only being used 12 times. The total usage time was 3 h, with 6 diary entries being recorded. The last family used it from 11 November to 5 January, and there were a total of 44 data entries, with a total usage time of 43 h.

We conducted in-person interviews with the GrandPad participants to understand general attitudes towards communication technology. We used the same interview questions as the uDraw study.

*3.3. Analysis*

During the research period, we immersed ourselves in the senior community and spent time talking directly with the participants and observing their lives and attitudes towards technology. We conducted an inductive thematic analysis [17]. This qualitative analysis focused on: (1) categorizing older adults to present the diverse attitudes towards interactive technologies; (2) identification of the factors of initial engagement in the use of interactive technologies. We focus on finding situations wherein older adults show emotionally positive affect related to use or discussion about interactive technology and finding situations where older adults become active and motivated by a desire to physically try to use technology. Two researchers met weekly to discuss the collected data of all activities, reflecting and iterating over the themes that lead our discussions, until a consensus was found. With the written field notes, video data analysis, direct observations, diary written by participants, and qualitative data, we extracted 5 case studies and 9 initial engagement values. Below, we present the results of the analysis, organized by themes.

## 4. Five Case Studies That Emerge from Empirical Observations of Initial Engagement with Technology

A total of 36 subjects are classified into five categories: positive about technology, negative about technology, social use of technology, diverse use of technology, and family oriented use of technology. By observing each participant over three months (the length of observation varies depending on participants, approximately from 10 days to 3 months for each participant), we consider six factors to define five case studies: family relationships, social contacts, general attitudes towards technology, need for technology, physical and cognitive health, and motivation.

*4.1. Positive (Active) about Technology*

Bob is a participant in the GrandPad study. Out of the three participants of the GrandPad study, Bob was the only one who had no problems with trying something new or using new functions of mobile technology. In the Diary study, Bob faithfully performed the daily tasks given, and overall, he did not report any difficulty or inconvenience in using the system. The three apps that Bob was most interested in and used the most were the reading, game, and music apps of the GrandPad. Bob has maintained a positive attitude toward the phone from the moment he first owned the mobile phone. When responding to his experience with technology, Bob often connected his experiences and memories of technology with people (See quotation in Figure 1), which reminds him of positive memories of that moment about mobile phones rather than remembering functions related to mobile phones.

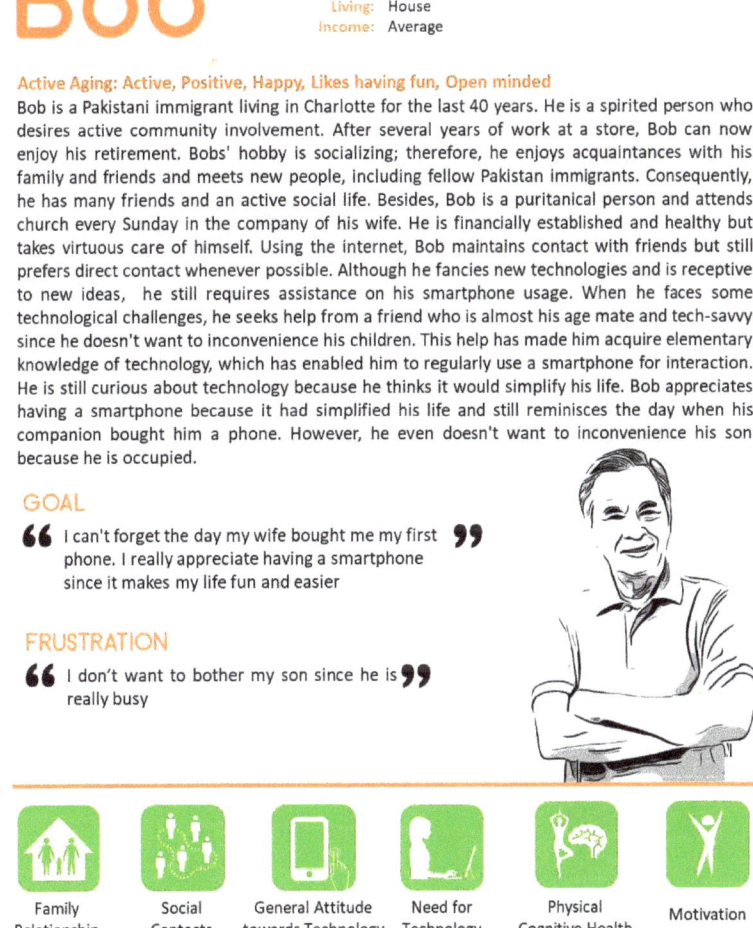

**Active Aging: Active, Positive, Happy, Likes having fun, Open minded**

Bob is a Pakistani immigrant living in Charlotte for the last 40 years. He is a spirited person who desires active community involvement. After several years of work at a store, Bob can now enjoy his retirement. Bobs' hobby is socializing; therefore, he enjoys acquaintances with his family and friends and meets new people, including fellow Pakistan immigrants. Consequently, he has many friends and an active social life. Besides, Bob is a puritanical person and attends church every Sunday in the company of his wife. He is financially established and healthy but takes virtuous care of himself. Using the internet, Bob maintains contact with friends but still prefers direct contact whenever possible. Although he fancies new technologies and is receptive to new ideas, he still requires assistance on his smartphone usage. When he faces some technological challenges, he seeks help from a friend who is almost his age mate and tech-savvy since he doesn't want to inconvenience his children. This help has made him acquire elementary knowledge of technology, which has enabled him to regularly use a smartphone for interaction. He is still curious about technology because he thinks it would simplify his life. Bob appreciates having a smartphone because it had simplified his life and still reminisces the day when his companion bought him a phone. However, he even doesn't want to inconvenience his son because he is occupied.

**GOAL**

" I can't forget the day my wife bought me my first phone. I really appreciate having a smartphone since it makes my life fun and easier "

**FRUSTRATION**

" I don't want to bother my son since he is really busy "

**Figure 1.** Case 1—Representative character to present positive attitude towards technology.

### 4.2. Negative (Passive) about Technology

John was also a participant in the GrandPad study. John had a negative attitude toward using technology (See Figure 2). He was not very interested in using the GrandPad during the research period except for the time that he explored mobile technology for his hobbies. Out of the three participants, John's total usage time was the lowest. He only used the GrandPad for 12 days in the first month of the study. Further, he did not complete the daily tasks very well, not because he faced technical difficulties but because he had no interest in the activities. However, the apps he used the most during the study were the magnifier app and the music app. John was relatively comfortable using the computer because he learned how to operate it when he was in the military before his retirement.

John often loses interests and complains about issues related to physical discomfort. For example, the mobility of his finger has deteriorated, so that a button cannot be properly clicked, and he found it difficult to read the screen due to poor vision. John has a very negative attitude to mobile phones, despite being experienced in using the technology.

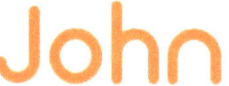

| | |
|---|---|
| Age: 70s | Family Status: One adopted daughter |
| Occupation: Retired | Lives with wife |
| Living: House | |
| Income: Average | |

**Passive Aging: Negative, Anxious, Inactive**

John is isolated despite having some acquaintances. However, he lacks close associates as he doesn't participate in sporting or group actions, although he habitually attends the church. Despite appreciating that he is healthy and alive, he is occasionally in solitude. Recently, his daughter has temporarily relocated to his residence due to childbirth, and John is delighted to stay with his daughter's family. John is healthy, but he has detected that age is catching up with him because of the little challenges that he encounters while performing household chores. John has no ear impairment but requires to use bifocals. He isn't curious about technology and contemplates that technology is unnecessary for his life, hence his deleterious perspective towards technology and his depiction of mobile phones as a form of disturbance. However, John owns a smartphone that he uses to perform limited tasks to the extent of not receiving calls; he only uses a zoom in the specification when viewing snapshots. Moreover, he has an interest in the restoration of old cars. Recently John took an image of a comprehensive design and zoomed in to resolve the wire connections; apart from this, a cellphone is unnecessary in his life. He asserts that he is complacent and only passionate about his hobby of restoring his car and gardening; therefore, he doesn't want to acquire smartphone usage knowledge.

### GOAL

" I want to stay in my comfort zone. I don't want to go outside. I am passionate about my hobbies. I like fixing my car and gardening "

### FRUSTRATION

" I don't want to learn how to use smartphone. I think they are not healthy to use, and difficult to use "

| Family Relationship | Social Contacts | General Attitude towards Technology | Need for Technology | Physical Cognitive Health | Motivation |

**Figure 2.** Case 2—Representative character to present negative attitude towards technology.

*4.3. Family Oriented Use of Technology*

Dorothy was the oldest of the participants in the GrandPad study. She was not able to use the GrandPad on her own and constantly needed her family's help. She is an example case that shows how negative attitudes towards technology can be changed in a positive direction. With the support of her family, however, Dorothy made great strides in using the technology's features during the study period. For her, family is an important factor in deciding to use technology (See Figure 3).

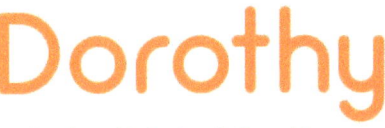

| | | |
|---|---|---|
| Age: 80s | Family Status: | Live alone |
| Occupation: Retired | | One daughter |
| Living: House | | One son |
| Income: Low | | |

**Family oriented Aging: Lonely, Forgetful**

Dorothy is socially isolated, with no other social associates besides her family. Her son calls her frequently and visits her every fortnight. Dorothy lacks a routine activity because she has minor dementia; hence she suffers from concentration hitches and memory loss. Due to this condition, shopping is a challenge such that she hardly remembers what she intended to purchase. However, her daughter, who resides by her household, ensures proper care because it is difficult for her to move effortlessly and tend to be unreceptive. Moreover, Dorothy has a mobile phone that she rarely uses due to her loose memory and worsened cognitive functions that make it difficult for her to use any technical device. This condition has forced her family to put up a speed dial to ensure she promptly calls the family when the need arises. However, she hasn't used it a lot. Dorothy isn't interested in acquiring technological knowledge and skills on phone usage due to her opinion that such devices are useless. Yet, her family actively seeks techniques to retain her in the societal and family relationship cycle. Nothing inspires her to use technology, but she attempts for her family; however, she enjoys remaining at home while watching TV. Dorothy has no interest in technology; therefore, she can't comprehend how they function, but her grandchildren still try to enlighten her. Despite the efforts to educate her, she is still preservative of her stance that she can't use a smartphone because it is too complicated, bearing in mind that she is old-fashioned and technology is contemporary. Besides, Dorothy prioritizes her family and maintains that she still misses her family.

**GOAL**

❝ My family comes first. I always did and always will miss my family ❞

**FRUSTRATION**

❝ My son wants me to use a smartphone. But I don't want to. It is too complicated for me. I am old fashioned and technology is too modern for me ❞

| Family Relationship | Social Contacts | General Attitude towards Technology | Need for Technology | Physical Cognitive Health | Motivation |

**Figure 3.** Case 3—Representative character to present family oriented use of technology.

### 4.4. Social Use of Technology

Gloria is described as a representative of the social use of technology, but two more participants named Peggie and Eva are also important in describing this case. All three were participants of the uDraw study. They participated in all five focus group discussions during the research period. Gloria visited the researcher at the designated time and additionally used the uDraw system twice. The other two participants did not use the system except during the focus group discussions and an initial training session. All three participants were not willing to use the system on their own, and the researcher's support was always required. They expressed difficulty when using the uDraw tablet but followed the researcher's instructions well. A characteristic of those described by this case is that they attend many activities at the community center to stay occupied (See Figure 4). In this case, we found that older adults' motivation for using technology was to maintain social relationships in a community center because they have a strong desire to engage and sustain others' interests.

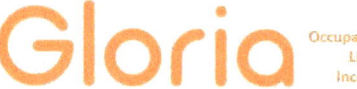 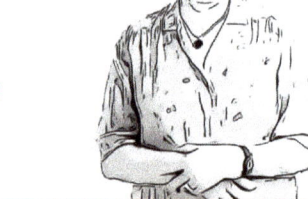

**Age:** 70s  
**Occupation:** Retired  
**Living:** Affordable Rental  
**Income:** Low  

**Family Status:** Live alone  
One son

**Social Aging: Active, Positive, Happy, Communicative**

Gloria is a dynamic and socially engaged person who adores life. Her son is living in the same city. They regularly come across each other or at least communicate via the phone numerous times a week. Her son frequently visits to check on her. Gloria attends all the facility's events to interact with her acquaintances, yet she is not interested in such platforms. However, she enthusiastically interconnects with staff members in her residence. Gloria was able to isolate herself for a long time. Recently, she faced some difficulties in performing daily tasks such as cooking and shopping, although not to a level of requiring help. She uses a flip phone and downplays the need to purchase a smartphone to connect with her social cycle as she lacks the necessary knowledge or prior experience in technology. However, Gloria is fond of trying such innovative things because she finds it fun when one is not engaged. Gloria observes that she wants to be positive and enjoy life as she participates in social undertakings because she can't live without her contacts. Gloria is interested in having more entertaining activities with her associates.

### GOAL

> I want to be positive and enjoy the rest of my life.
> I love participating in social activities

### FRUSTRATION

> I can't live without my friends. I want to engage in more activities to have fun with my friends

    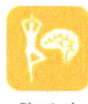 

Family Relationship | Social Contacts | General Attitude towards Technology | Need for Technology | Physical Cognitive Health | Motivation

**Figure 4.** Case 4—Representative character to present social use of technology.

### 4.5. Diverse Use of Technology

Michael was another participant in the uDraw study. He was the participant with the highest initial interest in the uDraw system. As in the case of Gloria, Peggie, and Eva, he also participated in five focus group discussions. In the beginning, he expressed high interest and engagement but could not sustain his engagement for three months. In the first month, he used the system by himself nine times. Of the four participants, Michael was the only one who used the system without any difficulty. He skillfully used the functions he had learned and experienced with the researcher, but he did not try new functions. Therefore, the range of functions that could be used was limited. He often visited the help desk and showed interests about new interactive technology such as Virtual Reality (VR), a voice-activated speaker, and a home robot (See Figure 5).

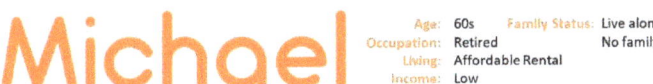

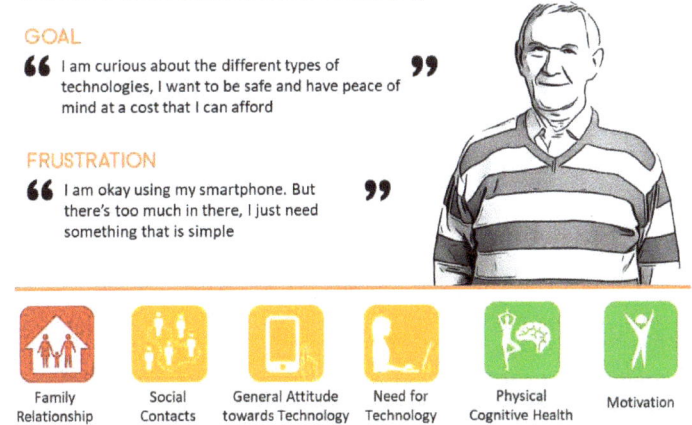

**Figure 5.** Case 5—Representative character to present diverse use of technology.

## 5. New Initial Engagement Values Emerging from Our Case Studies

In this section, we discuss new initial engagement values that have emerged from the five case studies. Under each factor, we compare to values that are discussed in existing literature as a way to support older adults' use of technology. We establish the meaning of each factor from the views of the participants with an understanding of their context and behavior during the observational period.

*5.1. Motivation (Desirability)*

Older Adults' Motivation Needs to Be Considered before Usability to Increase Initial Engagement for Older Adults

Most scholars have indicated that usability is a critical issue to help older adults to learn how to use the interactive systems independently [28,52,53]. Davis [60] identified the ease of use for interactive technology as a significant determinant of the adoption for an individual older adult. However, our study identified desirability should be considered before usability for engaging older adults. Whereas usability influence user's ability to complete a task [61], desirability means they have a pleasurable and engaging experience while using the system. Initial Engagement will increase when older adults have specific reasons or motivation to use interactive technology for having fun and engaging experiences. In the case of Dorothy, she does not like to use the mobile phone so usability was not the primary issue. When I asked about 'What do you like best about your cell phone?', Dorothy could not answer for a long time. Her daughter, Angela, encouraged her to answer.

> **Dorothy:** *"I don't really know how to answer you, if you want to know the truth ... Back again to being old fashioned, I'm not modern. There are some things that I don't understand. I put up with it, with help. Yeah, with help. I've had to rely on my son to guide me. And I don't know if I'll ever be much different from what I am now."*

We observed her attitude changes after we delivered the GrandPad to Dorothy and analyzed her usage through a diary study. When she received the GrandPad for the first time, the only thing she did was turn on the GrandPad and watch the photos posted by her children and granddaughter. Dorothy's children registered the Companion App to continue sending photos. Her family's efforts enabled her to appreciate the daily life of her grandchildren. The following quotes are the feedback of a diary study from her family members.

> *"Mom is still warming up to it. She looked at picture today"*

Dorothy needed help on how to use all the features except the ability to turn off the screen by herself. Five days after using GrandPad, she was able to send a text and picture through GrandPad with the help of Angela.

> *"Mom sent her brother a text/email this morning thanking him for the pictures that he sent her. Even though it was just 1 sentence, it overwhelmed her, but we will get her there."*

Sixteen days later (Nov, 28), we could see that Dorothy has finally figured out how to send a photo by herself. Then one day after (Nov, 29), we could get a response that she actually enjoys the GrandPad.

> *"Mom did a good job posting a photo of the Thanksgiving dinner that my sister is preparing. She seems to be enjoying GrandPad"*

Dorothy, who has no interest in using technology and feels that it's not a necessity in her life, comes to realize that it is possible to listen to any song she wants through technology a few days after using GrandPad. This case shows that Dorothy's attention to her family's photos using GrandPad leads to her motivation to learn how to listen to music on the Grandpad app. In the beginning of the Grandpad intervention, Dorothy could not use the app for a long time because it made her feel tired, but eventually she became motivated by family and then she was delighted to learn new features.

> *"Mom just sent me an email informing me that Choo Choo Ch' boogie by Louis Jordan is the song that she listened to today."*

This case shows that desirability should be given priority over designing technology rather than usability in the early phase of the design. Dorothy was engaged to listen to music and therefore was able to focus on the usability of the technology. This encouraged her to learn to use other features like games and puzzles.

*5.2. Social*

Creating the Opportunity to Build Social Relationships with a Technology Need to Be Considered Rather Than Supporting the Ability to Being Alone for Older Adults

As people begin to grow older, older adults become passive to participate in activities that are critical for their wellbeing [62]. Interactive technologies such as "aging in place" and "assisted technologies" assist with such activities or support older adults who are deficient and in need of assistance to execute them to promote their independence [39,63,64]. These technologies are expected to be used mainly in situations where older adults are alone. However, our study shows that Initial Engagement will increase when there is more opportunity to build a social relationship while using interactive technology.

We learn through the case of Gloria, Peggie, and Eva, how social relationships positively influence their interest in technology. Older adults show a preference for emotionally meaningful and positive relationships with others in the senior community [65,66]. Gloria enjoys investing in personal effort in keeping up her social relationships. We were able to see how socially active older individuals are changing the community. Gloria is a central part of social activities in the community. She constantly invites and encourages other residents to participate in activities provided by the community center. Looking at how Peggie and Eva participated in the focus group discussion, Gloria's prior experience had a positive impact on their persuasion and eventually played together. Initially, Peggie's social activities are heavily influenced by Gloria. Gloria always takes care of Peggie, who is not interested, and tries to socialize together. Peggie had a very negative attitude towards the uDraw system at the beginning.

> "I am so tired, you know that this is my nap time. Can I go back and take a nap?"

We were able to see her gradually growing through Gloria and gradually enjoying using the uDraw system. Older adults typically learn from their relationships about new products and activities, which may influence the perceived benefit of new technology. Playing games together is a meaningful social activity for them. Peggie frequently mentions how positively her best friend Gloria affects her life during an interview.

> "I like to spend time with my girl (Gloria), If I'm feeling down and out, I just come here and meet my best friend Gloria who's going to make me smile, or laugh, or whatever. I bet we'd make each other happy. Yeah, we communicate really well."

Our study points out that social value is important in encouraging older people to use technology. The benefits of engaging in using technology do not only include the learning of technology but also the engagement into a small group class, which can become an integral part of the social contexts of older adults.

### 5.3. Familiarity

Keeping a Familiar Lifestyle for Older Adults Instead of Forcing Older Adults to Use Technology for Convenience

Older adults are likely to adopt interactive technology to maintain their independence and convenience at the end of life. That is, they do not exclusively rely on caregivers to do all their activities of daily living (ADLs) [33,34] and live more conveniently at their homes [67]. In this study, we found that older adults are reluctant to change their daily routines or old habits to pursue convenience by using technology. Older people can be engaged more and can adopt technology into their lives when technology is integrated into their lives without interfering with older adults' basic routines. For example, Eva, Peggie, and Gloria use flip phones. Gloria shares information with her friends in a face-to-face manner rather than using technology. When being reminded about the upcoming events at the community center, they prefer to use the old-fashioned way.

> "Ok, can you write the day and time on the paper for me? I will mark it on the calendar when I go home."

From Eva's quotation, we can see that she does not use technology unconditionally because convenience is enhanced by using technology. Eva has mentioned once that she recognizes that using a calendar app can effectively manage schedules, but it is her old habit to write appointment dates on physical calendars. The participants did not feel the need to learn to use technology until they broke the way they'd been using it. Eva mentioned during the focus group discussion that she never forgets taking medication or an appointment at the hospital. In this case, Eva will not purchase a smartphone to use the reminder app. She will also not ask someone to download the app or spend time learning how to use it. Rather, it is more important for Eva to develop the ability to explore the technology without fear by familiarizing herself with the existing functions of her current mobile phone so that she can use them to her benefit. Therefore, we need to consider ways to help older adults become familiar with the technologies that are widely and easily found near their living environments.

### 5.4. Cognitive Activity

Providing the Opportunity for Cognitive Activities with Technology Rather Than Physical Activity

Staying physically active is important for older adults to use technology [3]. Many research and innovation in technology development for older adults specifically focused on health-related technology [68,69]. There are many ways in which ubiquitous and mobile technology can motivate people of all ages to be more physically active [35,36]. We found that older adults who participated in our study are more proactive when faced with cognitive challenges. They lose interest when they realize that they will not be able to overcome their physical issues.

We introduced two kinds of Wii games to our research participants. *Wii play* games require the use of physical ability, and *Wii brain* games require the use of the mental ability. In order to play *Wii Play*, older adults need to move fast. For example, while playing a table tennis game, Eva cannot keep up with the speed of the game because his body movement is slow. Additionally, although it is much more advantageous to stand and play the game than to sit on a chair, she feels a burden on standing for a long time. She has a very difficult time maintaining a normal rally in the table tennis game due to physical limitations. In this case, we can observe that she loses her confidence quickly and is reluctant to try other mini games. However, when playing the *Wii Brain* game, we can observe the changed attitude of Eva. If the time limit does not solve the assigned problem, she expresses the desire to challenge again. Besides, after the focus group was over and all discussion sessions were over, Eva remained for 30 min to continue playing. We found out participants are more engaged in playing cognitive games. The following is Eva's reaction after playing *Wii Play*.

> "You have to practice like anything else. We can do it if we practice. it's good, it's interesting, but sorry baby, this game is not for me"

However, Participants in the Focus group responded much more positively to the *Wii Brain* game. We learned that our participants are more likely to do cognitive activity than physical activity.

> **Michael:** "Mentally. Yeah. Give my brain a workout. We don't mind being challenged because we are challenged to everybody. It's (Wii Brain) a little more exciting than that other one (Wii Play). It's a fun activity, more have fun"

Through this case, we learned that we need to pay attention to how the attitudes of the participants change passively in physical activity and actively in cognitive activity. When performing cognitive activities, older adults show a willingness to overcome their limitations, and they become interested because of the sense of accomplishment they feel when they complete a task.

### 5.5. Peer Support

Providing Peer Interaction and in-Person Training When Introducing New Technology to Older Adults Rather Than Organizing Professional Group Training

Generally, many researchers believe that some of the difficulties that older adults face while using technology can be resolved to some extent through early training or education [37,70,71]. However, older adults need constant help until the interaction is over. Based on training experience through this study, group training unified to older adults is not suitable. While each individual uses the same system, their desired functions are clearly different. Providing training that satisfies an individual's expectations may increase the usability of technology and improve engagement.

> "Once you (facilitator) leave with that, I'm not going to think about that anymore. That's it. I'm going to learn this time, and the next time you come back, I'm going to know how to do it then"

Additionally, most older adults do not trust new technologies. Several studies have concluded that the mistrust is due to the lack of previous experience with technologies [28, 72]. This is an additional burden on older adults. Our participants are likely to commit their effort in learning or using the technologies [29]. In this situation, we found that peer support is needed to deliver the right information and to improve trust about technology to older adults. Bob mentioned that he finds himself far more comfortable when asking for help from friends within the Pakistani immigrant group rather than seeking assistance from their children.

> "I have a friend who uses the phone more than I do, so he's the one that actually taught me how to use the feature to do a video phone call. Yeah. So now, like I said, there are two groups that I'm connected with, actually there are three. So, we can video chat with each other. However, I don't want to bother my son, he is working at the department store. He is really busy"

A significant external factor that caused Bob to be positive about the use of technology was that his peer community was well developed. It also helped make his active attitudes more positive.

*5.6. Role of Grandkids*

Grandkids Are More Powerful to Encourage Older Adults to Use Technology Than Adult Kids

According to Courtney et al., [7] the family is the major determinant of whether an older adult would adopt a technology or not [39,40]. Many studies are conducted to reduce the burden on a family caregiver to take care of older adults [73,74]. Sometimes caregivers recommend the use of high-performance mobile technology for older adults for their convenience, but this can be a burden for them. Older adults feel sorry for the fact that children should pay a high price for devices, they have to learn new features they are not familiar with, and they have to ask for problem-solving whenever a problem arises. We found that the greatest stimulus for older adults emotionally is the participation of grandkids. In the case of the uDraw tablet, GrandKids are often referred to as the person they want to play with.

> "I'd actually like to bring my grandkids, one of them. To see what it would be like to have them and we all try to draw. You can leave some messages to your grandkids?"

The commercial focus needs to change from caregiver to grandkids. It is important to consider how to increase the intergenerational connection and how to increase the involvement of grandkids.

*5.7. Use of Existing Features*

Think a Way to Utilize the Existing Features According to the Needs of Older Adults Instead of Delivering New Ideas or Innovative Features

Much effort has been made to develop various innovative technologies for older adults for maximizing their physical, psychological, and environmental wellness [75]. Technological innovations have been set up for older adults such as high-tech wearable technology [41–43], voice-activated assistance [76,77], smart appliances, and even home robots [21,78]. However, we found that instead of creating innovations, it is better to integrate new features into the technology that is already in existence. In the case of John, he uses the mobile phone almost every day for repairing his old car, using it as a magnifier for small-size texts supported by the zoom-in function. Instead of looking for an innovative feature, John explored a basic feature and identified a way to meet his needs.

> "Like right here you got electrical, my clubhouse, I can take a look and see how the wires go and what wires go where, so I can hook it up better. I used it for that type of thing. Yeah, so I can read it. And it helps me when I'm working."

Another example as shown in the case of Michael, it is more effective to specify one familiar function more than to provide various functions of different kinds to older adults.

> "See? That's what I am talking about. I just need a simple, simple thing. I don't need all of these brushes, I don't need all of these options. Please get me a simple palette and canvas, that's it"

Even though there is a certain function of interactive technologies that improve the quality of life of older adults and support their daily activities more smoothly, we should be wary of putting older adults in the digitized context where older adults should learn something new continuously to adopt the technology. Rather than continuing to create new functions, it is necessary to consider in advance how to use the existing embedded functions of mobile phones or computers that are easily accessible to older adults.

### 5.8. Awareness

Make Older Adults Aware of the Opportunity to Use Interactive Technologies That Can Be Enjoyed Free of Charge, Regardless of Cost

Another factor that influences technology adoption to older adults is affordability [44,45]. For those not connected to technology, the start-up costs (both the financial costs and the learning costs) are so unattractive as to not make the service interesting. Besides, older adults are less aware of the importance or significance of the technologies, and they are not willing to spend money on something they do not understand [79]. Before considering affordable prices for older adults to adopt technology, our study shows that it is more important to make older adults available more frequently to various technologies. In the case of Michael, he emphasized the importance of awareness in the in-depth interviews and focus group discussions. He said that he would like to use the system once he fully understood when and how uDraw was available, what features of uDraw he could use, and how he could use the system without difficulty with his abilities and experience. In other words, he was ready to engage in something new and was interested in trying it, but he did not know the options available to him. Older adults thus need to be fully informed in advance before they attempt to use the system.

> "I would love learning new things, but I have never had the opportunity to actually learn."

The aging population is generally not aware of the new technologies and their utility. Therefore, there is a critical need for older adults to be enlightened about the new technologies that are potentially useful for their ADLs, since lack of awareness is a barrier to adoption. Older people think technology is expensive, so they are reluctant to try technology because they are afraid to pay for what they use. The more they do, the older they lose the chance to experience technology. Government programs should increase the chances of older adults accessing new innovative technologies for free in a community or senior centers. This process raises older adults' interest and pleasurable experience in technology and becomes an opportunity to reduce the initial barrier to technology.

### 5.9. One off Benefit

Focus on One Time for Fun Instead of Providing Continued Benefit to Use Interactive Technologies

Many studies focused on older adults have also identified usefulness as a key factor [80,81]. Studies have shown that older adults are attracted to technologies that provide utilities that are clear and are deemed to improve their current wellbeing [28,82]. Generally, researchers believe that regardless of the novelty of a technology or its popularity, older adults are more likely to adopt that which they perceive to have a potential benefit or might help them attain their desired convenience [28,75]. When designing technology for older adults, designers and developers consider sustaining the use of technology for older adults. However, our study shows that older adults have identified one-off usefulness or benefit as an important value. Participants mentioned that the uDraw system is not a system to be used continuously because our participants are not interested in drawing but are satisfied with using the uDraw system to enjoy time with friends. The following is a quotation showing their view of the uDraw system.

*"So it's something not going to use for a long time, it is just going to be for one time for fun, It's just something that relaxes us, that we just enjoy doing together. That's all."*

In the use of the uDraw system during the research period, our participants appreciate the opportunity to have time for fun, relieve stress, and connect to other residents. They do not want to use the system for a long period of time. Helping older people to have positive feelings about technology through one-time interests can also be effective in promoting the engagement of older adults in the use of interactive technologies.

## 6. Discussion

We present five case studies and identify nine factors that influence older adults' behaviors and engagement with two given systems. In this section, we present a new research direction on the topic of older adults: engagement. Then, we suggest a methodological direction for studying older adults to understand the context of aging in a digitized world.

*6.1. A New Research Direction on the Importance of Initial Engagement*

We claim that initial engagement is more important than need and usability and has different challenges for older adults based on their behavior with interactive technology. When designing interactive technology for older adults that are passive towards technology, consideration of the factor of initial engagements should precede the design of interactions or evaluation of usability issues in the early phase of interaction. In this study, we see that studying older adults' engagement in the use of technology is limited, and often used interchangeably with the notion of usability or user needs. Our understanding of the notion of initial engagement and need is that they are both cognitive processes of the user, but usability is a physical process that is more related to actual usage. Usability becomes critical and encompasses a lot of what the user feels after they decide to use the system. To distinguish between initial engagement and need, we need to understand what older adults want versus what older adults need. Older adults would be more engaged in using technology when they want rather than the technology that designers think they need. For example, wearable technology may be a "required" system for older adults, but it might not be the system "wanted" by older adults. Since the initial engagement is part of user experience and helps significantly the user has a more positive experience. We should understand that initial engagement is as important as usability and user needs. More research is needed to distinguish the difference between initial engagement, usability and needs. Initial engagement values that we present here are not completely new, but these values deserve more attention when considering the older adults' user experience of technology. These findings serve as a focus to inspire new research directions for future Human Computer Interaction (HCI) research.

*6.2. A Methodological Direction for Studying Older Adults's Use of Technology*

In this study, we experienced difficulties in conducting research with older adults in the context of technology. The difficulties are centered around recruiting enough participants and gathering sufficient data to generalize the results. While laboratory based studies make it easier to collect large amounts of data, and allow generalizations and significance testing, we learned that gaining insights from older adults in sufficient numbers in ethnographic studies is not reasonable or possible. Qualitative data, collected using the ethnographic approaches we adopted in this study to understand individual behavior, produce deep and valuable insights to understand the participants' engagement in the use of technology. Observing and evaluating the use of technology by older adults in an artificially created research setting can yield results that differ from the patterns used by older adults in real life situations. In our study we noticed that the older adults behaved differently when they knew they were being observed (for example in the focus group sessions) and when they were engaging with the technology on their own when the researcher was not present. By observing older adults' use of technology in their own community over 3 months, we were able to better understand and critically consider their responses and engagement with the technology interventions. This does not mean that ethnographic qualitative approaches are the only way to collect data about engagement with interactive technology, but more ethnographic studies are needed to comprehensively and holistically engage with older adults.

## 7. Future Work

There are two distinct avenues for future research. First, as a theoretical concept, the engagement factors can be used to measure older adults' initial engagement and to design engaging user experiences for older adults. We could test which factors directly affect older adults and increase their level of engagement with technology in the behavioral patterns of older adults, the use of technology, and cognitive aspects. Initial engagement has a huge influence on the mindset of older adults when they encounter new technology. Initial engagement is a phase that can be measured by time or by cognitive changes. Another research direction is to study the transition from initial engagement to regular use as a cognitive marker that indicates older adults have demonstrated certain behavior and cognitive changes when initial engagement changes to long term engagement.

Second, as a practical tool, the engagement factors can be used to evaluate engagement with specific applications. Due to the COVID-19 pandemic, older adults may be required to use technology to receive care that is related to health and survival or communicate with a loved one in a remote setting. One of the application areas of interest for future research is smart home devices and smart services for older adults. Therefore, we can study the effectiveness of initial engagement by older adults in different application domains.

## 8. Conclusions

Although older adults who acquire digital literacy are increasing, a significant number of older adults are still unable to initiate technology on their own without help. Therefore, we should not overlook the initial barrier of older adults in the use of technology, and more research should be conducted on how to overcome the initial barrier. Through a synthesis of past research, and a mixed method study with two technological interventions, this study provides a focus on understanding older adults' initial engagement that can change older adults' behavior toward technology from passive to active. Then, we identify the key factors that influence the initial engagement of older adults: Desirability, Social, Familiarity, Cognitive activity, Peer support, Role of grandkids, Use of existing features, Awareness, and One-off benefit. In terms of the research methodology, we presented an approach for a more comprehensive understanding of older adults when they face a new technology in the real context rather than conducting experiments and analyzing results based on a limited exposure and assessment focused on physical and cognitive characteristics. The initial engagement factors contribute to both researchers and practitioners working on the topic of older adults' engagement, adoption and use of technology, as well as those investigating ways to design and develop engaging technology for improving quality of life at old age.

**Author Contributions:** L.L. composed this study, conceived and designed the analysis, collected the data, performed the analysis and wrote the paper. M.L.M. provided supervision throughout the research, wrote, and reviewed the paper and contributed substantially to the analytical part of the research. Both authors have read and agreed to the published version of the manuscript.

**Funding:** The researcher was funded by a Graduate Assistant Support Program (GASP) at UNCC, and the Department of Software and Information Systems at UNCC provided the funds for the Grandpad subscriptions.

**Institutional Review Board Statement:** The study was approved by the University of North Carolina at Charlotte's Institutional Review Board. The uDraw study (IRB number: 19-0262) was approved on 4 November 2019. The GrandPad study (IRB number: 19-0356) was approved on 16 October 2019.

**Informed Consent Statement:** Informed consent was obtained from all subjects involved in the study.

**Data Availability Statement:** Data collected during this study is not available due to privacy issues. The detailed nature of the data collected during the ethnographic study means that the data cannot be edited to eliminate the possibility of re-identification.

**Conflicts of Interest:** The authors declare no conflict of interest.

# References

1. Schoenborn, N.L.; Janssen, E.M.; Boyd, C.; Bridges, J.F.; Wolff, A.C.; Xue, Q.-L.; Pollack, C.E. Older adults' preferences for discussing long-term life expectancy: Results from a national survey. *Ann. Fam. Med.* **2018**, *16*, 530–537. [CrossRef] [PubMed]
2. Blackman, S.; Matlo, C.; Bobrovitskiy, C.; Waldoch, A.; Fang, M.L.; Jackson, P.; Mihailidis, A.; Nyg\aard, L.; Astell, A.; Sixsmith, A. Ambient assisted living technologies for aging well: A scoping review. *J. Intell. Syst.* **2016**, *25*, 55–69. [CrossRef]
3. Peek, S.T.; Luijkx, K.G.; Rijnaard, M.D.; Nieboer, M.E.; van der Voort, C.S.; Aarts, S.; van Hoof, J.; Vrijhoef, H.J.; Wouters, E.J. Older adults' reasons for using technology while aging in place. *Gerontology* **2016**, *62*, 226–237. [CrossRef] [PubMed]
4. Hanson, G.J.; Takahashi, P.Y.; Pecina, J.L. Emerging technologies to support independent living of older adults at risk. *Care Manag. J.* **2013**, *14*, 58. [CrossRef] [PubMed]
5. Watanabe, K.; Niemelä, M.; Määttä, H.; Miwa, H.; Fukuda, K.; Nishimura, T.; Toivonen, M. Meaningful technology for seniors: Viewpoints for sustainable care service systems. In Proceedings of the 4th International Conference on Serviceology, ICServ, 2016: Special session: Meaningful Technologies for Seniors; Society for Serviciology, Tokyo, Japan, 6–8 September 2016.
6. Tsai, T.-H.; Chang, H.-T.; Wong, A.M.-K.; Wu, T.-F. Connecting communities: Designing a social media platform for older adults living in a senior village. In *Proceedings of the International Conference on Universal Access in Human-Computer Interaction, Orlando, FL, USA, 9–14 July 2011*; Springer: Berlin, Heidelberg, 2011; pp. 224–233.
7. Courtney, K.L.; Demeris, G.; Rantz, M.; Skubic, M. Needing smart home technologies: The perspectives of older adults in continuing care retirement communities. *J. Innov. Health Inform.* **2008**, *16*, 195–201. [CrossRef]
8. Conroy, K.M.; Krishnan, S.; Mittelstaedt, S.; Patel, S.S. Technological advancements to address elderly loneliness: Practical considerations and community resilience implications for COVID-19 pandemic. *Work. Older People* **2020**, *24*, 257–264. [CrossRef] [PubMed]
9. Figueroa, C.A.; Aguilera, A. The need for a mental health technology revolution in the COVID-19 pandemic. *Front. Psychiatry* **2020**, *11*, 523. [CrossRef] [PubMed]
10. Charness, N.; Boot, W.R. Aging and information technology use: Potential and barriers. *Curr. Dir. Psychol. Sci.* **2009**, *18*, 253–258. [CrossRef]
11. Czaja, S.J.; Lee, C.C. The impact of aging on access to technology. *Univers. Access Inf. Soc.* **2007**, *5*, 341. [CrossRef]
12. Chin, J.; Fu, W.-T. Age differences in exploratory learning from a health information website. In Proceedings of the SIGCHI Conference on Human Factors in Computing Systems, Austin, TX, USA, 5–10 May 2012; pp. 3031–3040.
13. Vines, J.; Pritchard, G.; Wright, P.; Olivier, P.; Brittain, K. An age-old problem: Examining the discourses of ageing in HCI and strategies for future research. *ACM Trans. Comput. Human Interact. (TOCHI)* **2015**, *22*, 1–27. [CrossRef]
14. Worden, A.; Walker, N.; Bharat, K.; Hudson, S. Making computers easier for older adults to use: Area cursors and sticky icons. In Proceedings of the ACM SIGCHI Conference on Human factors in computing systems, Atlanta, GA, USA, 22–27 March 1997; pp. 266–271.
15. Ziefle, M.; Schroeder, U.; Strenk, J.; Michel, T. How younger and older adults master the usage of hyperlinks in small screen devices. In Proceedings of the SIGCHI conference on Human factors in computing systems, San Jose, CA, USA, 28 April–3 May 2007; pp. 307–316.
16. Bailey, C.; Sheehan, C. Technology, older persons' perspectives and the anthropological ethnographic lens. *Alter* **2009**, *3*, 96–109. [CrossRef]
17. Braun, V.; Clarke, V. Using thematic analysis in psychology. *Qual. Res. Psychol.* **2006**, *3*, 77–101. [CrossRef]
18. Beer, J.M.; Smarr, C.-A.; Chen, T.L.; Prakash, A.; Mitzner, T.L.; Kemp, C.C.; Rogers, W.A. The domesticated robot: Design guidelines for assisting older adults to age in place. In Proceedings of the seventh annual ACM/IEEE international conference on Human-Robot Interaction, Boston, MA, USA, 5–8 March 2012; pp. 335–342.
19. Czaja, S.J.; Boot, W.R.; Charness, N.; Rogers, W.A. *Designing for Older Adults: Principles and Creative Human Factors Approaches*; CRC Press: Boca Raton, FL, USA, 2019.
20. Kappen, D.L.; Nacke, L.E.; Gerling, K.M.; Tsotsos, L.E. Design strategies for gamified physical activity applications for older adults. In *Proceedings of the 2016 49th Hawaii international conference on system sciences (HICSS), Koloa, HI, USA, 5–8 January 2016*; IEEE: Washington, DC, USA, 2016; pp. 1309–1318.
21. Lee, L.N.; Kim, M.J. A Critical Review of Smart Residential Environments for Older Adults with a Focus on Pleasurable Experience. *Front. Psychol.* **2019**, *10*, 3080. [CrossRef]
22. Peek, S.T.; Wouters, E.J.; Van Hoof, J.; Luijkx, K.G.; Boeije, H.R.; Vrijhoef, H.J. Factors influencing acceptance of technology for aging in place: A systematic review. *Int. J. Med. Inf.* **2014**, *83*, 235–248. [CrossRef] [PubMed]
23. Booker, C.G. Elderly Adults' Perceptions of Home Lifestyle Monitoring Technology. Master's Thesis, Ball State University, Muncie, IN, USA, 2011.
24. Nimrod, G. Technophobia among older Internet users. *Educ. Gerontol.* **2018**, *44*, 148–162. [CrossRef]

25. Sponselee, A.; Schouten, B.; Bouwhuis, D.; Willems, C. Smart home technology for the elderly: Perceptions of multidisciplinary stakeholders. In Proceedings of the European Conference on Ambient Intelligence, Darmstadt, Germany, 7–10 November 2007; Springer: Berlin/Heidelberg, Germany, 2007; pp. 314–326.
26. Forberger, S.; Bammann, K.; Bauer, J.; Boll, S.; Bolte, G.; Brand, T.; Hein, A.; Koppelin, F.; Lippke, S.; Meyer, J. How to tackle key challenges in the promotion of physical activity among older adults (65+): The AEQUIPA network approach. *Int. J. Environ. Res. Public Health* **2017**, *14*, 379. [CrossRef]
27. Hanson, V.L. Influencing technology adoption by older adults. *Interact. Comput.* **2010**, *22*, 502–509. [CrossRef]
28. Lee, C.; Coughlin, J.F. PERSPECTIVE: Older adults' adoption of technology: An integrated approach to identifying determinants and barriers. *J. Prod. Innov. Manag.* **2015**, *32*, 747–759. [CrossRef]
29. Berkowsky, R.W.; Sharit, J.; Czaja, S.J. Factors predicting decisions about technology adoption among older adults. *Innov. Aging* **2017**, *1*, igy002. [CrossRef] [PubMed]
30. Astell, A.J.; McGrath, C.; Dove, E. "That's for old so and so's!": Does identity influence older adults' technology adoption decisions? *Ageing Soc.* **2020**, *40*, 1550–1576. [CrossRef]
31. Maher, M.L.; Lee, L. Designing for gesture and tangible interaction. *Synth. Lect. Hum. Cent. Interact.* **2017**, *10*, i-111. [CrossRef]
32. Park, S. A study on affordance dimensions of digital services for the elderly through the analysis of senior adults' daily activities. *Archit. Res.* **2008**, *10*, 11–20.
33. Wickramasinghe, A.; Torres, R.L.S.; Ranasinghe, D.C. Recognition of falls using dense sensing in an ambient assisted living environment. *Pervasive Mob. Comput.* **2017**, *34*, 14–24. [CrossRef]
34. Yu, J.; An, N.; Hassan, T.; Kong, Q. A pilot study on a smart home for elders based on continuous in-home unobtrusive monitoring technology. *HERD Health Environ. Res. Design J.* **2019**, *12*, 206–219. [CrossRef] [PubMed]
35. Stefanov, D.H.; Bien, Z.; Bang, W.-C. The smart house for older persons and persons with physical disabilities: Structure, technology arrangements, and perspectives. *IEEE Trans. Neural Syst. Rehabil. Eng.* **2004**, *12*, 228–250. [CrossRef] [PubMed]
36. Yang, C.-C.; Hsu, Y.-L. A review of accelerometry-based wearable motion detectors for physical activity monitoring. *Sensors* **2010**, *10*, 7772–7788. [CrossRef] [PubMed]
37. Hickman, J.M.; Rogers, W.A.; Fisk, A.D. Training older adults to use new technology. *J. Gerontol. Ser. B Psychol. Sci. Soc. Sci.* **2007**, *62*, 77–84. [CrossRef] [PubMed]
38. Rogers, W.A.; Campbell, R.H.; Pak, R. A systems approach for training older adults to use technology. *Commun. Technol. Aging Oppor. Chall. Future* **2001**, 187–208.
39. Mynatt, E.D.; Rogers, W.A. Developing technology to support the functional independence of older adults. *Ageing Int.* **2001**, *27*, 24–41. [CrossRef]
40. Silver, H.J.; Wellman, N.S. Family caregiver training is needed to improve outcomes for older adults using home care technologies. *J. Am. Diet. Assoc.* **2002**, *102*, 831–836. [CrossRef]
41. Baig, M.M.; Gholamhosseini, H.; Connolly, M.J. A comprehensive survey of wearable and wireless ECG monitoring systems for older adults. *Med. Biol. Eng. Comput.* **2013**, *51*, 485–495. [CrossRef] [PubMed]
42. Mohler, M.J.; Wendel, C.S.; Taylor-Piliae, R.E.; Toosizadeh, N.; Najafi, B. Motor performance and physical activity as predictors of prospective falls in community-dwelling older adults by frailty level: Application of wearable technology. *Gerontology* **2016**, *62*, 654–664. [CrossRef]
43. Najafi, B.; Armstrong, D.G.; Mohler, J. *Novel Wearable Technology for Assessing Spontaneous Daily Physical Activity and Risk of Falling in Older Adults with Diabetes*; SAGE Publications: Los Angeles, CA, USA, 2013.
44. Ma, Q.; Chan, A.H.; Chen, K. Personal and other factors affecting acceptance of smartphone technology by older Chinese adults. *Appl. Ergon.* **2016**, *54*, 62–71. [CrossRef]
45. Mitzner, T.L.; Boron, J.B.; Fausset, C.B.; Adams, A.E.; Charness, N.; Czaja, S.J.; Dijkstra, K.; Fisk, A.D.; Rogers, W.A.; Sharit, J. Older adults talk technology: Technology usage and attitudes. *Comput. Hum. Behav.* **2010**, *26*, 1710–1721. [CrossRef] [PubMed]
46. Broady, T.; Chan, A.; Caputi, P. Comparison of older and younger adults' attitudes towards and abilities with computers: Implications for training and learning. *Br. J. Educ. Technol.* **2010**, *41*, 473–485. [CrossRef]
47. Olson, K.E.; O'Brien, M.A.; Rogers, W.A.; Charness, N. Diffusion of technology: Frequency of use for younger and older adults. *Ageing Int.* **2011**, *36*, 123–145. [CrossRef]
48. Birkland, J.L.; Kaarst-Brown, M.L. What's so special about studying old people? The Ethical, Methodological, and Sampling Issues Surrounding the Study of Older Adults and ICTs. In *Proceedings of the Cultural Attitudes Towards Technology and Communication (CATaC) 2010. Vancouver, BC, Canada, 15–18 June 2010*; Sudweeks, F., Hrochovec, H., Ess, C., Eds.; School of Information Technology Murdoch University: Murdoch, Australia, 2010.
49. Hu, X.; Dor, R.; Bosch, S.; Khoong, A.; Li, J.; Stark, S.; Lu, C. Challenges in studying falls of community-dwelling older adults in the real world. In Proceedings of the 2017 IEEE International Conference on Smart Computing (SMARTCOMP), Hong Kong, China, 29–31 May 2017; IEEE: New York, NY, USA, 2017; pp. 1–7.
50. Clawson, J.; Pater, J.A.; Miller, A.D.; Mynatt, E.D.; Mamykina, L. No longer wearing: Investigating the abandonment of personal health-tracking technologies on craigslist. In Proceedings of the 2015 ACM International Joint Conference on Pervasive and Ubiquitous Computing, Osaka, Japan, 7–11 September 2015; pp. 647–658.
51. Young, R.; Willis, E.; Cameron, G.; Geana, M. "Willing but Unwilling": Attitudinal barriers to adoption of home-based health information technology among older adults. *Health Inform. J.* **2014**, *20*, 127–135. [CrossRef]

52. Barnard, Y.; Bradley, M.D.; Hodgson, F.; Lloyd, A.D. Learning to use new technologies by older adults: Perceived difficulties, experimentation behaviour and usability. *Comput. Hum. Behav.* **2013**, *29*, 1715–1724. [CrossRef]
53. Czaja, S.J. Usability of technology for older adults: Where are we and where do we need to be. *J. Usabil. Stud.* **2019**, *14*, 61–64.
54. Harrington, C.N.; Hartley, J.Q.; Mitzner, T.L.; Rogers, W.A. Assessing older adults' usability challenges using Kinect-based exergames. In *Proceedings of the International Conference on Human Aspects of IT for the Aged Population, Los Angeles, CA, USA, 2–7 August 2015*; Springer: New York, NY, USA, 2015; pp. 488–499.
55. Apted, T.; Kay, J.; Quigley, A. Tabletop sharing of digital photographs for the elderly. In Proceedings of the SIGCHI conference on Human Factors in computing systems, Montréal, QC, Canada, 22–27 April 2006; pp. 781–790.
56. Kurniawan, S.; Mahmud, M.; Nugroho, Y. A study of the use of mobile phones by older persons. In Proceedings of the CHI'06 extended abstracts on Human factors in computing systems, Montréal, QC, Canada, 22–27 April 2006; pp. 989–994.
57. Bannon, L.J. From human factors to human actors: The role of psychology and human-computer interaction studies in system design. In *Readings in Human–Computer Interaction*; Elsevier: Burlington, VT, USA, 1995; pp. 205–214.
58. Lee, L. Creativity and Emotional Attachment as a Guide to Factors of Engagement for Elderly Interaction with Technology. In Proceedings of the 2019 on Creativity and Cognition, San Diego, CA, USA, 23–26 June 2019; pp. 664–669.
59. Lee, L.; Okerlund, J.; Maher, M.L.; Farina, T. Embodied Interaction Design to Promote Creative Social Engagement for Older Adults. In *Proceedings of the International Conference on Human-Computer Interaction, Copenhagen, Denmark, 19–24 July 2020*; Springer: New York, NY, USA, 2021; pp. 164–183.
60. Davis, F.D. Perceived usefulness, perceived ease of use, and user acceptance of information technology. *MIS Q.* **1989**, *13*, 319–340. [CrossRef]
61. Li, Q.; Luximon, Y. Older adults' use of mobile device: Usability challenges while navigating various interfaces. *Behav. Inf. Technol.* **2020**, *39*, 837–861. [CrossRef]
62. Anaby, D.; Miller, W.C.; Eng, J.J.; Jarus, T.; Noreau, L.; Group, P.R. Participation and well-being among older adults living with chronic conditions. *Soc. Indic. Res.* **2011**, *100*, 171–183. [CrossRef] [PubMed]
63. Cahill, J.; McLoughlin, S.; Wetherall, S. The design of new technology supporting wellbeing, independence and social participation, for older adults domiciled in residential homes and/or assisted living communities. *Technologies* **2018**, *6*, 18. [CrossRef]
64. Horgas, A.; Abowd, G. The impact of technology on living environments for older adults. In *Technology for Adaptive Aging*; National Academies Press (US): Washington, DC, USA, 2004.
65. Kamin, S.T.; Lang, F.R.; Kamber, T. Social contexts of technology use in old age. In *Gerontechnology. Research, Practice, and Principles in the Field of Technology and Aging*; Springer: New York, NY, USA, 2016.
66. Kwon, S. *Gerontechnology: Research, Practice, and Principles in the Field of Technology and aging*; Springer Publishing: New York, NY, USA, 2016.
67. Mostaghel, R. Innovation and technology for the elderly: Systematic literature review. *J. Bus. Res.* **2016**, *69*, 4896–4900. [CrossRef]
68. Estes, C.L.; Binney, E.A. The biomedicalization of aging: Dangers and dilemmas. *Gerontologist* **1989**, *29*, 587–596. [CrossRef]
69. Hassol, A.; Walker, J.M.; Kidder, D.; Rokita, K.; Young, D.; Pierdon, S.; Deitz, D.; Kuck, S.; Ortiz, E. Patient experiences and attitudes about access to a patient electronic health care record and linked web messaging. *J. Am. Med. Inf. Assoc.* **2004**, *11*, 505–513. [CrossRef] [PubMed]
70. Huber, L.; Watson, C. Technology: Education and training needs of older adults. *Educ. Gerontol.* **2014**, *40*, 16–25. [CrossRef]
71. Mitzner, T.L.; Fausset, C.B.; Boron, J.B.; Adams, A.E.; Dijkstra, K.; Lee, C.C.; Rogers, W.A.; Fisk, A.D. Older adults' training preferences for learning to use technology. In *Proceedings of the Human Factors and Ergonomics Society Annual Meeting*; SAGE Publications: Los Angeles, CA, USA, 2008; Volume 52, pp. 2047–2051.
72. Demiris, G.; Doorenbos, A.Z.; Towle, C. Ethical considerations regarding the use of technology for older adults: The case of telehealth. *Res. Gerontol. Nurs.* **2009**, *2*, 128–136. [CrossRef]
73. Madara Marasinghe, K. Assistive technologies in reducing caregiver burden among informal caregivers of older adults: A systematic review. *Disabil. Rehabil. Assist. Technol.* **2016**, *11*, 353–360. [CrossRef] [PubMed]
74. Miller, C.A.; Dewing, W.; Krichbaum, K.; Kuiack, S.; Rogers, W.; Shafer, S. Automation as Caregiver; the role of Advanced Technologies in Elder Care. In *Proceedings of the Human Factors and Ergonomics Society Annual Meeting*; SAGE Publications: Los Angeles, CA, USA, 2001; Volume 45, pp. 226–229.
75. Melenhorst, A.-S.; Rogers, W.A.; Bouwhuis, D.G. Older adults' motivated choice for technological innovation: Evidence for benefit-driven selectivity. *Psychol. Aging* **2006**, *21*, 190. [CrossRef] [PubMed]
76. Morris, M.E.; Adair, B.; Miller, K.; Ozanne, E.; Hansen, R.; Pearce, A.J.; Santamaria, N.; Viega, L.; Long, M.; Said, C.M. Smart-home technologies to assist older people to live well at home. *J. Aging Sci.* **2013**, *1*, 1–9.
77. Zajicek, M. Patterns for encapsulating speech interface design solutions for older adults. In Proceedings of the 2003 conference on Universal usability, Vancouver, BC, Canada, 10–11 November 2002; pp. 54–60.
78. Fasola, J.; Mataric, M.J. Using socially assistive human–robot interaction to motivate physical exercise for older adults. *Proc. IEEE* **2012**, *100*, 2512–2526. [CrossRef]
79. Heinz, M.; Martin, P.; Margrett, J.A.; Yearns, M.; Franke, W.; Yang, H.I.; Wong, J.; Chang, C.K. Perceptions of technology among older adults. *J. Gerontol. Nurs.* **2013**, *39*, 42–51. [CrossRef] [PubMed]
80. Heinz, M.S. Exploring Predictors of Technology Adoption among Older Adults. Ph.D. Thesis, Iowa State University, Ames, IA, USA, 2013.

81. Mitzner, T.L.; Savla, J.; Boot, W.R.; Sharit, J.; Charness, N.; Czaja, S.J.; Rogers, W.A. Technology adoption by older adults: Findings from the PRISM trial. *Gerontologist* **2019**, *59*, 34–44. [CrossRef] [PubMed]
82. Walsh, K.; Callan, A. Perceptions, preferences, and acceptance of information and communication technologies in older-adult community care settings in Ireland: A case-study and ranked-care program analysis. *Ageing Int.* **2011**, *36*, 102–122. [CrossRef]

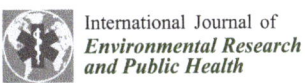 

*Article*

# Patient Clothing as a Healing Environment: A Qualitative Interview Study

Seonju Kam and Youngsun Yoo *

Department of Clothing and Textiles, Kyung Hee University, Seoul 02447, Korea; kamjoo@empas.com
* Correspondence: ysyoo@khu.ac.kr; Tel.: +82-2-961-0254

**Abstract:** Patients' emotional responses to the hospital environment can be considered as important as medical technology and equipment. Therefore, this study investigated their experiences to determine whether the pattern using hospital identity (HI) elements, a widely used design method for patient clothing in university hospitals, can affect their emotional response and contribute to healing. It aimed to identify whether controlling the motif characteristics, arrangement, and spacing in this pattern design, and the direction between motifs, could be a method to design patient clothing for healing. To investigate patients' emotional response and suggestions for patient clothing design, an interview-based qualitative approach was used. In-depth interviews were conducted with 12 patients discharged from Kyung Hee University Hospital Medical Center (KHUMC), Seoul. The interview questions consisted of two parts. One part featured questions about participants' emotional responses to the medical environment and their latest patient clothing experience, and the other featured questions about their emotional response to, and suggestions for, the healing expression of pattern design using HI. The results confirmed that the motif characteristics, arrangement, and spacing, and the direction between motifs, influenced patients' positive emotions and contributed to the healing effect. Therefore, when the HI elements of a medical institution are applied in the design of patient clothing with the characteristics of a healing design, patients perceive this as providing stability and comfort. The design of patient clothing becomes a medium that not only builds the brand image of medical institutions, but also enhances the quality of medical services centered on patient healing.

**Keywords:** hospitals; patients; clothing

## 1. Introduction

The current medical environment is rapidly changing with the development of advanced technology, but provider-oriented medical services are still causing unsatisfactory results for patients. Patient satisfaction is evaluated as an important factor in the quality of medical services [1–4]. The interior design of a medical institution, including its furniture, ornaments, lighting, sound, color, landscape, and physical environment, including factors such as patient clothing and the uniforms of the medical personnel, are important factors in creating a healing atmosphere by stimulating the senses of patients and staff and creating memorable experiences [5].

As a physical environmental factor, patient clothing facilitates treatment and helps the healing of both mind and body [6]. Patient clothing is part of the medical environment and influences patients' recovery. It also has a key role in building a rapport between patients and medical service [7]. Medical services are provided under conditions in which the patient and their family are physically and emotionally vulnerable, a fact that should be emphasized [8]. Healing requires the patient to recover physically and mentally, and can be approached using various characteristics related to human emotions, such as nature-friendliness, familiarity, stability, aesthetics, and relaxation [9]. A healing design for patient clothing can improve comfort and help patients to adapt to the treatment environment by

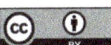

considering their sensibility and spirit. Patient clothing with a healing design can alleviate stress, soothe negative emotions, and even play a role in helping the patient's recovery by eliciting comfort, pleasure, and psychological and physiological stability.

Hospital identity (HI) is reflected in the hospital's logo, symbol, signature, and slogan, and represents the visual image of the organization. Patient clothing reflecting HI functions to represent the hospital's unique identity and differentiated brand image.

As existing patient clothing is mainly manufactured according to the HI plan, the hospitals' position has usually received more attention than considerations regarding patient healing. Thus, there are many cases in which the patient's psychological situation is not considered. This study aimed to identify a patient clothing design method that helps patients heal by modulating the motif of the pattern design associated with the HI factor. It investigated, through interviews, whether controlling the motif characteristics, arrangement, and spacing, and the direction between motifs in pattern designs using HI elements could be a method of designing patient clothing for healing.

## 2. Literature Review
### 2.1. Patient Clothing

Patient clothing originated in the 19th century when hospitals needed to improve hygiene and arrange suitable clothing for poor patients [10]. Patient clothing is the most important factor in maintaining a patient's dignity and well-being and is one of the first factors encountered during hospitalization [11]. In addition, patient clothing is a part of the treatment environment, along with medical technology and equipment, and wearing patient clothing becomes an active therapeutic medium in the relationship between medical staff and patients by recognizing it as an object in the treatment process [7].

A number of earlier studies have mentioned the uncomfortable emotions that patients feel when wearing patient clothing. These have stated that the worn-out appearance of patient clothing affects the patient's self-esteem [8] and causes discomfort by unintendedly exposing body parts [12]. Unnecessary exposure of the patient's body to medical staff leads to a decrease in relative status, and patients feel shame because their privacy is not guaranteed [13]. Patients experience reduced opportunities for self-expression and feel depersonalized when wearing uniformly-shaped patient clothing [14]. Khorshid et al. [6] reported that when patients suffered stress and physical constraints during hospitalization and the recovery phase, positive emotions about clothing were effective in improving their healing and self-esteem. Therefore, when considered in terms of the treatment process, patient clothing is required not only to have a physical function for convenience of treatment, but also to influence the patient's emotions by the quality of its design. Hospitals with a corporate system nowadays differentiate their brand value from their competitors by expressing the hospital's identity in the design of patient clothing. The design of hospital patient clothing in Korea reflects brand identity and image by utilizing logos and symbolic marks. Figure 1 shows hospital clothing designed with the hospital's logo and mark in a striped pattern, and Figure 2 shows clothing designed with a block repeat pattern. This was composed of an ordered image in which signatures and logos of the same size were arranged in repeating patterns. This seems to be related to the intention of most hospitals to promote favorable images such as trust, quality, and reputation. However, even if patient clothing reflecting HI can help differentiate hospitals at the point of contact with the customer, considering that the final goal of the relationship between the hospital and the patient is the patient's healing, a design plan that can offer physical and psychological comfort should be developed.

When designing patient clothing, an emotional approach is possible through the visual image of the clothing and its design elements [15]. In addition, a style that changes the angle or arrangement of logos or logos related to the hospital's visual identity can increase the awareness of movement and promote visual engagement by customers [15]. Moreover, the motif's line, shape, and size, and the spacing between the motif and the background determine the feeling when looking at the pattern [16]. In other words, it is possible to provide a quality service with a design that considers the patient's sensibilities and psychological state by changing the angle or interval of the pattern repeats while maintaining the same core design elements of HI. Patient clothing design can be promoted as a service that improves the psychological well-being of the patient while adding quality through design that considers the patient's sensibilities and dignity as well as the basic function of ease of treatment.

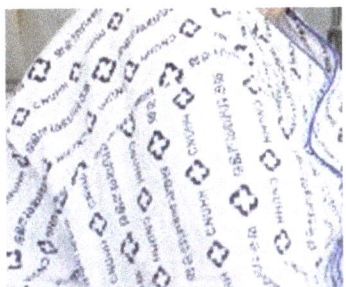

Figure 1. Striped pattern for patient clothing.

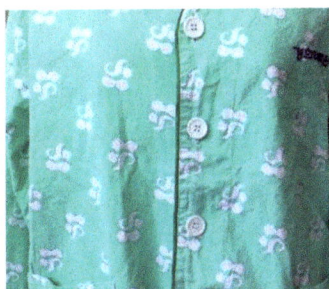

Figure 2. Block repeat pattern for patient clothing.

*2.2. Healing Design Approach*

Healing is a lively process that involves regaining physical and mental integrity, recovery, and rehabilitation. Healing takes place at several levels of the human system, including the mental, physical, emotional, and spiritual [17]. The care environment has the potential to reinforce an individual's inner strength, and a visually comfortable care environment has a positive effect on recovery after surgery [8,18]. The concept of healing design as a means of treatment is related to solving the patient's psychological and physical needs and improving the patient satisfaction [19]. The environment has the potential to reinforce an individual's inner strength and aid in healing by facilitating or enhancing the patient's behavior [17,20]. Many previous studies have mentioned that it is helpful to introduce a healing environment into physical design.

Healing design includes many aspects that positively influence people to achieve healing goals. It is mainly used in medical facilities, such as hospitals, sanatoriums, healing spas, and retiree homes, for a positive impact on mental and physical health. In the design of patient clothing, research is needed to consider the interconnection between the physical and mental factors that prioritize healing.

On investigating the literature on design approaches for healing roles, Harris et al. [5] reported that the physical environment has an important role in the hospital experience and causes hospitals to function as healing spaces, thus influencing patient satisfaction. In terms of interior design, comfortable and functional equipment and furniture provide home-like comfort, and aesthetically pleasing decoration, art, and a spacious layout to accommodate visitors were factors that increased the patient's satisfaction with the hospital. In addition, exposure to nature is said to combat mental fatigue and aid healing.

Timmermann et al. [21] found that positive sensory impressions in the hospital environment significantly affected mood and were largely obtained from maintaining patient identity and positive thoughts and emotions. In addition, they found that from the viewpoint of healing, natural and aesthetic decoration helps to maintain the patient's identity, and that patients who can see pleasant, scenic views of nature through their hospital window develop positive thoughts and emotions.

Schreuder et al. [22] mentioned spatial comfort, privacy, and safety among the important design elements for a healing environment. The spatial comfort of the patient relates to the personalization of space, an aesthetic interior design, and the access to nature; moreover, privacy, and safety affect the patient's well-being. Riisbøl et al. [23] studied a design method that provides healing architecture for patients, their relatives, and nurses. Sensory impressions are induced in patients through the atmosphere of the visit, the view of natural surroundings, and the provision of privacy. The aesthetics experienced in the wall decoration and the room color, as well as the atmosphere, influenced the experience of well-being and the quality of treatment; the resulting comfort gave patients a home-like familiarity and reduced the stress generated in the clinical hospital environment. Privacy is related to space, and the healing effect may improve on separating the space with a partition or curtain between patients.

Based on these studies, we explored theories related to "nature experience," "comfort," "aesthetics," and "relaxation" as elements for healing design. Figure 3 shows the design expression characteristics and the design methods that influence healing, which we identified through a review of the literature on the following four characteristics.

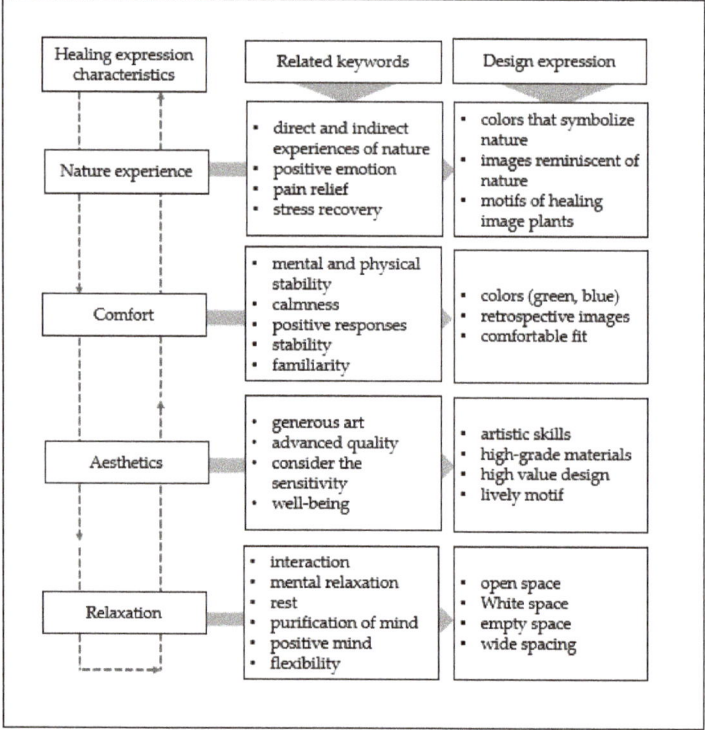

**Figure 3.** Summary of the design expression characteristics that influence healing through literature review studies.

### 2.2.1. Nature Experience

Contact with nature can benefit personal health, and patients tend to experience recovery by looking at the natural environment [18,24–26]. For patients, experiences of nature can influence healing by reducing anxiety, anger, or negative emotions and inducing positive emotions. Numerous previous investigations have shown that exposing patients to nature has a positive effect on pain relief and healing, and that a brief look at nature can lead to a quick and meaningful recovery from stress [27]. In a study of patients recovering from appendectomy by Park and Mattson [28], patients in hospital rooms with plants and flowers had a significantly reduced intake of analgesics after surgery than those in hospital rooms without plants and flowers. Blood pressure, heart rate, pain, anxiety, and fatigue were lowered, and positive feelings and satisfaction with the hospital room were higher. Ulrich et al. [9] confirmed that colors symbolizing nature and images reminiscent of nature sustain or increase positive emotions such as comfort and calm and reduce negative emotions that cause worry and stress. Totaforti [29] stated that plants (especially roses), natural ventilation, natural light, and environmental design that can contact nature improves the work efficiency and organizational ability of hospital workers as well as the well-being of patients. Cliff Goldman and Louise Russell attempted to combine textile design with a healing environment, and developed a "healing fabric" arranged in a repeating pattern using life-size images of healing plants such as eucalyptus, silver dollar plant, bamboo, and jasmine [30].

### 2.2.2. Comfort

Patients are likely to experience anxiety and feel vulnerable during hospital stays due to the unfamiliar sensations associated with the medical environment, which is mainly white color [23]. In addition, lack of visual or auditory privacy can cause discomfort [22]. In particular, patient clothes are often designed for medical treatment purposes and are in the form of pajamas or a gown for ease of treatment, which can cause anxiety about exposure if worn without underwear. For the safety of patients, patient clothing design must proper ease of access to enable comfortable treatment, but must also create a psychological environment that allows the patient to feel cared for and provides emotional comfort [6]. Color is an important design element and has a strong relationship with emotions [31]. Green, reminiscent of plants, and blue, reminiscent of the sky and water, are quiet and positive, and they encourage stability [32]. Emotional stability can be achieved by providing familiarity and comfortable environmental design. A study on the design of nursing homes found that elderly people preferred a retro-style flower design, which was able to bring memories of home and offered familiarity and comfort [33]. The design of patient clothing requires the development of patterns and the use of colors that can enhance psychological comfort, along with clothing design that avoids physical discomfort.

### 2.2.3. Aesthetics

An attractive environment has the ability to distract attention and help patients recover from mental fatigue. The patient's satisfaction with the hospital increases when the space they are in is aesthetically pleasing and comfortable [34]. An art-rich environment can be seen as therapeutic, providing a means to alleviate physical discomfort, emotional pain, and mental crises. Using art as a healing tool can improve the outcome and quality of treatment, and art plays an important role in rapid recovery [25]. The design of the elements comprising the physical environment that result in sensory stimulation, such as buildings, equipment, furniture, signboards, colors, art, landscapes, and clothing, is perceived to indicate a hospital's quality of care and can positively influence patient healing [35]. Since patients experience the patient clothing design directly, the aesthetics that can inspire positive emotions in them, such as images representing optimism, vitality, and humor, should be considered to improve the healing system [36]. Feodoroff, a designer who developed a functional patient suit "Original Healing Threads" for women with cancer, emphasized the importance of design considering the aesthetic sensitivity of patients by commenting that when you feel like you look good, you will get better [37]. For patient clothing designs, aesthetics should be addressed as a different concept from that of general fashion. Above all, patient clothing should be designed to help heal by adjusting design elements by reflecting the emotions and tastes of patients.

2.2.4. Relaxation

Lau et al. found that viewing an open space would clear the minds of users who want to relax, arouse positive attitudes, and relieve tense nerves [38]. The white space in advertising design leads users to interact with the design in a relaxed emotional state, increasing their favorable perceptions about product quality and reliability [39]. Relaxation is not only related to the comfortable fit of the patient clothing design, but also to the healing effect since it allows the patient to experience the emotion of comfort in the white space constituting the pattern design.

## 3. Methodology

### 3.1. Design and Interview Participants

The study was designed to explore user suggestions for patient clothing design using a qualitative approach that involved conducting individual in-depth interviews. Before recruiting participants, approval was obtained from the administrative department of KHUMC, Seoul. The target group of study participants was cured patients of KHUMC who had completed the discharge procedure. Potential participants and their families were informed about the purpose of the study and the interview method to be used. Subsequently, 12 participants voluntarily agreed to participate in the study. Their interviews were conducted from 1–30 December 2020.

### 3.2. Procedure

The stimulus was based on the patient clothing currently used by KHUMC (Table 1), which was designed by this research team with the support of the KHUMC Fund. To examine whether the current patient clothing pattern design using HI elements embodies the characteristics of the healing theory effectively, and to explore user opinions on what they would consider an improved healing design, the healing design was based on the shape and color of the current patient clothing. Six stimuli related to four characteristics were added.

Semi-structured questions were used in the interviews. Each interview lasted about 30–40 min. The interview questions consisted of two parts. One part had open-ended questions to explore the participants' emotional response to the medical environment and to the current patient clothing experience. The other part had questions on the participant's emotional response to, personal preference for, and suggestions regarding the healing expression of pattern design using HI; the stimulus was used along with the questions. The two-part questions were built around the keywords related to design expression characteristics that influence healing shown in Figure 3.

Figure 4 summarizes the questions used to elicit patients' feelings about the current medical environment and their clothing experience. The keywords in Figure 4 were alternately referred to as additional questions to facilitate the participant's answers during the interview process and to more accurately identify the emotions associated with healing characteristics.

The interview about the users' emotional response, personal preference, and suggestions for the healing characteristics of pattern design using HI were conducted by presenting a stimulus. During each interview, a tablet, which had a photograph of the current patient clothing, and a printed photograph of the patient clothing with manipulated patterns to reflect various healing characteristics, were used.

Table 1. Current patient clothing.

| Textile Design | Outfit |
|---|---|
| 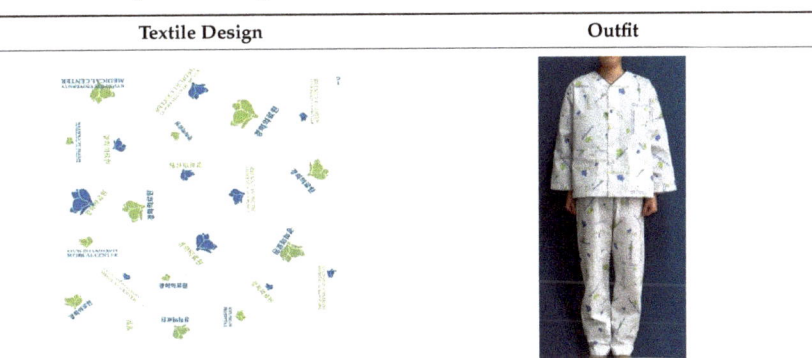 | |

Healing expression characteristics: A character mark symbolizing a magnolia flower, which is an element of HI, was introduced as a motif, and among the colors constituting the character mark, blue and green, noted to be related to psychological stability, were adopted as the colors of healing.
HI: The hospital's character mark and signature were used as the motif for the pattern design.
Protection of patient privacy: The neckline depth was 1.5 cm higher than that of existing patient clothing to reduce exposure during bowing the upper body. The existing patient clothing has a deep neckline for convenience when using medical devices such as stethoscopes. To reduce exposure from the gaps between the buttons, the overlapping part of the front fastening was made wider than that of the existing patient clothing.
Activity and sustainability: To better consider the patient's activity and comfort levels, the width between the shoulders was greater than that of the existing clothing and the height of the sleeves was lowered. This was taken from the flat pattern of Hanbok, and affects the order of sewing in mass production, improving economic efficiency and sustainability.
Hygiene management: A white background was chosen to easily deal with contamination.

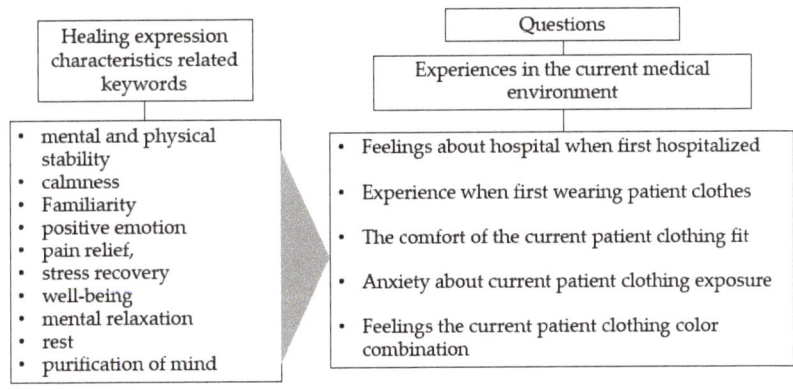

Figure 4. Questions used to elicit patients' feeling about the current medical environment.

Figure 5 shows the process used to elicit answers from the interviewees regarding their emotional response to pattern design using HI. The following are the four design directions used as a stimulus. Questions about plant motifs relate to the nature experience design direction. This design direction was based on the findings in the literature that images reminiscent of nature maintain or increase positive emotions and influence healing [9]. An image using only the pattern representing the hospital's brand identity was used, and tree trunks and leaves were added to create a stimulus that realistically expresses the nature image.

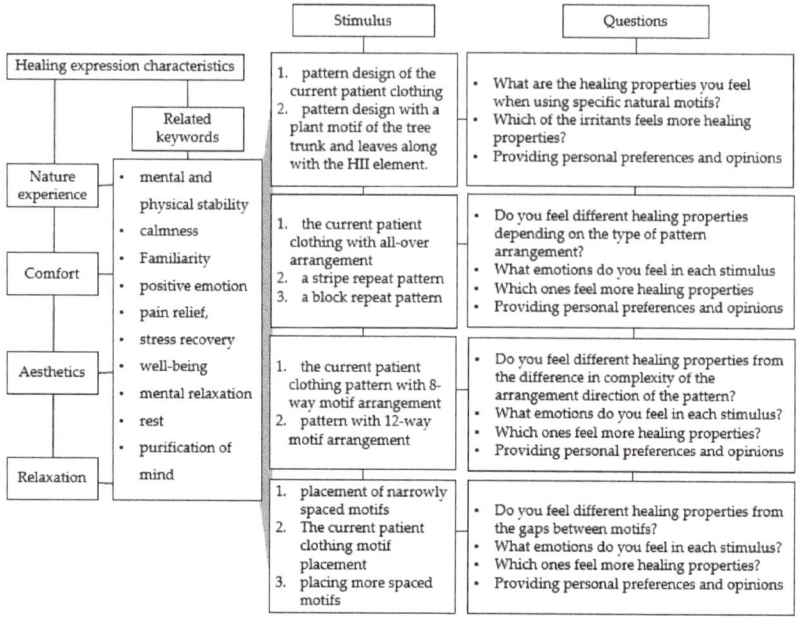

**Figure 5.** The question-extraction process for the patient's emotional response to pattern design using HI.

Regarding the second research direction, comfort, studies have shown that a familiar and comfortable design improves emotional stability [23]. While the all-over arrangement of patterned motifs is related to comfort, directional arrangements in which the motifs are repeatedly arranged along the length of the garment or in parallel have significant and influential psychological effects [15]. Additional stimuli were created with a striped repeat pattern and a block repeat pattern for comparison with the current patient clothing.

The third design direction is aesthetics. Designs that aesthetically apply humor or vitality can improve healing by creating positive emotions in the patient [36]. In pattern design, the angle at which a motif is placed can affect the patient's psychological vitality. We added the stimulus of the all-over pattern placed at 12 angles to compare its effect with those of the current patient clothing in the pattern placed at 8 angles.

The fourth design direction is relaxation. The white space in a design stimulates patients' sense of leisure, helping to calm the mind. Designs with wide margins around the motif can lead to a positive evaluation and image improvement [38]. To compare the differences between narrowly spaced pattern motifs and wider spaced motifs, we added three images with different margins, as stimuli.

## 4. Result

A total of 12 adults participated in the interviews, among whom 10 were working age, and two were aged 65 years or above. The male to female ratio was 2:10. Interviewees were assigned alphabets as initials to ensure anonymity.

### 4.1. Experiences and Opinions in the Medical Environment

A number of prior studies have emphasized the healing environment by mentioning patients' hopes for healing when hospitalized and their anxiety about an unfamiliar environment. In this study, most patients felt relief, expectation, and hope for healing as soon as they were hospitalized, and at the same time, there was fear or discomfort in the unfamiliar environment of the hospital. Most interview participants mentioned their hopes for healing and positive feelings.

"I'm relieved that the medical staff is taking care of me closely, but I'm nervous about the treatment. The treatment process could be painful, and it was unfamiliar because it wasn't home. But seeing the tidy room made me feel stable ... " (Interview Participant D)

Interview participants seemed to be trying to accept their anxiety about their disease and unfamiliar and uncomfortable feelings about the new environment with trust in the treatment staff, and they felt a sense of stability in a ward arranged as a healing environment.

In response to the question about their emotions when they first put on the patient clothing, most of the participants answered that they felt comfortable, clean, and comfortable to work. In contrast, one respondent answered that they were worried about the deprivation of their social status, while another worried about exposure when wearing patient clothes, but most of the interviewees mentioned the feeling of being cared for.

"The patient clothing was comfortable, clean, and pleasant, but it looked cheap." (Interview Participant A)

"When I wear patient clothing, I felt a little deprived of my self-esteem because my job doesn't appear anyway. But I felt more cared for." (Interview Participant K)

Most of the interview participants commented that the first feeling associated with wearing the patient clothing was that of being treated and that it was comfortable, and a clean and pleasant feeling was mentioned next. They were provided with fresh patient clothes on a regular basis and they could be replaced at any time in case of contamination.

Studies have identified that the problems with using conventional patient clothing are that it induces a feeling that their social status has reduced, anxiety about physical exposure, and negative emotions, such as shame, in patients. This was associated with negative feelings that privacy was not guaranteed. Most of the 12 interview participants were satisfied with the shape and structure of the patient clothing. However, there were a few interview participants who mentioned size-related discomfort, which was related to the length of the sleeves and pants.

"When wearing patient clothing, it's comfortable, but the ankles are exposed because the sleeves are short and the pants are short." (Interview Participant I)

In terms of shape, interview participants expressed satisfaction with the current clothing regarding their concerns about exposure and comfort, in particular for arm activity. This seems to have been improved by taking into account patient dissatisfaction through theoretical research.

In theoretical research, color is an important aspect of patient clothing because it can access the emotions, and certain colors influence common emotions. Most of the participants expressed the opinion that they felt clean and hygienic in clothing with a white background color. Some of the participants talked about the fact that any contamination was easily visible because of the white background, but this was different from the negative emotion provoked as a result of the contamination.

"Because the background color is white, contamination is easy to see. If there is still contamination, then you can replace it and wear clean clothes immediately." (Interview Participant C)

Most of the interview participants expressed positive opinions that the background color was white, and none of the participants mentioned that the clothes looked worn because of the color. As mentioned in previous studies, there were also opinions mentioning that white clothing looks cold. The blue and green colors used in the pattern motif are colors brought from the character mark representing the hospital's brand identity, and are reminiscent of natural images. During the interview, the most common opinions about these colors were about the clean and fresh feeling they were associated with.

"It's clean and fresh. That's why it seems to be the color used a lot in patient clothing." (Interview Participant I)

Interviewees K, J, and F mentioned emotions they felt in response to the colors.

"The colors of the pattern feel calm and gentle, and there are positive and hopeful feelings. It feels unfamiliar, but it also feels warm. The color saturation feels refined and luxurious." (Interview Participant K)

There were some participants who mentioned aesthetics as an expression of refinement and luxury as an expression of aesthetics.

"The color scheme is fresh." (Interview Participant J)

"I think the color scheme is tacky." (Interview Participant F)

Various opinions were expressed regarding the color scheme, but colors are most often encountered by the general public, and it seems that positive opinions were expressed regarding personal preferences and experiences. The color of the current patient clothing is the color of the natural images among the HI's character mark colors and aims to contribute to a healing effect.

*4.2. Opinions of the Healing Characteristics of the Hospital Identity Motif Design*

4.2.1. Nature Experience

In theoretical research, the pattern has an effect of reminiscent of images and has a psychological influence based on the images in the pattern. Images reminiscent of nature sustain or increase positive emotions, which has a healing effect. Stimulus A, using only the pattern extracted from HI, and Stimulus B, with the addition of tree trunks and leaves, were presented as realistically expressing a nature image (Table 2). Interview Participant F, who commented on the nature environment featured in the pattern, said that seeing the floral design made them feel alive. Interview Participant B said that he chose Stimulus A because he felt good when he saw both stimuli and the nature image.

**Table 2.** Nature experience healing characteristics: the patient clothing design stimulus.

| A | B |
|---|---|
| Current patient clothing: Magnolia character mark and signature used in HI | The magnolia character mark, signature and motifs in HI. Tree trunks and leaves symbolizing life form the pattern |

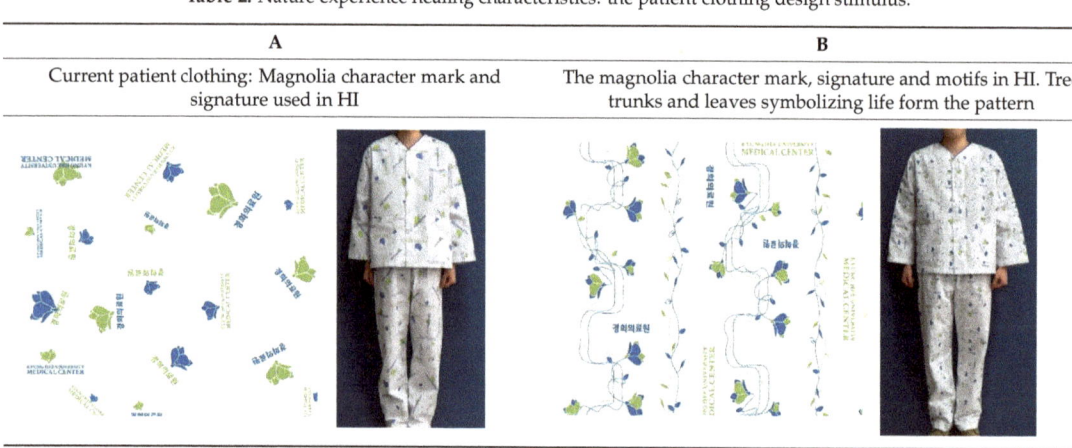

"I feel that Stimulus A is more stable. When I see the nature image in Stimulus B, it feels good, but it feels a bit distracting. It's nice to have a lively feeling, but I think that the patient clothing is stable." (Interview Participant B)

Interview participants preferred Stimulus A. Among the reasons for choosing Stimulus A, they stated that they felt familiarity, comfort, neatness, and stability when looking at the pattern.

"I think a neat and stable feeling makes me more comfortable." (Interview Participant K)

"Stimulus B has the shape of a tree trunk and leaves, so it looks lively, but it looks a little messy and distracts, so my eyes are tired." (Interview Participant F)

There were more reasons expressed by the interview participants to feel positive emotions and a familiar, stable, and comfortable feeling after seeing the nature image, and in some cases, the nature image gave them a lively and energetic feeling. The nature image motif was not affected by whether the form representing natural objects was realistic or metaphorical, but it positively influenced the interview participants.

Among the elements expressing HI, pattern design A using only the magnolia character and signature was better received than pattern design B, which added a natural object motif unrelated to HI. We presume that if used properly, this may influence the healing effect of the clothing. As described above, the nature experience design direction may have a healing effect by positively affecting patients' emotions. However, the introduction of excessive motifs hindered their emotional stability, and they perceived the image as cluttered. KHUMC's HI used magnolia graphics. Thus, if the HI has images of natural objects, then designing patient clothing using HI will yield successful results.

4.2.2. Comfort

In a theoretical study, a sense of being cared for comfortably and safely was positive for the patient [40]. Table 3 shows stimuli related to the arrangement of the pattern motifs. When interview participants talked about their preferences for the arrangement of the pattern motifs, the most important factor was comfort and stability. Most interview participants preferred the all-over arrangement, and none preferred the striped pattern often used in existing university hospitals.

**Table 3.** Comfort healing characteristics: patient clothing design stimulus.

| A | B | C |
|---|---|---|
| Current patient clothing: All-over arrangement | Stripe arrangement | Block repeat arrangement |

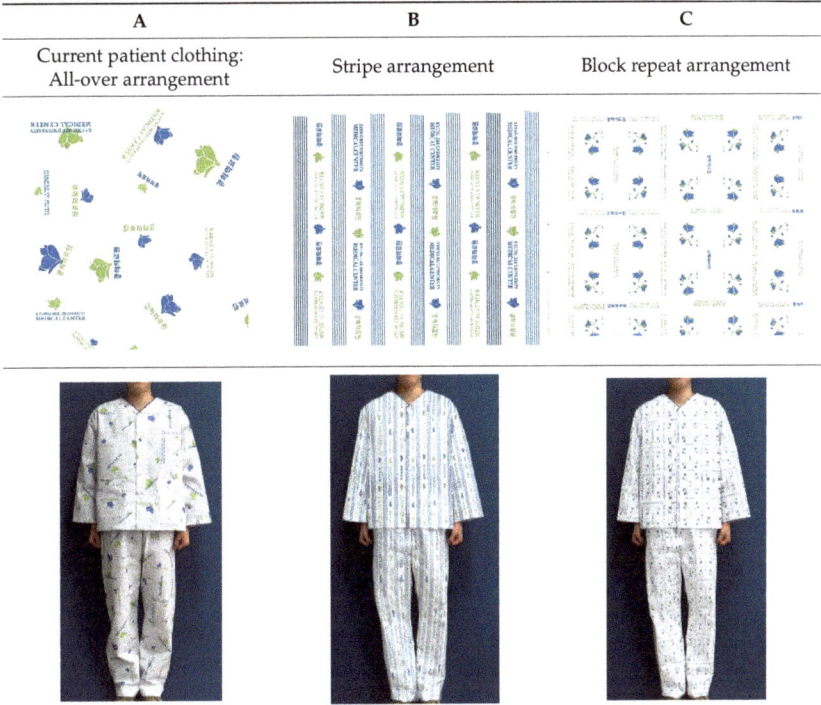

"I like the all-over arrangement. It looks good and gives a sense of stability and comfort." (Interview Participant C)

The participant who preferred the block repeat arrangement said that the reason for his preference was that it felt stable and comfortable because the floral pattern was more recognizable than the block repeat arrangement.

"I like the friendly floral pattern in a block repeat arrangement, so it looks comfortable." (Interview Participant E)

In addition, the interview participants wanted a comfortable feeling, but tried to feel liveliness or dynamism with comfort rather than a rigid or stagnant feeling. They said that they felt stable and comfortable when they saw the all-over arrangement.

"The grid pattern also looks comfortable, but I like the current patient clothes with the all-over arrangement because they don't feel stagnant. They feel lively." (Interview Participant L)

There was also a negative opinion of striped arrangement, because it gave a feeling of rigidity.

"The stripe pattern arrangement is like prison garb. The block repeat arrangement is distracting and it makes my eyes tired. The arrangement in all directions feels stable and my eyes are comfortable." (Interview Participant B)

"It's uncomfortable to arrange hard or complicated arrangements in patient clothing." (Interview Participant K)

Based on this, most interview participant felt stable and comfortable when wearing the all-over pattern arrangement, and the floral motif was related to this arrangement, so there was a preference for the block repeat arrangement.

In the case of motifs designed using HI expression elements, it is thought that healing properties can be exhibited by applying different pattern arrangement methods accordingly. In a previous study, as regards the arrangement method, the image of the rigid stripe and block arrangement was mentioned as a negative image [15]; however, some interview participants expressed the opinion that the flower motif was stable when used with the block arrangement. It is inferred that they felt this way because this arrangement induced in them a feeling of closeness with nature, and it was reflected as a healing characteristic.

4.2.3. Aesthetics

In previous studies, attractive patient clothing designs have been shown to give patients confidence. We investigated whether attractive and vibrant patterns are related to healing. Stimulus A is the all-over pattern placed at 8 angles, and Stimulus B is the all-over pattern placed at 12 angles Interview (Table 4). participants said that although they prefer moderate liveliness, motifs oriented in too many different directions feel more confusing than lively.

"B has too many tilt angles, so it looks uneasy. I like A because A has a stable angle." (Interview Participant H).

Interview Participant J said that the angles are so different that the pattern seemed rather complicated. Interview Participant K said that it while it was good to be all-over of a directional pattern, but too many varied angles make them feel dizzy.

Interview participants felt positive emotions with the direction of movement when there was some stability in the pattern direction, but distractions from too many angles produced negative emotions. Vibrancy can be used as a healing property that enhances patients' self-confidence, but if it is excessive, it can reduce patients' psychological stability. In this part of the analysis, it was also confirmed that the excessive use of elements in the pattern design of patients' clothing could hinder the healing effect. To suggest a more appropriate number of elements or a design method, a follow-up study that uses more different cases of stimulus needs to be conducted.

**Table 4.** Aesthetic healing characteristics: Patient clothing design stimulus.

| A | B |
|---|---|
| The current patient clothing pattern motif | More various angular directions than current patient clothing |

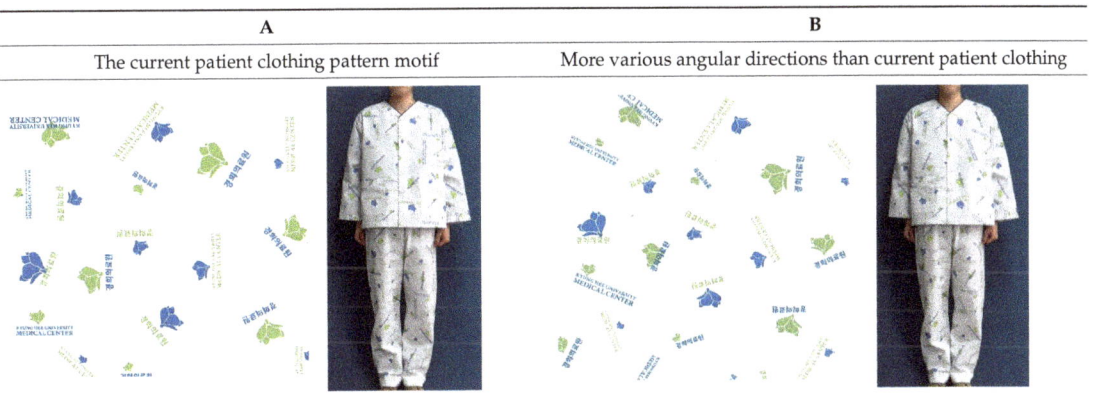

### 4.2.4. Relaxation

In previous studies, it was reported that blank space in an environment provides an opportunity for the user's emotions to intervene. In the design of clothes, it is possible to provide a relaxed feeling for patients by adjusting the spacing of patterns. Table 5 shows three images with different the spacing of patterns, as stimuli. The interview participants felt a sense of relaxation with the blank spaces in the clothing, and they felt frustrated and tense when the gap between the patterns was narrow. Half of the participants chose the Spacing B of the pattern motif they were currently wearing, and four participants chose Spacing C when the spacing of the pattern was wider. The reason they preferred the spacing of the motifs of the current patient clothing is comfort.

**Table 5.** Relaxation healing characteristics: patient clothing design stimulus.

| A | B | C |
|---|---|---|
| Narrow gap between pattern motifs | Current patient clothing pattern motifs | Wide space between pattern motifs |

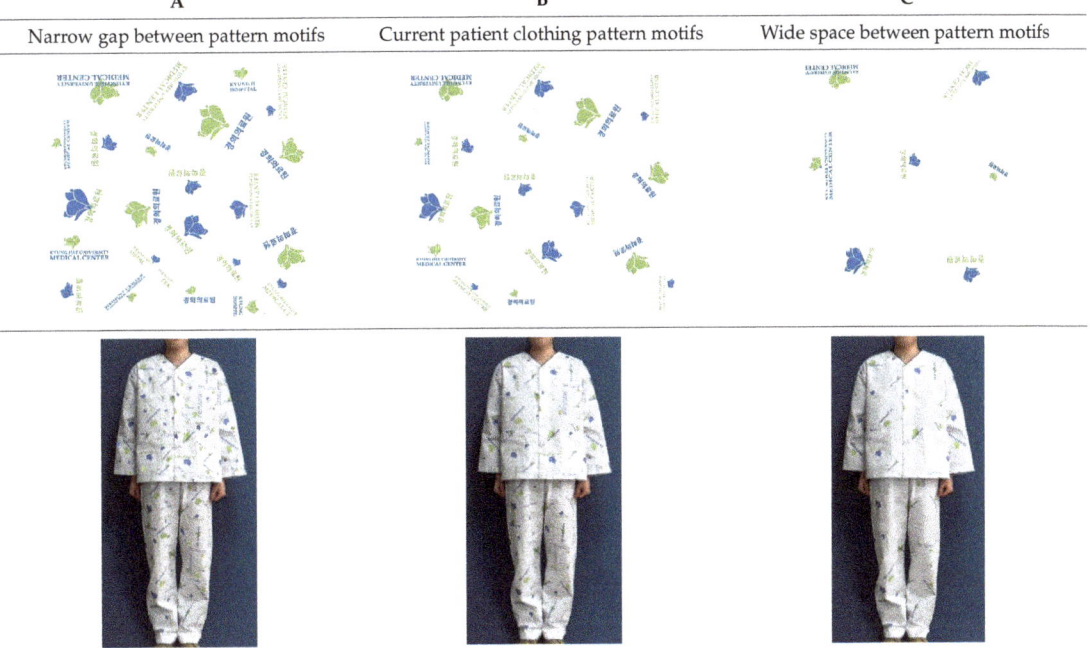

"If the spacing of the patterns is adequate, the viewer feels relieved. If it's narrow, it's frustrating." (Interview Participant K).

"It's stable because the pattern spacing is adequate. If it is too wide, it feels too relaxed, and if it is dense, it is complicated." (Interview Participant L).

If the gap between the patterns was narrow, interview participants felt frustration and a sense of complexity, and if the gap was too wide, they felt a feeling of looseness.

The preference for a pattern design with wide spacing between the motifs was common, and this may be related to previous studies indicating that the emotions felt in response to the blank spaces may be different for each individual. In previous studies, the space itself felt empty, and luxury was recognized in the blank spaces.

## 5. Discussion

This study attempted to identify methods of designing patient clothing that can contribute to patient treatment based on questions about the pattern design related to HI elements, the motif characteristics, arrangement, and spacing, and the direction between motifs. Through in-depth interviews, it was found that in patient clothing design, design adjustments such as the use of the motif characteristics, arrangement, and spacing, and the direction between motifs, influence the healing effect. This focuses on the characteristics of healing sensibility, such as nature experience, comfort, aesthetics, and relaxation. Interestingly, in the case of patient clothing design, the patient's emotional healing is an important factor, and appropriate adjustment of the size or quantity of the design motifs was required. First, the healing properties of nature experience can be employed by utilizing nature motifs such as flowers or leaves. We have confirmed that excessive use of many motifs with different characteristics hinders healing due to the complexity of the pattern. This finding is consistent with the theories that seeing nature induces positive emotions and reduces stress [9], but it contradicts the theory that predicts that the more immersed in environmental distraction that patients are, the greater is their pain reduction [41]. Second, the in-depth interviews revealed that the interview participants gained psychological stability through the all-over arrangement, which is consistent with the literature [15]. When using images of natural objects or HI expression elements, the all-round arrangement conveyed a sense of stability. The interview participants felt comfortable because the flower patterns in this arrangement gave them a sense of familiarity. This is connected with the fact that intimacy has an influence on comfortable emotions [33]. In addition, in the case of using a nature object image or using an HI expression element, the block repeat arrangement method can also provide stability via the nature property or arrangement. Third, a sense of stability is recognized when an appropriate number of angles are used in the design of the pattern direction. Various distracting angles create anxiety. The direction of the pattern expresses liveliness and can increase the confidence of patients by acting as a charming aspect of patient clothing design. Therefore, the direction of the pattern needs proper adjustment. This study showed that although visual distraction reduces both pain and anxiety stress [9], the degree of distraction requires appropriate adjustment and differs between the interview participants. Fourth, the middle-width spacing of the motifs was the most preferred among the three stimulus examples, followed by the widest space. Our results support the assertion that blank spaces allow for a sense of relaxation and are felt as luxuriousness or sophistication [42].

In a number of previous studies on patient clothing, shame due to exposure, poor clothing design, and reduced social status were mentioned as negative effects. These dissatisfaction factors were improved in the KHUMC patient clothing, but young patients were concerned about exposure as a result of white clothing. The use of white was requested by the medical provider to aid in hygiene management of patient clothing, but the fact that patient clothing should be user-centered needs to be considered when designing clothing in the future. Most of the participants felt positive about the patient clothing currently worn. This is thought to be because the design plan was made after referring to previous studies prior to the production of the patient clothing.

In this study, the perspectives of 12 people with experience in patient clothing were obtained through interview. This methodology may not be suitable for, or implemented in, other settings. However, we have shared an important finding, that designing patient clothing by analyzing their experiences can contribute to healing.

## 6. Conclusions

Most of earlier studies related to patient clothing have been conducted from the providers' point of view, so our understanding of users' requirements was insufficient. This study is meaningful in that it has gone through the process of confirming existing theory through in-depth interviews with patients using actual patient clothing. This study is significant in that it revealed that when designing patient clothing using HI elements, motif characteristics, arrangement, and spacing, and the direction between motifs, must be considered, since these positively affect patients' healing. In the future, we will apply the results of this study to patient clothing and develop and thoroughly review the designs in more case studies.

**Author Contributions:** Conceptualization, Y.Y.; investigation, S.K. All authors have read and agreed to the published version of the manuscript.

**Funding:** This research received no external funding.

**Institutional Review Board Statement:** Ethical review and approval were waived for this study because it was a sensory test conducted in compliance with safety standards without collecting and recording personally identifiable information for healthy people.

**Informed Consent Statement:** Informed consent was obtained from all subjects involved in the study.

**Data Availability Statement:** Data available in a publicly accessible repository.

**Conflicts of Interest:** The authors declare no conflict of interest.

## References

1. Marimon, F.; Gil-Doménech, D.; Bastida, R. Fulfilment of expectations mediating quality and satisfaction: The case of hospital service. *Total Qual. Manag. Bus. Excell.* **2019**, *30*, 201–220. [CrossRef]
2. Moliner, M.A. Loyalty, perceived value and relationship quality in healthcare services. *J. Serv. Manag.* **2009**, *20*, 76–97. [CrossRef]
3. Nekoei-Moghadam, M.; Amiresmaili, M. Hospital services quality assessment. *Int. J. Health Care Qual. Assur.* **2011**, *24*, 57–66. [CrossRef] [PubMed]
4. Jennings, S. What really matters to healthcare consumers. *J. Nurs. Admin.* **2005**, *35*, 173–180. [CrossRef]
5. Harris, P.B.; Ross, C.; McBride, G.; Curtis, L. A place to heal: Environmental sources of satisfaction among hospital patients. *J. Appl. Soc. Psychol.* **2002**, *32*, 1276. [CrossRef]
6. Vaskooi-Eshkevari, K.; Mirbazegh, F.; Soltani-Kermanshahi, M.; Sabzali-Poursarab-Saeedi, M.; Alipour, S. Customized patient clothing and patient satisfaction. *Int. J. Health Care Qual. Assur.* **2019**, *32*, 635–644. [CrossRef]
7. Topo, P.; Iltanen-Tähkävuori, S. Scripting patienthood with patient clothing. *Soc. Sci. Med.* **2010**, *70*, 1682–1689. [CrossRef]
8. Esposito, A. Hospital Branding in Italy: A Pilot Study Based on the Case Method. *Health Mark. Q.* **2017**, *34*, 35–47. [CrossRef]
9. Ulrich, R.S.; Zimring, C.; Zhu, X.; DuBose, J.; Seo, H.B.; Choi, Y.S.; Quan, X.; Joseph, A. A review of the research literature on evidence-based healthcare design. *HERD* **2008**, *1*, 61–125. [CrossRef]
10. Iltanen, S.; Topo, P. Ethical implications of design practices. The case of industrially manufactured patient clothing in Finland. In Proceedings of the Konstfack of the Conference, Stockholm, Sweden, 27–30 May 2007.
11. Rabin, J.M.; Farner, K.C.; Brody, A.H.; Peyser, A.; Kline, M. Compassionate coverage: A patient access linen system. *J. Patient Exp.* **2019**, *6*, 185–193. [CrossRef]
12. Karro, J.; Dent, A.W.; Farish, S. Patient perceptions of privacy infringements in an emergency department. *Emerg. Med. Australas.* **2005**, *17*, 117. [CrossRef]
13. Nayeri, N.D.; Aghajani, M. Patients' privacy and satisfaction in the emergency department: A descriptive analytical study. *Nurs. Ethics* **2010**, *17*, 167–177. [CrossRef] [PubMed]
14. Edvardsson, D. Balancing between being a person and being a patient—A qualitative study of wearing patient clothing. *Int. J. Nurs. Stud.* **2009**, *46*, 4–11. [CrossRef] [PubMed]
15. Davis, M. *Visual Design in Dress*, 2nd ed.; Prentice-Hall: Upper Saddle River, NJ, USA, 1987.
16. Kim, S.M.; Jeong, S.J. A Study of the Changes in Dress Wearers' Images in Relationto the Changes in the Size and Area Ratio of Polka Dots Relative to Coloration. *J. Korean Soc. Costume* **2008**, *58*, 54–68.

17. Jonas, W.B.; Chez, R.A.; Duffy, B.; Strand, D. Investigating the impact of optimal healing environments. *Altern. Ther. Health Med.* **2003**, *9*, 36–40.
18. Ulrich, R.S. View through a window may influence recovery from surgery. *Science* **1984**, *224*, 420–421. [CrossRef]
19. Stichler, J.F. Healing by design. *J. Nurs. Admin.* **2008**, *38*, 505–509. [CrossRef] [PubMed]
20. Leather, P.; Beale, D.; Santos, A.; Watts, J.; Lee, L. Outcomes of environmental appraisal of different hospital waiting areas. *Environ. Behav.* **2016**, *35*, 842–869. [CrossRef]
21. Timmermann, C.; Uhrenfeldt, L.; Birkelund, R. Cancer patients and positive sensory impressions in the hospital environment—A qualitative interview study. *Eur. J. Cancer Care* **2013**, *22*, 117–124. [CrossRef] [PubMed]
22. Schreuder, E.; Lebesque, L.; Bottenheft, C. Healing environments: What design factors really matter according to patients? An exploratory analysis. *HERD* **2016**, *10*, 87–105. [CrossRef]
23. Riisbøl, M.F.; Timmermann, C. User consultation and the design of healing architecture in a cardiology department—Ways to improve care for and well-being of patients and their relatives. *Nord. J. Arts Cult. Health* **2020**, *2*, 8–21. [CrossRef]
24. Wilson, E.O. Biophilia and the conservation ethic. In *Evolutionary Perspectives on Environmental Problems*; Routledge: Abingdon, UK, 2017; pp. 263–272.
25. Ulrich, R.S.; Gilpin, L. *Healing Arts. Putting Patients First*; Jossey Bass: San Francisco, CA, USA, 2003; pp. 117–146.
26. Kozarek, R.A.; Raltz, S.L.; Neal, L.; Wilbur, P.; Stewart, S.; Ragsdale, J. Prospective trial using virtual vision as distraction technique in patients undergoing gastric laboratory procedures. *Gastroenterol. Nurs.* **1997**, *20*, 12–14. [CrossRef] [PubMed]
27. Malenbaum, S.; Keefe, F.J.; de Williams, A.C.C.; Ulrich, R.; Somers, T.J. Pain in its environmental context: Implications for designing environments to enhance pain control. *Pain* **2008**, *134*, 241–244. [CrossRef] [PubMed]
28. Park, S.-H.; Mattson, R.H. Effects of flowering and foliage plants in hospital rooms on patients recovering from abdominal surgery. *HortTechnology* **2008**, *18*, 563–568. [CrossRef]
29. Totaforti, S. Applying the benefits of biophilic theory to hospital design. *City Territ. Arch.* **2018**, *5*, 1–9. [CrossRef]
30. Carroll, R.A. Applying design and color to healing. *Nurs. Homes* **2005**, *54*, 48–52.
31. Güneş, E.; Olguntürk, N. Color-emotion associations in interiors. *Color Res. Appl.* **2020**, *45*, 129–141. [CrossRef]
32. Elliot, A.J.; Maier, M.A. Color and psychological functioning. *Curr. Dir. Psychol. Sci.* **2016**, *16*, 250–254. [CrossRef]
33. Stevens, K.; Fröis, T.; Masal, S.; Winder, A.; Bechtold, T. Design and colour preferences for older individuals in residential care. *Res. J. Text. Appar.* **2016**, *20*, 87–101. [CrossRef]
34. Urlich, R.; Zimring, C.; Quan, X.; Joseph, A.; Choudhary, R. *The Role of the Physical Environment in the Hospital of the 21st Century: A Once-in-a-Lifetime Opportunity*; The Center for Health Design: Concord, CA, USA, 2004; pp. 1–69.
35. Steinke, C. Assessing the Physical Service Setting. *HERD* **2015**, *8*, 31–42. [CrossRef]
36. Ingrid, E.; Pavla, G.; Martina, M. Healing and therapeutic Landscape Design—Examples and experience of medical facilities. *ArchNet-IJAR* **2018**, *12*, 128.
37. Greenberg, J. Spirited sisters heal with fashion. *WWD* **2005**, *190*, 8.
38. Lau, S.S.Y.; Gou, Z.; Liu, Y. Healthy Campus by Open Space Design: Approaches and Guidelines. *Front. Archit. Res.* **2014**, *3*, 452–467. [CrossRef]
39. Douglas, O.G.; Pracejus, J.W.; O'Guinn, T.C. Print Advertising: White Space. *J. Bus. Res.* **2012**, *65*, 855–860.
40. Campbell, D.E. Interior Office Design and Visitor Response. *J. Appl. Psychol.* **1979**, *64*, 648. [CrossRef]
41. McCaul, K.D.; Malott, J.M. Distraction and Coping with Pain. *Psychol. Bull.* **1984**, *95*, 516–533. [CrossRef] [PubMed]
42. Sharma, N.; Varki, S. Active White Space (AWS) in Logo Designs: Effects on Logo Evaluations and Brand Communication. *J. Advert.* **2018**, *47*, 270–281. [CrossRef]

*Article*

# Problems and Implications of Shelter Planning Focusing on Habitability: A Case Study of a Temporary Disaster Shelter after the Pohang Earthquake in South Korea

**Mikyung Kim [1], Kyeonghee Kim [1] and Eunjeong Kim [2],***

[1] Department of Housing and Interior Design, Chungbuk National University, 1 Chungdaero, Cheongju, Chungbuk 28644, Korea; mkmkkim@chungbuk.ac.kr (M.K.); rlarudgml721@naver.com (K.K.)
[2] Dodam Design and Research, #101-904, Hangangdaero 211, Yongsan-gu, Seoul 14322, Korea
* Correspondence: dodam.design.research@gmail.com

**Abstract:** Habitability is an essential concept for shelter planning in terms of supporting victims' right to life with dignity and recovering from what they suffered. The study aimed to identify problems and needs in shelter spaces and suggest measures to improve shelter space plans by conducting a case study in South Korea. The temporary disaster shelter in Pohang built right after the earthquake (2018) was selected as a case subject. From the literature review, a framework consisting of four concepts of habitability (safety, health, sociality, comfort) and four shelter zones (entry, residential, service, special needs zone) was developed for the in-depth interviews and analysis. The field study and in-depth interviews with victims, staff, and volunteers were conducted to collect problems and needs regarding shelter space planning. The results showed that the entry zone needed improvements in 'protection', 'prevention', 'sanitation', 'accessibility', 'area', and 'privacy'. The residential zone lacked 'area', 'privacy', and 'indoor environmental quality'. The service zone problems were mainly seen in the categories of 'area' and 'privacy'. The special needs zone was less habitable in the categories of 'protection' and 'area'. To appropriately respond to victims' urgent needs, the temporary shelter planning should secure enough space beyond the legal minimum standards, provide sanitation and indoor environmental quality management, and separate spaces by function and user type.

**Keywords:** temporary disaster shelter; habitability; shelter planning

## 1. Introduction

A 5.4 magnitude earthquake struck Pohang, South Korea in November 2017, which led to large-scale destruction with nearly 1300 people left homeless in the wake of the disaster. The evacuation was prolonged and people were housed in a temporary disaster shelter prepared hastily in a gymnasium. Due to the frequent aftershocks, residents had to stay in the temporary shelter for over two years, suffering in unhealthy conditions both in the cold winter and the extreme heat of the summer. This led to physical illness and severe psychological anxiety. Tents were provided for survivors to protect their privacy, but this led to various problems such as the tents being too narrow for people to live in and they did not block external noise.

A temporary shelter should be safe from external potential physical risk factors and provide stability for those living there to regain their physical health and mental security [1–3]. Prior studies emphasized that the concept of habitability should be applied to temporary disaster shelters [4–6]. Habitability means suitability as a residence, and suitability implies the provision of a shelter, heating system, sanitary condition to prevent infection, indoor quality (noise, smoke, drugs, etc.), and the drinking water supply. It also includes the broader aspects such as a close association with local communities, people's will to recover, and consideration of various needs based on individuals' physical and emotional states [6]. Therefore, as an essential concept for building and managing a shelter to accommodate those who survived a disaster, habitability should not be seen as a minimum standard for survival but be viewed as a building a soft environment that can be respected and dignified as a human. In this aspect, to better support the concept of habitability, temporary shelter for disaster survivors should provide a physically and psychologically stable living environment that considers health, safety, hygiene, and a prolonged recovery stage in various disaster situations.

The Ministry of the Interior and Safety in South Korea issued formal guidelines [7] for supporting survivors in temporary disaster shelters during the early stage (within 24 h), emergency stage (3–5 days), and recovery stage (more than 5 days), depending on the period. In the early stage, the guidelines include indoor and external facility inspections, guidance on initiating shelter operations, and preparing plans for prolonged evacuation. The emergency stage involves the preparation of (a) registration forms for disaster survivors and (b) spatial zoning and arrangement according to function and needs within the shelter environment. In the recovery stage, for better response to prolonged evacuation, the required spaces and facilities are checked and service types and qualities expanded.

Recently, temporary shelters have seen many improvements in their operation and management. However, specific details regarding shelter planning for a stable living environment considering the physical and psychological health of disaster survivors have not been fully examined and reflected in the guidelines issued in South Korea.

A temporary shelter houses people for the short term after a disaster. To provide survivors better service and a decent quality of life, it is important to build a physically and psychologically stable living environment. For this, one needs to view the situation on-site and understand survivors' direct and indirect needs. Against this background, this study aims to identify problems and actual needs for each space within the shelter and suggest potential measures to improve the shelter space plan for habitability. For the field research, data were collected from the H indoor gymnasium in Pohang, where the largest number of survivors were temporarily housed after the 2017 earthquake.

## 2. Literature Review

### 2.1. Habitability in Temporary Disaster Shelters

Habitability is an essential concept for establishing and managing temporary shelters. It ensures they can live safely over the long term. It is a humanitarian response toward creating an environment that considers the quality of life, health, welfare, and recovery from the crisis [3,8]. People can live a healthy life and prepare for a future disaster only by securing a safe and appropriate living space [8]. To this end, reflecting on survivors' opinions regarding a safe environment, comfort, adaptability, sanitation, community connections, privacy, and functionality could help build an environment that increases a person's will to recover [3,4,9–11].

The concept of temporary shelters' habitability can be confirmed through prior studies. Um et al. [12] suggested protection, privacy, safety, psychological stability, health services in the form of medical support, and hygiene and pollution management as crucial factors affecting habitability. The American Red Cross [13] mentions safety, cleanliness/hygiene, consideration toward vulnerable people, diversity, and privacy, while Bashawri et al. [5] explains it through environmental aspects (external environment response, safety, hygiene) and sociocultural aspects (cultural differences, security, and communication). Sphere [8] suggests each family affected by the disaster needs to be provided with adequate space for basic living, and that local culture and lifestyle should be considered to accommodate the diverse needs of family members for sleeping, food preparation, and meals. The Sphere handbook also explains that physical security, privacy, protection from the weather, optimal lighting conditions, ventilation, heat, and comfort should be addressed to achieve adequacy for an affordable, habitable, culturally acceptable, and accessible and usable shelter environment. Moreover, the residential areas should be safe for cooking, toileting, laundering, bathing, living, socializing, and recreation, ensuring victims' privacy.

Choi, Kim, and Kim [6] developed a shelter planning guide for temporary shelters in South Korea. The authors classified the concept of habitability into four aspects to build a research framework, and based on the analytic framework, 46 shelter planning guidelines were developed after conducting literature reviews and interviews. They suggested a framework consisting of 4 main categories (safety, health, sociality, and comfort) and 10 sub-categories (protection, prevention, sanitation, medical support, vulnerable people, accessibility, community, area, privacy, and indoor quality) to conduct interviews and develop guidelines. In this study, we adopted the framework as a part of an analysis method and explanation of the concept of habitability as shown in Table 1. The category of main and sub-concepts was borrowed, but the slight explanations were added or modified in the description part. The adopted framework (category of habitability) was combined with the shelter zones which were classified by the authors, and the analysis matrix with the x and y-axis was introduced in the analysis section.

Table 1. Critical concepts of habitability in temporary shelters for disaster survivors.

| Main Concept | Sub-Concept | Mark | Description |
|---|---|---|---|
| Safety | Protection | Sa1 | - Protection from additional disasters<br>- Protection from bad weather conditions and potential danger<br>- Provision of a storage system for personal items |
| | Prevention | Sa2 | - (Emergency) lighting system for movement<br>- Firefighting equipment considering the emergency type<br>- Evacuation routes and exits for additional disasters<br>- Installation of information boards on the evacuation route |
| Health | Sanitation | He1 | - Drinking water facilities<br>- Garbage disposal space and living area<br>- Sanitary facilities such as toilets and showers<br>- (Portable) sanitary facility considering the disabled and sex<br>- Hand washing table for hygiene management<br>- Laundry and drying space |
| | Medical support | He2 | - Medical support space<br>- Psychological counseling space |
| Sociality | Vulnerable people | So1 | - Privacy for breastfeeding and childcare space<br>- Privacy for the children's space<br>- Convenient movement<br>- Simplified lifts and small ramps for wheelchairs and strollers<br>- Information signs considering foreigners and the hearing impaired<br>- Accessible toilets and living areas for the vulnerable<br>- Evacuation space for companion animals |
| | Accessibility | So2 | - Distance and travel time from the disaster area<br>- Parking and drop-off areas for survivors and managers<br>- Access to community facilities from the temporary shelter<br>- Move flow for wheelchair users<br>- Signs for temporary shelter locations and routes |
| | Community | So3 | - Community space for watching TV, exchanging information, and eating<br>- Communication devices such as bulletin boards and broadcasting facilities that deliver relief information |

Table 1. *Cont.*

| Main Concept | Sub-Concept | Mark | Description |
|---|---|---|---|
| Comfort | Area | Co1 | - (Minimum) area for each person considering relief supplies and disability<br>- (3.3 m² per person by the law)<br>- Community space<br>- Staff managers area<br>- Installation of portable sanitation facilities and relief tents |
| | Privacy | Co2 | - Space for individual or family unit<br>- Configurable dividers and tents<br>- Separate changing room for men/women |
| | Indoor quality | Co3 | - Proper cooling and heating system<br>- Ventilation to maintain good air quality<br>- Secure daylights<br>- Proper humidity management |

Table 1 introduces the critical concepts of habitability which play important roles to build a suitable shelter as a residence. The concept of "safety" involves protection from potentially dangerous situations such as additional disasters, bad weather conditions, and trespassers, etc., and the provision of secure storage areas. "Health" includes hygiene and medical assistance facilities and services for survivors' physical and psychological health. "Sociality" refers to the connectivity of the temporary shelter to neighborhood facilities, the absence of pedestrian obstacles, and its location and accessibility. "Comfort" refers to personal space for privacy, minimum living area, natural/artificial lighting, heating, ventilation, and other indoor environmental factors related to survivors' living space.

*2.2. Zoning for Temporary Disaster Shelters Focusing on Habitability*

A temporary disaster shelter requires various functional space types, such as a residential space for daily living, a public area for medical treatment and administrative services, meals, and communication, and a dedicated employee space to accommodate diverse users.

Regarding shelter zoning, The Department of Justice (DOJ) [14] included entrance spaces (boarding/unloading, parking lots, sidewalks, entrances, corridors), living spaces (sleeping areas, toilets, showers, public telephones, drinking fountains, dining areas), and others (personal/family toilets, medical care room, temporary toilets). FEMA [15] classified shelter spaces like a parking lot, space for pick-up and drop-off, waiting, registration, residence, children and family, pet, snack bar, dining, medical care, resting, staff, management, and warehouse based on accessibility and functional support. The US Centers for Disease Control and Prevention (CDC) [16] proposed a separate isolation area in case of an outbreak of infectious disease by emphasizing the maintenance of a sanitary environment for sustainable living in the temporary shelter. Of particular importance is ensuring hygiene in public areas such as entrances, dining spaces, medical care spaces, pet areas, and children's playrooms to prevent the spread of infection [17,18].

Based on the functional spaces mentioned above, the spaces in a temporary shelter can be divided into four categories: entry zone, residential zone, service zone, and special needs zone. The entry zone includes parking spaces, entrances, registration/waiting spaces, and it should be accessible by emergency vehicles and survivors' vehicles. People who are unable to walk or have disabilities should be able to easily access these spaces. Besides, since the entry zone is marked by the constant movement of people in and out, thorough hygiene management should be planned in this zone. A hand washstand or hand disinfection system should be installed near the entrance, and a separate independent waiting area for people with infectious diseases should be provided. Along with the hygiene issue, plans must be made for protecting survivors' safety and privacy. For this, an access security checkpoint should be provided right in front of the entrance to screen outsiders or reporters.

The residential zone includes the living space, toilet, shower room, laundry area, dining and meal-preparation area, and rest area. The appropriate area per person should be secured considering the composition of the various personnel, the number of survivors staying in the shelter, types of family/individuals, gender, and special needs for vulnerable people. The space layout for the residential zone should be planned to minimize noise from the outside, passages, or public areas such as lounge, dining room, playrooms, etc. Physical obstacles should be removed from passages to provide people a barrier-free environment. Besides, it is important to provide a pleasant and hygienic living environment by maintaining a proper temperature, humidity, and lighting. Hand washstands or hand sanitizers should be placed at regular intervals.

The service zone covers the management space of employees and medical/isolation spaces. An adequate area for employees and managers should be secured for both work and rest. Separate entrances and paths for staff should also be considered. Medical care and isolation spaces, accessibility, hygiene, and privacy should be considered.

The special needs zone includes rooms for children, women (pregnant/nursing mothers), and pets. For convenience, rooms for children and pregnant/nursing women should be adjacent to the toilet and hand washstand. These spaces should also ensure all practices involving safety, hygiene, and privacy by removing barriers, managing hygienic cleaning systems, and providing partitions. The space for pets should be planned in isolated or separate spaces away from the residential zone considering the dimensions, distance, drainage facilities, and the species and size of the pets.

Table 2 shows the classified hierarchy of temporary shelter zones by their functions. The shelter zones are divided into four different areas, and each zone has a public or private character depending on the function it performs involving various stakeholders such as victims, managers, and volunteers.

Table 2. Classification of temporary shelter zones.

| Main Zone | Sub-Area |
| --- | --- |
| Entry zone | Parking area/entrance/registration area |
| Residential zone | Living (sleeping) area/sanitary area/laundry and dry area/meal and prep area/rest area (lounge) |
| Service zone | Staff area/medical (isolation) area |
| Special needs zone | Childcare area/nursing area/pet area |

### 2.3. Research Method

The research questions for this study are: (1) How is a temporary shelter space in South Korea organized for vulnerable people right after a disaster occurs?; (2) What are the main problems identified for each zone in the temporary shelter regarding habitability?; (3) What can be improved to better support the shelter space planning?

For this study, qualitative research methods were applied. We selected a temporary shelter located in Pohang for the study and visited the place to conduct in-depth interviews with people who lived through the disaster. The interviews were conducted twice: (1) the first interview focused on the identification of people's overall needs, and the shelter's physical environment and atmosphere; (2) the second interview collected more voices from the field, specifically from vulnerable people. The interviews were based on the semi-structured questionnaire which was developed from the literature review.

This study examines a temporary shelter, an indoor gymnasium, in Pohang (South Korea) in the aftermath of the earthquake that occurred in 2017. The shelter accommodated 430 survivors at that time. In-depth interviews were conducted with survivors, volunteers, and staff who stayed and worked in the shelter. We also examined the original floor plan of the gymnasium to identify how the gym's indoor space was organized as a shelter and how survivors responded to the indoor environment.

Data were mainly collected from the interviews due to the strict access restrictions at the shelter. The first interview was conducted on 27 January 2018, and the second interview was conducted on 27 March after the 4.6 magnitude aftershock on 11 February. Access to the inside of the shelter was strictly regulated for visitors, and accordingly, articles and broadcast materials were collected to analyze the inner space plans and environment.

In-depth interviews were conducted in the (a) first interview with 20 survivors, four volunteers, and two managing staff who stayed in the shelter for more than a month and (b) a second interview with 12 survivors, one volunteer, and one staff manager who had spent more than three months in the shelter. A total of 40 people participated in the in-depth interviews. The interviewees were discreetly approached by researchers and selected based on the period of shelter stay, user type (survivors/volunteers/staff), and their willingness to participate in the study. The interviewees were asked to informally describe their experience in the shelter based on the questionnaire's framework, and the problematic issues regarding the environment's space were discussed in-depth. Each interview was recorded with the permission of the interviewee, and after the interview, the data were transcribed and analyzed by finding concepts in meaningful words or phrases related to the research subject.

The questionnaire for the interview consisted of 30 questions (entry zone (9), residential zone (12), service zone (3), the special needs zone (6)) as shown in Table 3. The researchers asked people questions based on the questionnaire but allowed people to talk freely instead of following the format of the questionnaire. The questions did not proceed in order but varied according to the situation so that the flow of the interview was not disturbed.

Table 3. Semi-structured questionnaire framework.

| Main Zone | Sub-Area | Question |
|---|---|---|
| Entry zone | Parking area | (1) Are parking areas planned and identifiable?<br>(2) Is it easy to access the shelter building from the parking space?<br>(3) Is there a parking space for emergency vehicles and cars for vulnerable people to get on and off near the main entrance? |
| | Entrance | (1) Are protruding obstacles removed and the area sufficiently secured?<br>(2) Can the door be opened easily from the inside?<br>(3) Is the entrance planned to be easily identifiable?<br>(4) Is it wheelchair accessible? |
| | Registration area | (1) Is it located near the entrance?<br>(2) Is there enough space reserved for privacy protection? |
| Residential zone | Living (sleeping) area | (1) Were various personnel compositions considered?<br>(2) Has the minimum area per person been secured?<br>(3) Are temperature and lighting properly adjustable?<br>(4) Is natural light secured?<br>(5) Is a storage space for personal items provided? |
| | Sanitary area | (1) Are toilets and showers sufficiently secured in consideration of the number of people, sex, and vulnerable people?<br>(2) Regarding privacy, the toilets and showers are separated by sex, and shower curtains are installed? |
| | Laundry and dry area | (1) Are there separate laundry and drying spaces? |
| | Meal and prep area | (1) Is it located in a separate place from the living space?<br>(2) Is a hygienic environment secured?<br>(3) Are there preparation spaces for meal supply and distribution? |
| | Rest area (lounge) | (1) Is it located in a place with low noise? |

Table 3. Cont.

| Main Zone | Sub-Area | Question |
|---|---|---|
| Service zone | Staff area | (1) Are entrances and movement flows secured separately for managers and volunteers? |
| | Medical area | (1) Is it separated from the living space for privacy protection?<br>(2) Has the minimum area per person been secured? |
| Special needs zone | Childcare area | (1) Can children access the space?<br>(2) Are separate spaces provided for children to play safely? |
| | Nursing area | (1) Are toilets separated by sex?<br>(2) Are changing rooms, nursing spaces, and childcare spaces provided? |
| | Pet area | (1) Have other people staying in the shelter been considered?<br>(2) Has the area, isolation distance, and drainage facilities been secured in consideration of the type and size of companion animals? |

## 3. Results

### 3.1. Floor Plan and Physical Environment of the Shelter

#### 3.1.1. Entry Zone

The parking area was used as a space for providing snacks, meal booths, laundry vehicles, etc. There was insufficient parking space for disaster survivors as staff vehicles and ambulance vehicles occupied the area. The main entrance was the only passage open for disaster survivors after the first earthquake, but with the aftershock that occurred, the emergency exit was opened in case of an emergency evacuation. The registration/waiting space was located between the main entrance and the lobby; it also functioned as the management space and as a mobile phone charging station.

#### 3.1.2. Residential Zone

In the living (sleeping) area on the 1st and 2nd floors, tents were set up for each person or a family. Sanitary space for toilets, showers, and changing rooms was planned on the first floor. Survivors could also use the facilities in the nearby town office and a bath ticket to use the public bath nearby. This showed that hygiene management was considered important in the planning and management system with diverse options for people. The laundry/drying space was not planned, but laundry vehicles provided laundry and drying services. Dining/meal-preparation space comprised meal vehicles and dining booths were planned in the parking space, but as the shelter stay continued, four dining spaces were later reduced to one. The dining area was used as a lounge for information communication and watching television except during mealtimes. There was no separate resting space planned inside the temporary shelter, and accordingly, the space between tents in the living area was used as an informal lounge.

#### 3.1.3. Service Zone

The management space was planned in the entrance lobby at the main entrance and was furnished with tables and chairs for registration and access confirmation. A separate resting area was not provided for staff and volunteers. The volunteers spent most of their time in booths located in parking spaces. Medical services were located in the pulpit area in the hall, which was divided into a treatment space and waiting area using partitions for privacy.

#### 3.1.4. Special Needs Zone

There was a separate designated space for children inside the shelter for their medical treatment and for psychological counseling for those who had been affected by the trauma of the earthquake. No separate room was allocated for infants and toddlers, or pregnant or nursing mothers; thus, inconveniencing them. There was also no planned pet area.

## 3.2. Problems Pertaining to Habitability

### 3.2.1. Entry Zone

From the interviews and field study, it was identified that the parking lot was planned mainly for service spaces such as dining booths and parking laundry vehicles. There was no secure parking space for survivors and, therefore, poor access to the shelter. Furthermore, garbage was treated in the parking lot, causing an odor and public sanitation problem. The emergency exit was open only after the aftershock, but survivors were not aware of its location, thus causing bottlenecks at the main entrance initially. The door handles were easily contaminated by multiple users, resulting in problems such as safety and sanitation. The doubling up of the registration/waiting space as a management space and as a mobile phone charging station resulted in privacy issues such as leaking personal information due to insufficient space (Table 4).

**Table 4.** Problems identified in the entry zone.

| Category | Mark | Main Problems |
|---|---|---|
| Parking area (En1) | e-1 | Lack of parking space for survivors because of snack bars, dining booths, and laundry vehicles in the parking space |
| | | Keywords: lack of parking space for survivors |
| | e-2 | Garbage disposal in the parking lot increasing congestion, causing an odor, and thus, an unsanitary environment |
| | | Keywords: garbage disposal and odor, congestion |
| | e-3 | No separate sidewalk provided in the parking space exposing the survivors to a potential accident |
| | | Keywords: no separate sidewalk, potential car accident |
| Entrance (En2) | e-4 | A bottleneck at the main entrance during the evacuation after the aftershock; no signage provided for accessing the emergency exit |
| | | Keywords: bottleneck at the main entrance, no signage for accessing emergency exit |
| | e-5 | Contamination of entrance door handles and surfaces due to the frequent use resulting in an unsanitary environment |
| | | Keywords: door contamination |
| | e-6 | Narrow entrance causing congestion when many people use it at the same time |
| | | Keywords: narrow entrance width, congestion |
| Registration area (En3) | e-7 | Shared space arrangement with management space and a cell phone charging station in the crowded entrance lobby; no protection of privacy during the registration process in this open space |
| | | Keywords: space sharing, privacy |

This led us to understand that parking spaces must be planned to secure accessibility for survivors. The parking lot shared space with relief services. However, if not for everyone, it was necessary to provide parking spaces for older adults, the disabled, and families with children. A separate garbage disposal space plan was required to maintain cleanliness and hygiene. If the main entrance is the only access point, an emergency exit should be considered as a sub-entrance because of safety and hygiene. A hand washstand or hand sanitizing system should be provided at the entrance.

*"After dismantling the service booth, parking for disaster survivors was allowed in the parking space near the entrance. Before that, parking around the shelter was not allowed for survivors, and even older adults had to walk up outside the shelter, which made it difficult for them."* (survivor, 60s, woman).

*"Since many people use the same entrance door every day, it becomes dirty and sticky. So, sometimes I wipe it with a wet tissue to clean the handles and door surface."* (survivor, 70s, woman).

*"Even when there was an emergency exit open to the public after the aftershocks, people still flocked to the main entrance door making it more dangerous."* (survivor, 40s, man).

### 3.2.2. Residential Zone

In the living space, the survivors were provided a tent for two persons, and storing personal items securely in the tent became difficult; size options were not considered for a family unit (more than three persons). Family members had to live apart during the shelter stay and store personal items in public lockers located far away from the residential zone. Some survivors continued to go back to their damaged houses to bring personal necessities left in the house. These experiences brought up issues of privacy and protection. Besides, the passage between tents was narrow, making it difficult for people to pass through. People did not sleep well at night due to the noises, and these experiences were related to the sustainable aspects of accessibility and indoor quality.

Those who lived on the 2nd floor had poor accessibility to the toilets and the mobile phone charging stations that were on the 1st floor. Older adults were reluctant to go toward toilets or shower rooms if the spaces were far from their living area. The careless arrangement of sanitary spaces without considering sex, such as having a male toilet next to women's shower rooms or a women's toilet next to male shower rooms made people uncomfortable whenever they used these spaces. These revealed the need for the rearrangement of spaces for accessibility (Table 5).

**Table 5.** Problems identified in the residential zone (1).

| Category | Mark | Main Problems |
|---|---|---|
| Living/Sleeping area (Re1) | r-1 | Lack of storage space for personal items; storage space far from the tents exposes theft risk |
| | | Keywords: lack of storage for personal items, potential theft risk |
| | r-2 | Narrow space between tents made people uncomfortable |
| | | Keywords: a narrow passage |
| | r-3 | Potential exposure to a secondary disaster when survivors periodically return to damaged houses to bring stuff owing to lack of storage space for necessities (clothes, toiletries, etc.) |
| | | Keywords: secondary disaster exposure, lack of storage for personal items |
| | r-4 | Uniform tent size with no consideration for family size, personal characteristics (sex, height, etc.), and number of personal items |
| | | Keywords: same-sized tent with no flexibility |
| | r-5 | Sleep disturbance caused by excessive noise (walking, coughing, etc.) heard across narrow gaps between tents |
| | | Keywords: narrow gaps between tents, excessive noise |
| | r-6 | Bedding becoming wet or moldy due to condensation on the floor of the tent |
| | | Keywords: wet/moldy bedding, condensation on the tent floor |
| | r-7 | Open structure in the center causing dust generated on the 1st floor to rise and affect people's health staying on the 2nd floor; stinging sensation in the eyes and neck |
| | | Keywords: ventilation and dust care, open space |
| | r-8 | Survivors staying on the 2nd floor have poor accessibility to mobile phone charging stations and laundry vehicles on the 1st floor and have to use stairs |
| | | Keywords: stair use for facility access |
| | r-9 | Tent arrangement with no consideration for sex and family units, resulting in privacy issues |
| | | Keywords: no optional tent sizes and structures, privacy |
| | r-10 | Low humidity due to excessive heating during winter causing health problems such as colds and rhinitis |
| | | Keywords: excessive heating, low humidity, health issues |
| | r-11 | Residential space on the second floor adjacent to a window leading to exposure to cold weather |
| | | Keywords: living area at the window side, exposure to cold weather |

There was no drying space planned for laundry. Personal laundry when dried outside the tent was exposed to others, and when dried inside, increased the humidity causing an odor. Women especially had difficulty finding proper drying space for their underwear. This situation was highly related to aspects of privacy and sanitation.

Since the dining/meal-preparation space was in the parking lot outside the shelter, people had poor access, especially when it rained or snowed, and they became exposed to the cold. The rest area had privacy problems, such as noises and conversations overheard through the empty spaces between tents, which were used as a temporary lounge. From this, it was understood that in the living space, tents of various sizes and types should be provided for storing personal items and protecting family units. A storage plan such as prefabricated storage furniture is needed to safely store personal items (Table 6).

**Table 6.** Habitability problems identified in the residential zone (2).

| Category | Mark | Main Problems |
|---|---|---|
| Sanitary area (Re2) | r-12 | Sanitary space arrangement without considering sex and privacy |
| | | Keywords: space arrangement without considering sex, privacy |
| | r-13 | Discomfort among older adults as the toilets were far from their living space |
| | | Keywords: long distance and poor access to toilets, older adults |
| | r-14 | Privacy infringement due to absence of shower compartments |
| | | Keywords: no shower compartment provided, privacy |
| | r-15 | Insufficient hot water supply considering the number of survivors, causing people to use external facilities |
| | | Keywords: insufficient hot water supply |
| Laundry/Drying area (Re3) | r-16 | Lack of drying space, personal laundry exposed to others if dried outside the tent |
| | | Keywords: no laundry drying space, privacy |
| | r-17 | Drying personal laundry inside the tent causes high humidity, odor, respiratory infections, etc. |
| | | Keywords: underwear drying inside a tent, poor indoor quality |
| | r-18 | Personal laundry, such as underwear, is washed in a public washstand, causing exposure to an unsanitary environment |
| | | Keywords: no place for hand wash laundry, sanitary environment |
| Dining/Meal-prep. Area (Re4) | r-19 | Dining area in the parking lot exposed survivors to extreme weather conditions (rain, snow, strong wind) |
| | | Keywords: dining area location, no protection for people from extreme weather conditions |
| | r-20 | Dining spaces reduced to one after a prolonged shelter stay, lack of dining space for survivors |
| | | Keywords: insufficient dining area |
| | r-21 | Problems with freezing food materials stored in the outdoor meal preparation area |
| | | Keywords: no separate refrigerator for public use |
| Rest area (Re5) | r-22 | No separate resting area provided indoors resulted in people sitting on the floor, occupying empty spaces, talking loudly, and exposing private conversations and information |
| | | Keywords: no separate resting area provided |
| | r-23 | Space sharing in the dining area caused congestion |
| | | Keywords: space sharing in the dining area, congestion |

From the identifications mentioned above, it can be interpreted that the sanitary space arrangement plan should consider sex and accessibility, particularly for older adults, by planning the residential zone near sanitary spaces. Besides, the dining area should preferably be located inside the shelter, and if it is difficult to secure an indoor space, it is necessary to consider installing a refrigerator to keep people's food fresh. A place to relax must be mandatorily provided for people to converse and to ensure their emotional wellbeing. The scale and size of the lounge may be small considering the need to protect personal or family unit privacy.

> "The tent size is so small that it is uncomfortable to change clothes inside. My husband stays in a relative's house and I stay alone here for convenience. I don't have enough space to keep my stuff, and hence, I always carry all valuable items with me, and I frequently visit my home to bring other stuff whenever I need something." (survivor, 60s, woman)

> "I stay on the second floor, and I try not to drink water in the evening. The shower is close, but the toilets are in the opposite direction, and I have to go all the way around to get there. Whenever I use the toilet during the night, I can't sleep again." (survivor, 60s, woman)

> "The dining area is outside, and it is a temporary tent instead of a solid building or a room. When it is windy, rainy, or cold outside, it is cumbersome to move back and forth to eat." (survivor, 50s, man)

> "We do not have a separate drying room for laundry on the second floor. We hang socks and towels on a chair to dry, and our underwear is often placed in tents or hung on a sink." (survivor, 50s, woman)

### 3.2.3. Service Zone

The management space did not include a separate resting area for staff and volunteers, and they had to share the dining area and residential zone with survivors. This made communication between staff and volunteers difficult as survivors could overhear their conversations. Thus, room sharing between staff and survivors resulted in community and privacy issues. In the medical space, another privacy issue emerged. The designated space for medical treatment was small, and the distance between the consultation room and waiting area was too close to maintain patients' privacy (Table 7).

Table 7. Problems identified in the service zone.

| Category | Mark | Main Problems |
| --- | --- | --- |
| Staff area (Se1) | s-1 | No separate resting area for managers and volunteers; difficult to protect privacy due to space sharing |
| | | Keywords: no separate resting area for staffs/volunteers, privacy |
| Medical area (Se2) | s-2 | Privacy infringement in psychological counseling space as it is separated by a narrow space from the waiting area; not enough space in the medical treatment area |
| | | Keywords: a small area for medical care, privacy issue due to close spacing |

Therefore, from the interviewees' experiences mentioned above, we inferred that the resting area should be planned in a separate space and should not be shared in common. Sufficient distance was required between the treatment space and waiting space in the medical care area by preferably providing separate rooms for each function or installing partitions between spaces.

> "When taking a break, it's very hard for us because we don't have our own private space. The rest area in the parking space is mainly used by the disaster survivors, and hence, we can't just go there and sit and have conversations or take rest amid them." (Volunteer, 50s, woman)

> "The medical treatment room is very small. When I am waiting to receive psychological counseling, I am often embarrassed and uncomfortable because I can hear the other people's counseling conversation, and I become worried that other people would hear my story as well." (survivor, 50s, woman)

### 3.2.4. Special Needs Zone

Space for pregnant/breastfeeding women and pet areas were not included in the space plan for the shelter in Pohang. Families with infants and toddlers did not have any place to nurse babies and hence, had to return to their damaged house periodically to feed the babies. People with pets also went back to their houses to care for pets despite the danger of secondary disaster risks such as aftershocks, collapse, fire, etc. (Table 8). This showed the urgent need to provide spaces for special needs in the shelter and can be interpreted that the space plan should include areas for women to nurse their babies and pet so that infants, women, and pets can stay comfortably in the temporary shelter.

> "Because many people live together, there are hygiene issues and we are all anxious about it. Women who have babies cannot stay in the shelter because of the sanitation problem. In the beginning, there was a two-year-old baby in the shelter, but the mom and the baby left here soon." (survivor, 70s, woman)

> "I have dogs that have lived with me for 10 years, and the shelter does not provide a room for pets. So, I have no choice but to come home regularly and take care of them." (survivor, 50s, woman)

**Table 8.** Problems identified in the special needs zone.

| Category | Mark | Main Problems |
|---|---|---|
| Nursing area (Sp1) | sn-1 | No room provided for nursing babies in the shelter and families with infants and toddlers returned to their damaged houses to nurse babies, thereby risking exposure to a secondary disaster |
| | | Keywords: no separate space, secondary disaster exposure |
| Pet area (Sp2) | sn-2 | No space plan for pets in/around the shelter; people with pets return to their damaged houses to take care of pets with a risk of secondary disaster exposure |
| | | Keywords: no separate space, secondary disaster exposure |

### 3.2.5. Analysis

The following Table 9 is a comprehensive analysis matrix of habitability problems examined in the temporary shelter by zone. Most problems were pointed out in residential zones, especially in terms of comfort. In the entry zone and special needs zone, various aspects of habitability appeared relatively evenly, and the service zone lacked comfort.

**Table 9.** Analysis matrix.

| Category | Zone | Entry Zone | | | Residential Zone | | | | | Service Zone | | Special Needs Zone | |
|---|---|---|---|---|---|---|---|---|---|---|---|---|---|
| | | En1 | En2 | En3 | Re1 | Re2 | Re3 | Re4 | Re5 | Se1 | Se2 | Sp1 | Sp2 |
| | Sa1 | e-3 | - | - | r-1<br>r-3 | - | r-16 | r-19 | - | - | - | sn-1 | sn-2 |
| | Sa2 | - | e-4 | - | r-2 | - | - | - | - | - | - | - | - |
| | He1 | e-2 | e-5 | - | r-6<br>r-7 | r-15 | r-16<br>r-17<br>r-18 | - | - | - | - | sn-1 | - |
| | He2 | - | - | - | - | - | - | - | - | - | s-2 | - | - |
| | So1 | - | - | - | r-4<br>r-8 | r-13 | - | - | - | - | - | sn-1 | sn-2 |
| | So2 | e-1 | - | - | r-2<br>r-8 | r-13 | - | r-19 | - | - | - | - | - |
| | So3 | - | - | - | - | - | - | - | - | - | - | - | - |

Table 9. Cont.

| Category | Zone | Entry Zone | | | Residential Zone | | | | | Service Zone | | Special Needs Zone | |
|---|---|---|---|---|---|---|---|---|---|---|---|---|---|
| | | En1 | En2 | En3 | Re1 | Re2 | Re3 | Re4 | Re5 | Se1 | Se2 | Sp1 | Sp2 |
| Co1 | | - | e-6 | e-7 | r-1<br>r-2<br>r-3 | - | r-16<br>r-17 | r-20<br>r-20 | r-22<br>r-23 | s-1 | s-2 | sn-1 | sn-2 |
| Co2 | | - | - | e-7 | r-2<br>r-4<br>r-5<br>r-9 | r-12<br>r-14 | r-16 | - | r-22 | s-1 | s-2 | - | - |
| Co3 | | - | - | - | r-5<br>r-6<br>r-7<br>r-10<br>r-11 | - | r-17 | - | - | - | - | - | - |

## 4. Discussion

Examining the temporary shelter's spatial problems from the perspective of habitability revealed that each zone needed improvement in the same or different categories when compared to other zones.

In the entry zone, all four aspects (safety, health, sociality, comfort) of habitability were evenly mentioned. This implied that the entry zone was not limited to a specific factor, as the entry zone was the starting point of the building's access, crowd control, and shelter experience, so the overall aspect should be considered. In particular, "sanitation" and "area" were evaluated as relatively important elements in the entranceway. This was a place used by many people at the same time and frequently, so it required sufficient area and an effective width and supports the importance of sanitation management. The entrance door frequently used by all should open wide and the space around the door should be left free and uncrowded to support different activities such as waiting, passing, asking for help, applying for registration forms, etc.

In the residential zone, comprising personal area and public area, problems were identified in the categories of "protection/prevention" (safety), "sanitation" (health), "vulnerable people/accessibility" (sociality), "area/privacy/indoor environment quality" (comfort). Among them, it was found many comfort-related problems existed such as "area", "privacy", and "indoor environmental quality". Moreover, it was emphasized that improvement was necessary for hygiene management. In the end, this fact was summarized as a problem for the qualitative management of the area and indoor environment. If the space provided to individuals is not sufficient, privacy issues will follow. If the basic indoor environment such as noise, air, light, and heat is not properly managed, an unsanitary environment is created. Therefore, space where the survivors spend most of their time, whether personal or public, should be provided with a sufficient area per individual, and the quality management of the indoor environment was closely related to promoting habitability and wellness.

In personal living spaces, the biggest problem was uniform accommodations without considering the family composition of survivors. Failure to consider sex, disability, number of family members, age, etc., eventually leads to invasion of privacy, and the provision of insufficient space also caused a great inconvenience in long-term living. This uniform space plan and minimum area standard eventually resulted in poor indoor living quality and negatively affected survivors' physical health and psychological stability due to privacy violations.

Therefore, for personal living spaces, it is essential that (1) the area and arrangement of individual accommodations are first planned, and (2) the characteristics of members living in the accommodation must be carefully grasped in advance. Furthermore, it is legally necessary to establish a generous standard that takes into account psychological stability, without providing a minimum physical standard when arranging private accommodations or living space.

In public spaces, it was observed that the biggest problem was sharing multiple functions in one space without separating the space for each function or planning independently. Space sharing infringed on privacy between users. Therefore, when planning a public space, it is desirable to divide and provide space for each function. Besides, it is important to consider the diversity of various users. In the shelters in Pohang, there was a large shortage of dedicated spaces for managers and volunteers, and most of the space plans focused on survivors. Since this has an important relationship with the building and providing a better quality of environment for the survivors, it is necessary to consider the needs of all shelter users such as children, older adults, the disabled, managers, and volunteers.

Service zone problems were mainly seen in the categories of "area" and "privacy" in the aspect of comfort. It was identified that these problems were mainly caused by the fact that a dedicated space for managers and volunteers other than survivors was not prepared. Because a separate rest area was not provided, a privacy invasion occurred while taking a break in the corridor or using the same space as survivors. Given this fact, to improve the habitability of the service zone, it is necessary to ensure space is provided for all shelter users. Additionally, it may increase the satisfaction of shelter users and improve wellness by planning separate spaces by users or functions rather than sharing the same space for multiple purposes.

Last, the special needs zone was less habitable in the categories of "protection" (safety) and "area" (comfort). These problems were caused by the fact that hygiene, safety, and privacy were not secured because separate, independent spaces for infants, pregnant women, and nursing mothers were not provided. In the end, this problem was understood as the fact that dedicated spaces for children, pregnant women, and companion animals were not sufficiently provided. If a dedicated space was not planned, hygiene management may not be carried out thoroughly, and privacy may be infringed, making it difficult to obtain survivors' overall welfare. Therefore, it is necessary to plan separate spaces for survivors with special needs such as children, pregnant women, and companion animals.

In summary, highlights from the findings are as follows:

- Habitability should take into account all four aspects of safety, health, sociality, and comfort, and it is essential to achieve human wellness even in the planning of a temporary disaster shelter;
- Since the entry zone is a place where a large number of users move frequently, it is necessary to secure a sufficient area and thoroughly manage hygiene;
- The residential zone is key to providing a generous space by adjusting the area provided per user above the legal minimum standard, and to thoroughly manage indoor environmental factors such as light, noise, humidity, and ventilation. In particular, in a personal living space, a plan for private accommodation that considers family members is required, and in a public space, it is necessary to separate spaces for each function;
- For service zones and special need zones, it is important to separate spaces for each function and user.

These highlights provide important insights, including:

1. Secure enough space (secure space beyond the legal minimum standards);
2. Provide sanitation and indoor environment quality management;
3. Separate spaces by function and user.

These insights are deeply related to securing the physical health of shelter users, such as survivors, managers, and volunteers, and obtaining psychological stability and privacy. They are also related to the quality and satisfaction of human life.

Since the results of the above study were conducted for one temporary housing facility in Pohang, South Korea, it is difficult to generalize the results from the temporary disaster shelter's spatial plan. It will be necessary to add temporary shelter cases located in South Korea and expand the disaster types to floods, fires, and infectious diseases in addition to earthquakes. Furthermore, the follow-up task is to gradually increase the number of interviewees to accumulate more reliable data. These follow-up studies will help inform shelter design so that survivors acquire and maintain physical and psychological health without continuing to lose their dignity in preparation for increasing disasters.

## 5. Conclusions

The problems within the temporary shelter set up in an indoor gymnasium in Pohang revealed the need to improve the space planning and operation in terms of safety, health, sociality, and comfort to better support victims' needs. The following are some of the recommendations based on the main research results.

First, to better support the survivors' shelter stay, daily living activities must be performed with ease. Therefore, in preparation for various disaster situations, rather than simply switching the gym to a temporary shelter, it is necessary to review the designation and use of various types of temporary shelters carefully, such as mobile homes, welfare facilities, and lodging facilities in addition to public facilities such as gymnasiums and town halls.

Second, most of the disaster survivors staying in the temporary shelter in Pohang were older adults, and accordingly, problems such as reduced accessibility due to lack of parking spaces and frequent use of stairs to access the shelter were observed. There was also insufficient consideration for the disabled. When planning a temporary shelter, facilities and space plans for older adults and the disabled must meet the necessary standards with barrier-free access.

Third, the temporary shelter in Pohang was originally a gymnasium that was prepared for a temporary stay of one month. However, from the second field study, it was confirmed that the survivors stayed in the shelter for more than 4 months on average. Therefore, in the future, various types of disaster shelters should be developed considering the possible evacuation period, such as an emergency shelter for 2–3 days or a temporary shelter capable of supporting daily activities for a long evacuation period.

Fourth, in terms of habitability, the most important thing when planning a temporary shelter is to provide sufficient space by demarcating appropriate areas and independent spaces for each function. When spaces are shared for multiple functions, secondary problems such as accessibility, privacy, sanitation, indoor quality, and lack of protection may arise. Therefore, priority should be given to necessary functions and secure independent areas for each accordingly. Additionally, the composition and arrangement of space should consider different people's needs based on sex, age, and user type (staff/volunteers/survivors). By ensuring concepts of habitability such as safety, health, sociality, and comfort, the temporary shelter can provide survivors with both physical health and psychological stability during a disaster.

The study was based on a case in South Korea in which a gymnasium was converted into a temporary shelter. This could be helpful in exploring the different types of shelters in the world and collecting related data. In the light of previous studies, the result of the lack of detailed and specific guidelines regarding habitability stays on the same line with previous studies. However, it can be distinguished that the research process was focused on interacting with victims, staff, and volunteers on-site instead of analyzing the literature. It is difficult to generalize the guidelines of shelters as they all have different issues by country, region, and type of disaster. Thus, examining several cases and accumulating related issues can be meaningful for the long-term development of shelter planning.

**Author Contributions:** Conceptualization, M.K.; methodology, E.K.; validation, M.K. and E.K.; formal analysis, E.K. and K.K.; investigation, K.K.; resources, M.K.; writing—original draft preparation, K.K. and E.K.; writing—review and editing, M.K. and E.K.; visualization, E.K.; supervision, M.K.; project administration, M.K.; funding acquisition, M.K. All authors have read and agreed to the published version of the manuscript.

**Funding:** This research was funded by the National Research Foundation of Korea (NRF), the Ministry of Education, grant number NRF-2015R1D1A1A01060882.

**Institutional Review Board Statement:** Ethical review and approval were waived for this study, due to the reasons below. The investigation (interview with a questionnaire) of our study was conducted in early 2018. This study did not go through the procedure for issuing an official exemption certificate, because, in the case of research conducted to evaluate public welfare or service programs as national R&D, IRB review was not required at this time. However, we recognized the importance of ethical issues and specified (1) the purpose of the study, (2) an explanation of the guarantee of anonymity, (3) interview content to be used for research purposes only in the guide of the questionnaire. Additional explanation was given to interviewees so that the purpose and content of the interview could be fully understood. Those who responded to the interview expressed deep sympathy for this study and gave voluntary consent. To ensure anonymity and to speak more freely, we only asked their approximate age and the period of shelter stay without asking their names or contact information. For this reason, they gave voluntary consent verbally instead of signing the formal consent form. Contents that can directly or indirectly verify the identity of the interviewees were excluded from the question, and only the spatial issues were discussed rather than personal issues during the interviews.

**Informed Consent Statement:** Informed consent was obtained from all subjects involved in the study verbally for the reasons mentioned earlier.

**Conflicts of Interest:** The authors declare no conflict of interest.

# References

1. Quarantelli, E.L. Patterns of sheltering and housing in US disasters. *Disaster Prev. Manag. Int. J.* **1995**, *4*, 43–53. [CrossRef]
2. UNISDR. *Guidance Note on Recovery: Shelter*; UNISDR: Kobe, Japan, 2010.
3. Sanderson, D.; Burnell, J. *Beyond Shelter After Disaster: Practice, Process, and Possibilities*; Routledge: New York, NY, USA, 2013; pp. 24–35.
4. Iwasa, A.; Hasegawa, T.; Shinkai, S.; Shinozaki, M.; Yasutake, A.; Kobayashi, A. A Practical Approach to Temporary Housing for Disaster Victims. *J. Asian Archit. Build. Eng.* **2012**, *11*, 33–38. [CrossRef]
5. Bashawri, A.; Garrity, S.; Moodley, K. An Overview of the Design of Disaster Relief Shelters. *Procedia Econ. Finance* **2014**, *18*, 924–931. [CrossRef]
6. Choi, Y.R.; Kim, E.J.; Kim, M.K. A Planning Guide for Temporary Disaster Shelters Focusing on Habitability. *Indoor Built Environ.* **2020**, *29*, 1412–1424. [CrossRef]
7. Ministry of the Interior and Safety (MOIS). *2018 Disaster Relief Planning Guidelines*; Ministry of the Interior and Safety: Sejong, Korea, 2017.
8. Sphere. Humanitarian charter and minimum standards in humanitarian response. In *The Sphere Handbook*; Sphere Association: Geneva, Switzerland, 2018. Available online: https://spherestandards.org/wp-content/uploads/Sphere-Handbook-2018-EN.pdf (accessed on 20 June 2020).
9. Kronenburg, R. *Architecture in Motion: The History and Development of Portable Building*; Routledge: London, UK, 2013.
10. Kim, M.K.; Kim, E.J. Current Status and Implication for the Planning of Emergency Shelter Considering Users' Habitability. *Korean Inst. Int. Des. J.* **2016**, *25*, 23–31. [CrossRef]
11. Global Shelter Cluster. Shelter Projects 2015–2016: Case Studies of Humanitarian Shelter and Settlement Responses. 2017. Available online: http://shelterprojects.org/shelterprojects2015-2016/ShelterProjects_2015-2016_lowres_web.pdf (accessed on 20 June 2020).
12. Um, A.Y.; Oh, K.E.; Shin, Y.J.; Kang, B.K. A Study of Design Direction for Safety and Relief: Temporary Living Support Systems. *J. Korean Soc. Des. Cult. KSDC* **2014**, *20*, 393–407.
13. American Red Cross. *Mega-Shelter Planning Guide*; International Association of Venue Managers, Inc.: Coppell, TX, USA, 2010.
14. U.S. Department of Justice. ADA Checklist for Emergency Shelters. 2007. Available online: https://www.ada.gov/pcatoolkit/chap7shelterchk.pdf (accessed on 20 June 2020).
15. Federal Emergency Management Agency. *Shelter Field Guide*; Federal Emergency Management Agency: Washington, DC, USA, 2015.
16. Centers for Disease Control and Prevention (CDC). Infection Control Guidance for Community Evacuation Centers Following Disasters. Available online: https://www.cdc.gov/disasters/commshelters.html (accessed on 20 June 2020).
17. APIC Emergency Preparedness Committee. *Infection Prevention and Control for Shelters During Disasters*; APIC Emergency Preparedness Committee: Arlington, VA, USA, 2007.
18. Kim, M.K.; Jang, E.H.; Kim, E.J.; Choi, Y.R. Case Analysis of the Overseas Planning Guidelines to Develop the Domestic Temporary Shelter Planning Guideline. *Korean Inst. Int. Des. J.* **2018**, *27*, 3–13. [CrossRef]

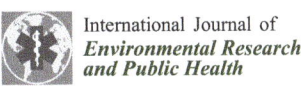

*Article*

# Toward the Biophilic Residential Regeneration for the Green New Deal

Eun Ji Lee [1] and Sung Jun Park [2,*]

1. Department of Architecture, Keimyung University, Daegu 42601, Korea; yej@stu.kmu.ac.kr
2. Department of Architectural Engineering, Keimyung University, Daegu 42601, Korea
* Correspondence: sjpark@kmu.ac.kr; Tel.: +82-53-580-5765

**Abstract:** As climate changes and species extinction accelerate, the global community focuses on Green New Deal plans to promote economic development based on environmental sustainability. The Green New Deal should encourage sustainable resilience in the environment and strengthen the community's innate ties with natural resources and biodiversity. This study describes biophilic design for sustainable and resilient residential regeneration from the perspective of the Green New Deal, and suggests potential possibilities for these approaches on a residential regeneration scale. A case study clarifies the applicable features of biophilic design in various fields, such as architectural planning and design, technology, and services, and is subdivided according to the scale of residential regeneration (unit, building, and complex). The results of this study suggest new values for existing Green New Deal policies and contribute to the segmentation of residential regeneration projects and the expansion of related industries.

**Keywords:** Green New Deal; climate change; biophilia; biophilic design; residential regeneration; sustainable resilience

## 1. Introduction

The acceleration of global warming has caused severe climate change that led to environmental pollution, drought, extreme cold and heat waves, and frequent natural disasters, threatening human health and welfare. In particular, along with climate change, the aging and decline of the population in modern society, the economic downturn, and the increase in decrepit housing are accompanied by an imbalance and qualitative decline in cities around the world [1]. With growing concerns over climate change, efforts to promote economic development based on environmental sustainability have been made around the world, and various proposals for the Green New Deal have been raised internationally [2,3]. The Green New Deal means environmental and human-centered sustainable development and focuses on the eco-friendly transformation of the energy supply and demand system, everyday life, and industrial infrastructure [4,5]. As a result, discussions are actively underway on the regeneration of urban and residential areas, and specific planning measures are required to integrate the welfare and environmental protection of local residents and economic growth.

The recent residential regeneration project presents a vision that considers the direction of economic regeneration, focusing on green remodeling, the application of green technology, and the new and renewable-energy industry. However, it also focuses on how to minimize human environmental impact, without considering various social issues such as the aging population and the quality of life of residents. Therefore, for existing environmental regeneration businesses to become more sustainable and resilient, it is important to secure neighborhoods and communities through the restoration of human-nature relations.

Humans evolved in response to the stimulus of the environment and were adapted to live in a natural environment. In fact, this is supported by research results and empirical evidence that the natural environment is preferred much more than the urban environment or built environment [6–8]. The Biophilia hypothesis conceptualizes it as a human biological trait, based on the premise that the stimulation of the natural environment induces a genetically positive response [9]. Specifically, biophilia cannot be explained by a single instinct, and it can be achieved by learning rules and iterative experiences to cultivate and effectively function biological tendencies [10]. Biophilia is applied to the architectural environment through biophilic design. The ultimate goal of the biophilic design is to restore a healthy relationship between humans and the natural environment, leading humans to a positive natural experience, offsetting negative environmental factors and creating a relaxed psychological state [11]. In the field of architecture, various classification systems have been proposed to apply biophilic design; it is divided into patterns of biophilic design [12], experiences and attributes of biophilic design [13], depending on the perspective of the researcher. Recently, biophilic design has highlighted health effects and economic benefits when they are applied to work, medical, and educational environments, which are discussed with the expectation of not only the quality living environment but also the economic revitalization of the community [14,15]. The design method utilizing the characteristics of the natural environment supports active physical activities and healthy mental states [11,12]; it also contributes to the securing of natural resources and the creation of new green jobs by cultivating various species in the urban area [14,16]. It is also advantageous because it promotes communication with a sentiment of social belonging to form community integration and a positive sense of society [10,17].

This study focuses on the similarities between the goals and directions pursued by the concept of the Green New Deal and biophilia and proposes the application of biophilic design and its value as a strategy for residential regeneration in response to climate change. The detailed goals of this study are as follows:

- First, it presents a theoretical basis for integrating the concepts of the Green New Deal and biophilia for the regeneration of residential areas in response to climate change and resilience;
- Second, it discusses the potential value and need for regeneration of biophilic design-based dwellings in health, economic, and social aspects;
- Third, through literature reviews, it derives the characteristics of the biophilic design considering the Green New Deal and proposes a biophilic residential regeneration strategy based on the scale of application.

This study covers not only the developments of theories that correspond to the purpose of the study, but also other areas and variables that do not fall within the scope of the subject.

Figure 1 shows the method and scope to achieve the goals of the study, and the details are as follows. First, it proposes a theoretical basis for the relationship between humans, nature, and the economy and sustainable resilience by considering theories related to the Green New Deal and biophilia concepts. Second, it discusses the health, economic, and social benefits of applying biomedical design by considering prior research related to biophilic design. Third, a case study of biophilic design applications that was conducted in the architectural planning, design, and technology and service industries, which are key areas of the Green New Deal's environmental regeneration project, is explored. The scope of the survey covers applications of related literature and preceding research, such as urban and residential areas; technologies, including architecture; and service industries, through keyword search. This is to derive a residential regeneration strategy from an integrated and comprehensive perspective. It was conducted using major academic databases, including Scopus, IEEE XPLORE, SpringerLink, ScienceDirect, and PubMed. The details are described in Section 3. Finally, based on the results of the case study, we propose a plan to regenerate the biophilic residential area. The housing regeneration plan proposed in this study is limited to the scope of unit scale, building scale, and complex scale in consideration of the possibility and usability of future applications.

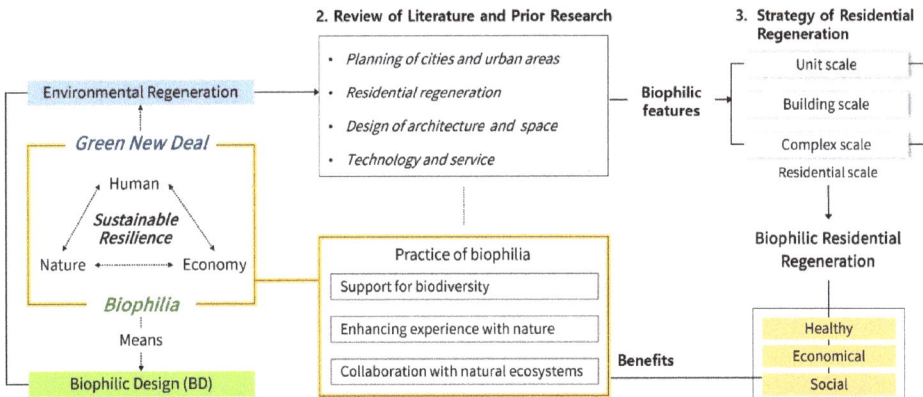

Figure 1. Research scheme.

To date, research on environmental regeneration for the Green New Deal has focused on environmental and energy sustainability and community and policy support [18–21]. However, it is insufficient to consider restoring the relationship between local residents and local ecosystems or to provide support for daily experience with nature. Discussions on biophilic urbanism have been taking place recently, with the emphasis on the impact of the regeneration of urban and residential areas on public health [22,23], but research suggesting a plan for specific applications considering the size and environmental characteristics of a region is lacking. Previous research has also focused on a limited scope, such as the restoration of public facilities and ecosystems, so that it is necessary to discuss economic and technological links, such as Green New Deal projects and smart industries. Amid the rapidly growing demand for the Green New Deal plan, this study discusses the direction of residential regeneration for healthy communities and residents and proposes various applications and the potential value of biophilic design as a key strategy. The results of this study indicate the possibility and need for a link between the Green New Deal project and the biophilic design strategy. Moreover, the results expand the understanding of residential regeneration and the application of biophilic design from the perspective of the Green New Deal. They also contribute the worth of segmenting residential regeneration projects on various scales, the potential utilization of biophilic architecture, and the development of related technologies.

## 2. Green New Deal and Biophilic Design
### 2.1. Climate Change and Green New Deal

Discussions on global weather phenomena and climate change aim at global and national strategic responses to changes in the global environment, including food, soil, energy, and health. Global warming prevents the planet from functioning properly by directly weakening the Earth's environmental services or disabling them, which inevitably has direct and indirect impacts on various areas, including human life, industrial structure, and the ecosystem [24]. In other words, rapid climate change is expected to pose the most serious threat to the world's economic, social and environmental stability, requiring continued access to essential goods such as clean water and air, and healthy food and housing.

Climate change is not an independent issue but is closely linked to the growth of the human population, energy, and everyday working and living environments. The fifth evaluation report by the International Panel on Climate Change (IPCC) explains how risks from [25] climate change can adversely affect the human living environment. The impact on the ecosystem may worsen social problems, such as diseases, and resource problems related to human life, such as food scarcity. It is estimated that an increase in average temperature and precipitation will lead to changes in the life cycle, geographical distribution, and species composition of plants and animals. The increase in carbon dioxide levels will have a serious impact on the marine ecosystem; the increase in temperature will cause natural disasters such as floods due to rising sea levels and erosion, accompanied by human casualties [26]. The impact on ecosystems soon leads to social and economic impacts, such as the decline in overall food production due to problems with water supply and demand and the change in the structure of energy supply due to the surge in demand for heating and cooling, increasing the emissions of secondary air pollutants. The system of such a vicious circle is also expected to be prominent in accelerating population migration, with flooding to high-altitude inland areas and an influx of the rural population into cities, which could lead to an imbalance in land use and food supply and demand [27]. Finally, the most serious threat of climate change is health problems, as they create favorable conditions for the spread of diseases, especially among the socially vulnerable. This will deal a heavy blow not only to developing countries but also to all cities suffering from aging populations worldwide. In this context, the living zone concentrated in the urban environment of modern society is expected to suffer huge losses. It is, thus, necessary to improve the quality of the environment and support human health and well-being through environmental management plans, policies, and technology to protect the environment from disasters caused by human activities.

Recently, every country has been pushing for a Green New Deal policy to form a win-win relationship that benefits both by integrating economic growth and environmental protection, which have been perceived as conflicting relations [28,29]. The direction of the New Deal policy in the global era is the convergence of the Digital and the Green New Deal [30], emphasizing the establishment of smart infrastructure in response to the Fourth Industrial Revolution and climate change, discussing environmental and economic responses through the development of green environment and green technologies, and job creation [27,29,31]. The fundamental solution to the problem of climate must be accompanied by extensive academic and industrial efforts, and the construction sector needs to first produce specific countermeasures at the minimum scale of the environment closest to our lives. Whereas the Green New Deal is a hot topic of debate, we are fully aware that the socially vulnerable, animal and plant species, and future generations around the world are already seriously damaged [32]. We should respond to this threat quickly.

The Green New Deal has once again called for an integrated and comprehensive perspective on the issue of residence, as the past way of life, which prioritized progress and development, has changed in a way that values today's quality of life. In particular, attention is being paid to how to "restore "or "replay" so that each function of "people," "community," "nature," and "economy" can be fulfilled efficiently and effectively [33]. Residential regeneration shall practice regional regeneration considering the identity and environment of the region, and infrastructure shall be established for the city and local community to grow continuously. Therefore, this study focuses on exploring approaches and methodologies to "resilient" residential regeneration, in which the development of residences, nature, and communities can circulate organically to cope with climate change.

*2.2. Biophilia, from the Point of View of the Green New Deal*

The Green New Deal is the coordination of social, ecological, and economic systems in response to current or anticipated climate change and its impact [34], in other words, to build a mutual developmental relationship between humans, nature, and the economy. The approach to the Green New Deal is discussed in convergence with the precautionary aspect, encompassing a multidisciplinary analysis, in which the production and use of energy is a combination of natural scientific perspectives [25,35–37]. The preventive approach focuses on "safe management rather than regret", a precautionary principle that is irreversible in the event of losses caused by climate change [25]. This study deals with the regeneration of residential areas for the Green New Deal and discusses the link with the concept of biophilia in consideration of the direction of preventive and convergent approaches.

Biophilia refers to the instinctive love for life and natural systems and promotes the restoration of nature and human relations based on human emotional partnerships in natural life [10]. Edward O. Wilson, who popularized the biophilia hypothesis, suggests that the most serious disaster of climate change is the loss of genetic diversity due to natural habitat destruction [38]. This is because being alive and staying healthy when activating the love of life within [39], especially exploring and feeling close to life, is an essential and positive process for mental health [10]. In other words, humans and society cannot be completely healthy in a modern urban environment that lacks access to nature and should provide a more renewable and resilient environment through the restoration of natural and human relations. Resilience is the ability of a system to derive profits by absorbing and utilizing psychological disturbances and changes and has a sustainable structure [40]. The resilience of a city based on biophilia requires a shift in the idea of recognizing natural resources and biodiversity as the basis of support for survival, and it is important to strengthen local residents' instinctive attachment to nature. In this context, this study focused on the similarity between the Green New Deal goals and the biophilia hypothesis, seeking benefits through positive ties between humans and nature, and drew a theoretical basis for applying and integrating residential regeneration. Figure 2 shows its link with the biophilia hypothesis from the Green New Deal perspective.

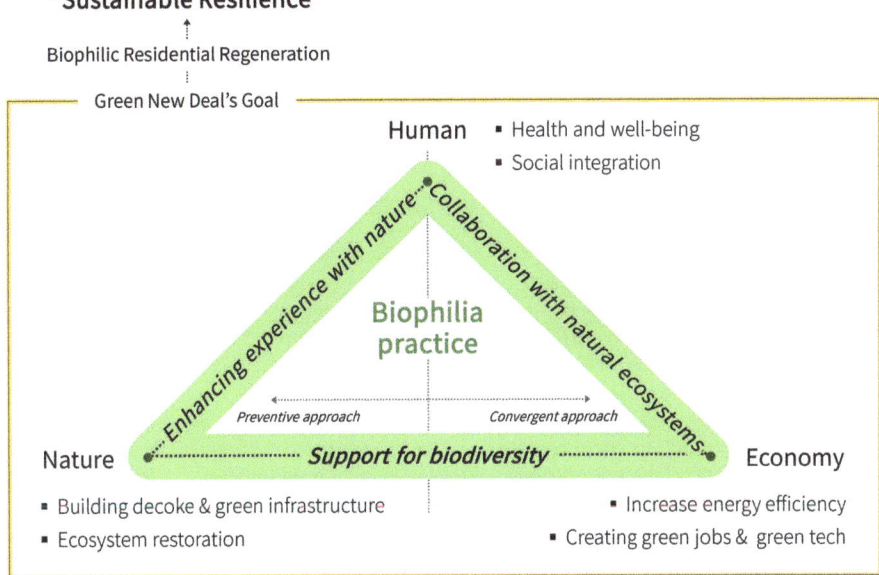

**Figure 2.** The link between the Green New Deal and Biophilia.

The Green New Deal is being discussed in terms of humanity, nature, and economy, and this study derived three concepts for the practice of biophilia from the perspective of the Green New Deal. The first is "support for biodiversity". The clearest common thing in the practice of the Green New Deal and biophilia is the preservation of the ecosystem, specifically an active attitude toward securing various species. Securing biodiversity supports diverse experiences with nature and contributes to enhancing the competitiveness of the community by assuring the evolution and specificity of indigenous creatures. In other words, biodiversity based on bioethics serves as an organism of a complete ecosystem by inducing continuous well-being of the individual and economic society of the city. The second concept is "enhancing experience with nature," which is to improve the bond between humans and nature through human physical, physiological, and mental characteristics that respond positively to nature and further ensure the health and healing of local residents. Prior studies related to human responses to nature have provided convincing evidence in a wide range of fields in which interaction with nature is related to inducing healing and recovery, improved understanding of learning, and reduced social hostility and aggression [13,17,41–43]. Recently, the architectural community has discussed planning and technical measures to maximize the experience with nature to build a healthy physical environment and a high-quality living environment through the effects of biophilia [44]. The third and last concept is the "collaboration with natural ecosystem", which is to recognize that all-natural resources are finite and pursue a cooperative relationship between humans and nature rather than a one-sided collection of resources. This needs to be considered in the Green New Deal plan, regarding the concept of biomimicry [11], which derives innovative ideas by imitating the principles of biology and creating new technologies and values in implementing eco-friendly buildings. The approach from collection to collaboration has a structure in which mutual benefits are generated in the process of utilizing resources, and this mutual benefit further strengthens access and relationship to nature.

From the perspective of the Green New Deal, biophilia provides interaction-based benefits through a complex process and ultimately ensures a healthy life for local residents, which can give new value to the existing Green New Deal strategy. Therefore, it is necessary to discuss specific linkages when building an urban and residential environment.

*2.3. Residential Regeneration and Biophilic Design*

Individual emotions and perceptions related to environmental preference are based on the characteristics of places where people can view the landscape and discover resources or hide themselves from dangers or threats [45–47]. The human mind, structure, and capacity, were formed through the process of living in the natural world, and its senses and tendencies developed according to the environmental characteristics of nature and way of life [48]. In just a few decades, the population of cities around the world has soared, leading to continued construction processes focused on efficiency and convenience, leaving humanity far from nature. Considering the history of lifestyles from an evolutionary perspective, biologically, there is not enough time for humans to fully adapt to a city. In this context, a plan to build an environment to promote and strengthen human interaction with nature was required. In architecture, biophilic design is being explored as a strategy to interpret biophilia and introduce it to the architectural environment. Eco-friendly and sustainable architecture and, recently, resilient living environments are discussed as major planning techniques [49–51].

Beatley [52] developed the "Nature Pyramid" as a metaphorical tool for suggesting nature's recommendation and diversity of experience depending on the scale of the environment. It emphasizes that "everyday neighborhood nature" is very important in conveying the essence of a happy and healthy life. Although international and national-scale Mother Nature, at the top of the pyramid, guarantees a high level of values and rewards, it does not guarantee equal access; it is often difficult to experience and cannot be included in a natural diet of all scales. In other words, the application of the biophilic design should take into account contact with the nature around us, and it is important to restore the ecosystem on the residential scale and secure the biodiversity in the local environment. For example, if multi-family housing or apartment types are generalized depending on the population distribution, geographical characteristics, and scale limitations of each region, the experience with nature can be further weakened, so a detailed plan according to the scale of the residential area is required.

This study regards residential regeneration considering biophilic design for residential environments that are closely connected to daily life, and details on the scale and scope of residential regeneration are as shown in Table 1.

**Table 1.** Range of residential regeneration.

| Scale | Range |
| --- | --- |
| Unit | Unit space in a house, including interior environmental planning (living room, bedroom, kitchen, etc.) and intelligent residential services |
| Building | A plan for energy management and shared space (piloti, lobby, rooftop garden, etc.) considering multi-family housing and apartment types |
| Complex | A plan for joint facilities (parking lots, parks, etc.) and access road & street for residents of nearby houses (building) |

As mentioned previously, it is important to understand the role and potential value of biophilic design from the perspective of the Green New Deal to regenerate residential areas responding to climate change and urban problems. This study analyzed the expected effects of biophilic design considering the Green New Deal and the benefits of biophilic design for residential regeneration. The benefits were summarized in view biophilic characteristics and biophilia practice through consideration of the literature and prior research related to biophilic design. Table 2 shows the characteristics and benefits for the expected effects of biophilic design.

**Table 2.** Characteristics and benefits of the biophilic design.

| | Expected Effect | Biophilic Design Characteristics | Biophilia Practice | Benefits | Resource |
| --- | --- | --- | --- | --- | --- |
| Healthy | Physical | A walk in the park and woods | Ee | Improved walking and balance; reduced falls | [53,54] |
| | | Natural material; green wall | Ee | Reduced respiratory diseases; relieved headaches and dizziness | [55,56] |
| | Physiological | A walk in the park and woods; visual exposure to nature | Ee | Reduced blood pressure and heart rate; decreased sympathetic nervous system activity | [41,57,58] |
| | | Plant cultivation; gardening activities; indoor garden | Ee | Promoted neuroendocrine system and stress recovery | [11,59] |
| | | Daylight | Ee | Improved life cycle and biorhythm | [60,61] |
| | | Green space close to homes | Sb | Improved average life span | [62] |
| | Psychological | Visual exposure to nature | Ee | Improved subjective satisfaction; reduced anxiety and tension, frustration, boredom, and fatigue | [63,64] |
| | | A walk in the park and woods | Ee | Improved observation, attention-inducing, concentration, and problem-solving skills | [53,65,66] |
| | | Natural color and pattern; Nature sound | Ee | Improved creativity and emotional recovery; reduced loneliness | [67–69] |

Table 2. Cont.

| Expected Effect | | Biophilic Design Characteristics | Biophilia Practice | Benefits | Resource |
|---|---|---|---|---|---|
| Economical | Healthcare savings | Biodiversity | Sb | Decreased disease rate and number of visits to medical institutions | [8,64] |
| | | Visual exposure to nature | Ee | Decreased hospitalization and pain medication doses | [48,70] |
| | | Daylight | Ee | Reduced sick leave and absence of students and workers | [71,72] |
| | Reduced energy consumption & maintenance costs | Green building system; green wall | Cn | Increased natural purification; reduced building maintenance costs | [14] |
| | | Rainwater recycling and solar heat energy | Cn | Secured renewable energy; reduced energy consumption | [14,44] |
| | | Microbial culture; community farm | Cn; Sb | Reduced waste disposal costs; secured food resources | [73,74] |
| | Revitalizing local economy | Urban forest restoration; forestry; urban agriculture | Cn; Ee | Created jobs for local residents; secured regional competitiveness | [74] |
| | | Water space; daylight | Ee; Cn | Increased local store sales and real estate value | [14,75] |
| Social | Enhancing community | Green space close to homes | Sb | Increased frequency of use of public spaces and regional community | [76,77] |
| | | Gardening activities; foodscaping; animals | Ee | Improved conversations, affinities and preferences | [78,79] |
| | Urban vulnerability reduction | A walk in the park and woods; nature sound | Ee | Reduced crime rate, aggressiveness, violence, and fear | [17,77,80] |
| | | Roadside trees; vertical greening | Sb | Reduced traffic accidents; revitalized communities | [51] |

Note: Sb = Support for biodiversity, Ee = Enhancing experience with nature, Cn = Collaboration with natural ecosystems.

The biophilic design has expected health, economic, and social effects, and offers a wide range of benefits through direct and indirect contact with nature, a level of awareness of biophilia, and interactions with animals and plants. The design method of promoting experience with nature should support active physical activities and healthy mental conditions and create job positions for securing natural resources and managing the ecosystem. It should also respond to the vulnerability of the community, reducing hostility and aggression by promoting a friendly atmosphere and social interaction. In particular, the development of smart technology related to the cultivation of urban agriculture and microorganisms expands the residents' understanding about biophilia and contributes to enhancing biophilic tendencies. The specific benefits of biophilic design for health contributes to the well-being of local residents and public health and provides economic and social benefits through biologically positive responses. This leads to the stabilization of economic and social structures, thereby maintaining the quality living and contributing to the formation of a healthy and resilient community.

## 3. The Biophilic Design for Residential Regeneration

### 3.1. Methodology of Study

This study analyzed literature and preceding research on biophilic design in a wide range of areas, including urban planning and residential regeneration, architectural planning and design, housing technology, and residential services to identify the features of biophilic design for the residential regeneration in various aspects. Table 3 summarizes the keywords used in this study.

**Table 3.** Keyword for literature review.

| Keyword & Criteria | | Contents |
|---|---|---|
| Keyword | City and urban planning | "Biophilic city", "Biophilic urbanism", "Urban greening", "Urban generation" |
| | Residential regeneration | "Biophilic residence", "Biophilic residential environment", "Biophilic community", "Biophilic living", "Residential generation" |
| | Design of architecture and space | "Biophilic design", "Nature-based design", "Biophilic architecture", "Biophilic building", "Biophilic indoor environment" |
| | Technology and service | "Biophilic technology", "Sustainable technology", Biophilic service", "Biophilic design industrial", "Nature immersive", "Smart-home technology", "Smart-home service" |

The information was collected through major academic databases, and the collected data examined the relevance and applicability by referring to the biophilic design elements and patterns presented in the referenced study. Figure 3 shows the literature review process.

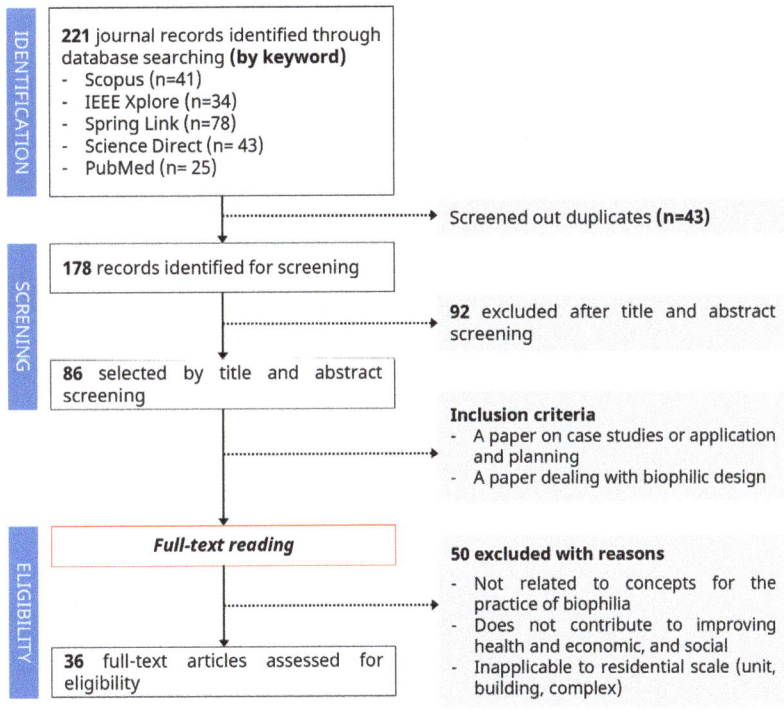

**Figure 3.** Literature review process.

This study prioritized whether the biophilic characteristics and cases proposed by literature and articles are related to the three biophilia practice concepts. In addition, we valued the characteristics and cases that can provide health, economic, and social effects from the perspective of the Green New Deal and reviewed the applicability and application plan considering the scale of residential regeneration proposed in this study. The literature and articles collected through keyword searches were first selected through title and abstract screening after excluding redundancy; the final 36 papers were selected according to the analysis criteria after full-text review.

### 3.2. Results of Biophilic Design Features

This study analyzed the main characteristics and related examples of the application of biophilic design presented in the literature and previous studies according to the concept of three biophilia practices considering the Green New Deal. The biophilic feature considers the characteristics of planning elements and case objects that are common in literature, and includes five for support for biodiversity, five for enhancement of the experience with nature, and two for collaboration with natural ecosystems.

As a result of the literature review, the application of biophilic design in the field of planning and design varies depending on the use and size of a building and the perspective of the researcher. In particular, policy efforts depending on the size of the city are being made to preserve or utilize the environmental characteristics of the region, such as mountainous and coastal areas, but there is a lack of research on specific criteria for the application of biophilic design. In addition, the application of biophilic design for housing and residential areas is insufficient due to the concentration of public facilities and ecological tourism. In the field of technology and services, the development of new technologies has improved the availability of biophilic design. However, the development of immersive technology centered on the games, and entertainment, and the smart home industry focused on energy efficiency and sustainability needs to be directed to a more positive experience of humans and nature.

#### 3.2.1. Support for Biodiversity

The support for biodiversity guarantees and manages the right to survive for all species, creating an ecosystem of cities where both terrestrial and aquatic species coexist. Table 4 shows the literature and prior research analysis related to support for biodiversity.

Table 4. Biophilic features related to support for biodiversity.

| | Biophilic Feature | | Biophilic Examples | Resource |
|---|---|---|---|---|
| A | Ecology park | Nature-Park Sudgelande, Berlin, Germany (2000) | Creation of a nature reserve through the participation of local residents to preserve the biodiversity around the closed Sudgelande Railway; used as parks and exhibition spaces for local residents and artists | [13,74,81,82] |
| | | Greenways for Pittsburgh program, USA (1980) | Open space for excellent management and conservation of ecology; creation of walkways and bike paths for local residents; creation of local jobs for environmental monitoring and maintenance | |
| B | Green rooftops | Podium Green Roof, Toronto, Canada (2009) | Utilization of modular systems comprised of indigenous species; plant species placement taking into account site conditions such as daylight and shade; habitat provision for insects and birds | [74,83–86] |

Table 4. Cont.

| | Biophilic Feature | | Biophilic Examples | Resource |
|---|---|---|---|---|
| C | Vertical gardening | Optima Camelview Village, Arizona, USA (2007) | Townhouses; creation of a variety of vegetation and green spaces on bridges and balconies connecting buildings; the provision of a series of landscapes throughout the complex | [13,15,51,83,86,87] |
| | | Bosco Verticale, Italy (2014) | Residential towers; provision of tree planted on balconies in each unit space; arrangement of tree species according to the height and direction of each building | |
| | | Façade of Quai Branly Museum, France (2006) | Support for the reproduction of various organisms, such as moss and insects; used materials such as green wall façades, stones, and trees | |
| D | Pocket park | Parklet, California, USA (2005) | Green spaces and pocket parks using parking spaces in creative ways for each residential complex; access to residential complexes and roads through green areas | [16] |
| E | Greening road & street | Green street program Portland, USA (2007) | Management of rainfall runoff through public facilities including planting; prevention of illegal parking through planting expansion facilities on roads and street pots; increase of superior infiltration surface | [13,16,74,84,88–90] |
| | | Wildlife passages, Canada (2007) | Creation of movement routes for animals, avoiding roads to connect animal habitats; construction around the upper part of tunnels, underground parking lots, and roads to protect protection local animals and ecosystems | |

The continuous landscape of the entire habitat through green rooftops and vertical gardens helps the dispersal of animals and plants. Securing native species in the residential environment encourages local residents to bond and creates new jobs to preserve the ecosystem. In addition, small ecosystems help reducing maintenance costs in residential complexes by forming circular structures, ultimately contributing to securing regional competitiveness.

3.2.2. Enhancing Experience with Nature

Enhancing experience with nature is about creating opportunities and inducing contact with nature in a variety of ways. Nature is divided into direct, indirect, and vicarious (symbolic nature), according to the type of contact [91]. Direct nature is in direct contact with the natural environment, and the more you touch, feel, and look, the higher its value. Indirect nature is a controlled environment that can be experienced in aquariums and museums and is in contact with processed nature, such as indoor gardens and botanical gardens. Finally, vicarious nature is a scene that expresses or describes nature, and is expressed in a realistic or metaphorical way, depending on the situation. Currently, vicarious nature includes smart-home technology for experiencing multisensory nature or immersive technologies such as VR (virtual reality) and AR (augmented reality). Table 5 shows the literature and prior research analysis related to enhancing experience with nature.

The greening of community space for enhancing experience with nature enhances access to nature and affects social friendship and integration, responding to social vulnerabilities, such as reduced crime rates, increased consideration, and altruistic behavior. In particular, the link between biophilic design and smart-home technology can maximize direct contact with natural factors, such as daylight, wind, and climate change, and if it actively utilizes technologies that promote experience with nature inside [44], it can ease physical space constraints and improve the living environment and the quality of health and welfare of residents.

Table 5. Biophilic features related to enhancing experience with nature.

| | Biophilic Feature | Biophilic Examples | | Resource |
|---|---|---|---|---|
| F | Community garden & farm | Paley Park, New York, USA (1967) | A small park between buildings in the city; an ivy, a tree canopy, and artificial waterfalls to increase the sounds of nature and reduce the noises in the city | [16,48,92,93] |
| | | Phipps Conservatory, Pittsburgh, USA (1893) | It plays the natural recorded sound of Pittsburgh through 12 speakers in the main atrium; autoplay based on seasonal and climate conditions | |
| | | Via Verde, New York, USA (2012) | Multi-family housing; terraced residential complexes to create walkways by height and communal gardens and to induce exploring experiences of vicarious nature | |
| G | Atria & green courtyards | Khoo Teck Puat Hospital, Singapore (2010) | An indoor garden with waterfalls; a city farm on the roof of a building; provision of a shared space for local communities | [13,16,94,95] |
| | | Victoria Park Villas, Singapore (2018) | A courtyard that can be viewed from any unit; the provision of natural light and airflow in the interior through skylight and louver; the provision of a transparent window for the privacy and view of the courtyard | |
| H | Indoor daylit & ventilation | One Central Park, Australia, Sydney (2013) | Residential towers; secured natural lighting of shaded areas through heliostats installed between two buildings | [16,44,96] |
| | | LS skylights; HC moons (CeoLux) | Artificial lighting display systems; the use of LED technology to recreate the spectrum of real sunlight and moonlight; virtual appreciation of the sky and climate changes | |
| | | Prolouver (Pergola) | Environmental sensor + controller + actuator coupling unit; provision of an optimized indoor environment, according to rainwater, light, and wind direction; provision of comfort and stability from the natural environment | |
| I | Natural analogs | Ekouin Nenbutsudo Temple, Japan (2013) | The use of natural materials such as trees and stones in every space; the use of colors and patterns to symbolize nature | [13,97] |
| | | Aqua Tower, Chicago, USA (2007) | An organic building in the shape of waves; prevention of collisions between buildings and birds through the shape of glass finishes and curves | |
| J | Virtual nature | Maplewood Senior Living, Westport, USA (2017) | Provision of "sky lounge" with immersive displays and audio, videos, and images of nature; support of real-time communication with friends and family | [44,96,98] |
| | | Undersea Project (Magic Leap) | Implementation of elements of nature's environment through technologies of augmented reality and mixed reality; support for experiences with living things based on virtual natural environments (dolphins, birds, etc.) | |
| | | Komorebi (LESLIE NOOTEBOOM) | A project lamp that generates shapes and shadows of virtual light; provision of the properties of light reflected in water or reflected between leaves | |

### 3.2.3. Collaboration with Natural Ecosystems

Collaboration with natural ecosystems focuses on the symbiotic relationship between humans and nature rather than the collection of resources [73,99], promoting a mutual benefit from the development of architecture and technology. The development of sectors and technologies in the industries involved has unlimited potential and can lead to innovations in technology and profits to the community. Inspired by biological systems, collaborating with various species benefits both corporate and local ecosystems and residents, and it is an effective way to meet global needs. Table 6 shows the literature and prior research analysis related to collaboration with natural ecosystems.

Table 6. Biophilic features related to collaboration with natural ecosystems.

| | Biophilic Feature | | Biophilic Examples | Resource |
|---|---|---|---|---|
| K | Enhanced environment | Supertree Grove in Gardens by the Bay, Singapore (2012) | Public structures with technologies that mimic the ecological functions of trees; shades, solar energy, and rainwater recycling; provision of habitats for insects and birds | [88,100–102] |
| | | Nedlaw Living Walls (Biofilter company) | Provision of indoor air quality and humidity control through wall recording; reduction of >90% of energy compared to existing HVAC [1] systems; provision of optimal plant cultivation conditions using automatic irrigation systems | |
| | | Smart Aquarium; Smart Plants Growers (Multiple companies) | Devices for fishery harbor and plant management using the Internet of things; creation of an optimal growth environment with minimal management; provision of living conditions and related information; contribution to strengthening biophilia propensity | |
| | | Termite Humidity Damping Device (Terrapin Bright Green) | Passive humidity damping device based on fungal combs in termite mounds; stabilization of humidity in buildings and reduction of energy demand | |
| L | Waste and energy management | Microbial Home (Phillips design, 2011) | Generation of bacteria and biogas energy through the decomposition of food and plastic waste; biogas energy utilization for cooking or cultivation of food, indoor lighting, etc. | [73,103–105] |
| | | Aquaponic Systems (Multiple companies) | Hydroponics and fish farming based on symbiotic relationships between fish and plants; fish waste provides nutrients to plants, who filter the water for fish | |
| | | Biolytix (Biolytix) | Household wastewater treatment systems that rely on worms and other organisms to filter water and break down sewage; exclusion of toxic chemicals; 90% energy saving compared with conventional sewage treatment system | |
| | | Pilus Cell (Pilus Energy) | As modified bacteria break down organics in wastewater, producing electricity, treated water, and useful chemical compounds | |
| | | Latro Lamp (Mike Thompson) | A lighting device that extracts electricity during photosynthesis of the lamp's algae through sunlight, $CO_2$, and water | |

Note: [1] HVAC: heating, ventilating, and air conditioning.

Examples showing collaboration with natural ecosystems are applied to a wide range of areas ranging from environmental planning and design of architecture to technology and services; the tendency of biophilia can be strengthened by helping local residents understand and feel nature and biological systems, as they are closely related to their daily lives.

## 4. Biophilic Residential Regeneration for the Green New Deal

### 4.1. Integration of Residential Regeneration and Biophilic Features

This study derived a total of 12 biophilic features for residential regeneration and was divided into features of planning and design and features of technology and services, based on a review of the literature. The biophilic features of planning and design include elements and expression techniques of biophilic architecture, such as green rooftops, vertical greening, and natural analogs. The features of technologies and services include technologies of immersive experiences that support experiences and relationships with nature, such as virtual nature, improved environment, and waste and energy management, and elements of smart-home services. Based on the analysis, this study proposes a path to integrate the biophilic design and regeneration of residential areas; details are as shown in Figure 4.

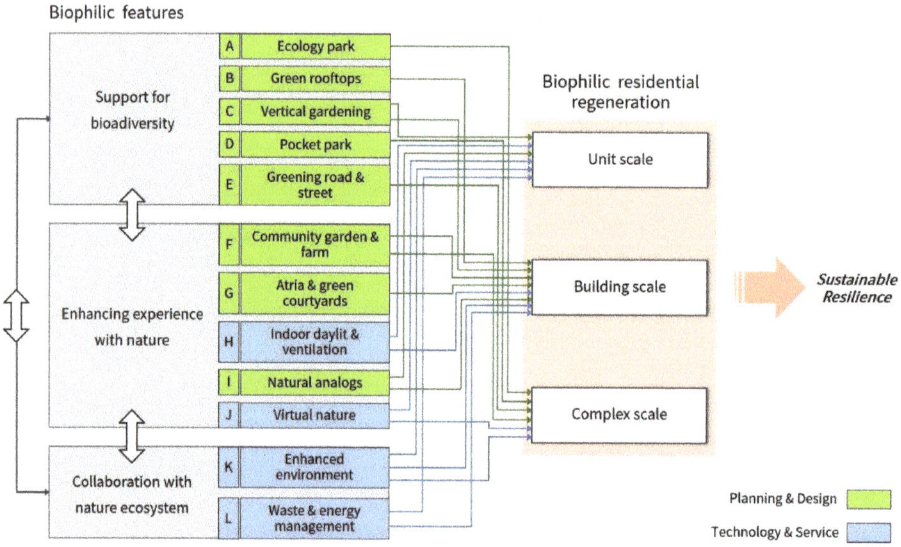

**Figure 4.** Integration pathways of biophilic design features considering the scale of residential regeneration.

This study classifies biophilic features according to the concept of biophilia practice; however, each feature is closely related to each other and forms a sustainable and resilient structure through a complementary relationship. Restoring wild nature and inducing life's habitats around us to support biodiversity leads to opportunities for contact with nature in our daily lives, strengthening a positive natural experience. Activities to strengthen experience with nature promote biodiversity and require collaboration with the natural ecosystems for sustainable experiences. In addition, being inspired by nature or collaborating with the natural ecosystem is based on biodiversity, which requires a balanced approach to the three concepts of practice, and it is important to lay the foundation by applying it to a small environment first.

### 4.2. Strategies of Biophilic Residential Regeneration

Based on the literature and case studies, this study explored the application of biophilic features (A-L) considering the scale of residential regeneration, through which we propose a biophilic residential regeneration strategy. Table 7 shows the biophilic residential regeneration strategy and its associated benefits.

Table 7. Biophilic residential regeneration strategy and benefits.

| Scales | Biophilic Features | Strategies | Specific Benefits | Common Benefits |
|---|---|---|---|---|
| Unit | C | Balconies of each unit of housing for vegetation | Biodiversity; enhancing access to nature | • Improved health and well-being<br>• Reduced building energy demand<br>• Reduced illness<br>• Increased productivity<br>• Increased property value<br>• Increased food security<br>• Extended infrastructure longevity<br>• Reduced UHI [1]<br>• Improved air quality<br>• Enhanced water quality (filtration)<br>• Residential regeneration<br>• Encouragement physical activity<br>• Provided recreation<br>• Increased regional competitiveness<br>• Increased community sense |
| Unit | C | Bio wall (green wall) with built-in automatic irrigation system | Improved indoor air quality | |
| Unit | H | Automatic actuator (louver; curtain; window; etc.) according to daylighting and wind direction | Improved indoor air quality; maximization of daylight; | |
| Unit | I | Interior design using natural shapes and patterns | Reduced stress; emotional stability | |
| Unit | I | Using of natural colors and materials | Reduced stress; emotional stability | |
| Unit | J | Smart-home device that provides virtual nature (3D object; video; etc.) | Enhancing access to nature; reduced stress | |
| Unit | K | Smart aquarium; smart plants growers | Enhancing access to organism; reduced stress | |
| Unit | L | Waste treatment system through microbial culture | Reduced waste disposal costs | |
| Building | B; F | Green rooftops and foodscaping considering indigenous species | Improved space efficiency; securing food | |
| Building | C; K | Façade greening and vertical greening system using rainwater | Improved water management and energy efficiency | |
| Building | C | Green corridors between buildings | Improved visual amenity; biodiversity | |
| Building | G | Nature-friendly sharing space in atria and courtyards | Promotion of communication | |
| Building | G; H | Heliostate for solar path tracking and daylight streams | Maximization of daylight | |
| Building | I | Organic building shapes and forms for bird protection | Improved visual amenity; biodiversity | |
| Building | L | Water treatment and energy management system based on microorganisms | Reduced waste disposal costs; improved energy efficiency | |
| Complex | A | Linkage between ecological parks and residential complexes; participation of residents for ecological management and operation | Promotion of communication; creates employment | |
| Complex | D | Parklet utilizing parking space | Biodiversity; improved visual amenity | |
| Complex | E | Shade planting for buildings placed to remove heat load | Prevention of heat load | |
| Complex | E | Green permeable sidewalks; plantation expansion facilities | Prevention of flooding | |
| Complex | F | Community parks that include artificial waterfalls, fountains, and sounds of nature | Promotion of communication; enhancing access to nature | |
| Complex | J; K | Public design considering the habitats of urban creatures and virtual nature | Biodiversity; enhancing access to nature | |

Note: [1] UHI: Urban heat island.

The unit scale is important to maximize direct and indirect contact with nature in limited indoor spaces. This requires housing technologies and services that can sense and respond organically to external natural environments. In addition, it is necessary to induce a visual or tactile connection with the indirect nature by utilizing the colors and materials of interior elements such as walls, ceilings, and floors. With the recent development of immersion technology, it is possible to simulate natural environments [44], and the construction of a natural immersive environment in a house using this innovation can be an original means to improve access to nature. The unit-scale biophilic strategy actively contributes to the improvement of residents' health and well-being and helps reinforce the residents' biophilia propensity to nature.

Biophilic strategies for building scale can support a continuous landscape outside and inside a building, while enhancing the functionality of the building and communication among residents. It is important to tend to indigenous species through rooftop landscaping to form small community farms and establish a self-sustaining system of buildings through natural resources and microbial culture environments. This increases the efficiency of building energy and space promotes social exchange and contributes to securing food resources.

Biophilic strategies for the complex scale is a strategy for residential activation and community awareness, including residents' participation in managing ecosystems near residential areas. The extensive greening of the complex, such as pedestrian paths, and street and pocket parks, improves water treatment and circulation systems and has a positive effect on the improvement of the microclimate. In addition, public design and community parks in residential complexes that take into account biodiversity protection and virtual nature contribute to building biological knowledge, strengthening community awareness, and revitalizing residential areas. Biophilic residential complexes support the sustainability of biophilic units and buildings, while also providing the foundation for biophilic cities.

## 5. Discussion

The healthy environment required by the Green New Deal can be strengthened by biological characteristics based on the relationship between humans and nature and, ultimately, contribute to the sustainable health and well-being of local residents. Prior research on biophilic design has played a significant role in shaping the biophilic system, emphasizing the role of the architectural environment for health and well-being. However, we often tend to overlook everyday places in the urban environment; in particular, there should be sufficient discussion about the minimum natural level or approach for local residents and neighbors. There is also a lack of consideration for technical and smart methodologies to enhance bio-friendliness. Therefore, from a multifaceted and long-term perspective, the biological investment for public health of the community is a very important research topic. This study deals with how to respond to climate change and urban vulnerabilities and apply biophilic design as a strategy for residential regeneration for quality residential life.

Interaction of people with nature promotes the recovery and well-being, acting as a preventive factor related to everyday stress. This can promote climate stabilization and regional competitiveness by driving meaningful interactions for the health and sustainability of communities. It also contributes to public health by ensuring equal access of residents to nature. Therefore, the government-led Green New Deal project needs a residential regeneration strategy that strengthens the organic linkage of biophilic design and maximize the effectiveness of financial expenditure in the long term.

To support biodiversity in continuous landscaping of various sizes, from indoors to buildings to residential complexes and cities, all creatures should coexist through strategies tailored to the biogeographic characteristics of the region. The experience with nature should be discussed in various aspects, and technical services should be provided in the scale of the unit and building for the equality of natural contact. In this process, companies can not only obtain innovative ideas but also have to develop sustainable products and processes, which would serve as an opportunity to respond to external and internal environmental vulnerabilities.

Finally, the concept of biophilia practice proposed in this study is a complementary relationship, taking into account the characteristics, housing type, and scale of each local environment to secure biodiversity, strengthen experience with nature, and facilitate collaboration with the natural ecosystems. In unit scale, it is necessary to utilize various technologies to bring the external natural environment indoors and to develop the contents of the user's experience. Moreover, considering the improvement of the health and energy efficiency of residents can be a cost-effective alternative in the long term. Building scale shall provide residents with experiential opportunities of nature through rooftops and public spaces and shall establish a system of buildings to support the cultivation of microorganisms and the utilization of natural resources. This contributes to the provision of a certain amount of healthy food and to the improvement of building efficiency. On a complex scale, it is important to create small green spaces and a bio-friendly ecosystem. Services and contents indicating indigenous plant species and surrounding environmental characteristics in the residential complexes continuously maintain and promote bio-friendly units and buildings and contribute to the improvement of the residents' community awareness.

## 6. Conclusions

A key premise of this study is that there is a close link between biophilia or biophilic residential regeneration and recovery-resilient communities and healthy residents, where specifically, the former helps develop the latter. The extent to which local residents can be termed 'bio-friendly' depends on their preference for the natural environment around them, the level of participation in their experience with nature, or the social attitude that supports them. In other words, the biophilic residential environment should help residents actively interact with nature, enjoy nature, and take care of it. However, more efforts and research are needed in the future for biophilic residential regeneration. For example, short-term economic costs for green roofs and building systems can hinder the creation of a bio-friendly environment. Whilst implementation of these strategies requires policy investment and management, it also leads to long-term cost savings. In addition, to provide biophilic services, it is necessary to provide indicators to understand and measure specific environmental factors favored by local residents, as well as change the modern lifestyle that relies on the means of living indoors and transportation.

The study emphasizes that the Green New Deal project should focus on linking essential relationships rather than on the superficial mutual development of human, natural, and economic benefits. In addition, various methods to apply a bio-friendly design in residential regeneration were explored. The biophilic residential regeneration proposed in this study is worthy of use as a series of indicators that contribute to the Green New Deal and the resilience of the community. This contributes to expanding the understanding of biophilic design and residential regeneration from the perspective of the Green New Deal and provides insight into the conversion of biological ideas into the market in architectural planning and technology development. This study deals with the developed domain of existing theories about the topic of the study and has a challenging value in that it takes into account the linkage with other related variables.

However, by utilizing the few categories presented in the literature and previous studies, this study is limited in comparing and analyzing specific applications, taking into account the characteristics of the local environment and residents and in buildings on clear criteria for the application of biophilic design. This is because the concept of biophilic design is often ambiguous and hardly defined as a single analytical standard, as it is diversified and complex based on the respective researcher and the field and scale of the application. Nevertheless, this study proposes a meaningful theoretical basis for integrating the concepts of the Green New Deal and biophilia, and proposes a detailed plan considering the scale of residential regeneration, along with the features of biophilia based on the concept of biophilia practice. In future research, it is important to establish a system of guidelines that can ease constraints and limitations in the use of biophilic residential regeneration strategies. It is further necessary to specify a strategy for biophilic residential regeneration by considering the cultural characteristics of local residents, the environmental features of local ecosystems, and the level of technology.

**Author Contributions:** Conceptualization and methodology, E.J.L. and S.J.P.; Formal analysis and investigation, E.J.L.; Resources and data curation, E.J.L.; Writing-original draft preparation and visualization, E.J.L.; Writhing-review & editing and supervision, S.J.P. All authors have read and agreed to the published version of the manuscript.

**Funding:** This research was funded by National Research Foundation of Korea (NRF) under the Korean Government Ministry of Education, Science and Technology (MEST), grant number 2018R1C1B6008735; This research was funded by Basic Science Research Program through the National Research Foundation of Korea (NRF) funded by the Ministry of Education, grant number 2020R1A6A3A13077228.

**Conflicts of Interest:** The authors declare no conflict of interest.

## References

1. Martinez-Fernandez, C.; Audirac, I.; Fol, S.; Cunningham-Sabot, E. Shrinking cities: Urban challenges of globalization. *Int. J. Urban Reg. Res.* **2012**, *36*, 213–225. [CrossRef] [PubMed]
2. Klein, N. *On Fire: The (Burning) Case for a Green New Deal*; Simon & Schuster: New York, NY, USA, 2019.
3. Mayors Announce Support For Global Green New Deal; Recognize Global Climate Emergency. Available online: https://www.c40.org/press_releases/global-gnd (accessed on 27 January 2021).
4. Bhuyan, R.; Wahab, S.; Park, Y. A green new deal for social work. *Affilia* **2019**, *34*, 289–294. [CrossRef]
5. Luke, T.W. A green new deal: Why green, how new, and what is the deal? *Crit. Policy Stud.* **2009**, *3*, 14–28. [CrossRef]
6. Kaplan, R.; Kaplan, S. *The Experience of Nature: A Psychological Perspective*; Cambridge University Press: Cambridge, NY, USA, 1989.
7. Herzog, T.R.; Bryce, A.G. Mystery and preference in within-forest settings. *Environ. Behav.* **2007**, *39*, 779–796. [CrossRef]
8. Korpela, K.M.; Ylén, M.; Tyrväinen, L.; Silvennoinen, H. Favorite green, waterside and urban environments, restorative experiences and perceived health in Finland. *Health Promot. Int.* **2010**, *25*, 200–209. [CrossRef]
9. Wilson, E.O. *Biophilia*; Harvard University Press: Cambridge, MA, USA, 1984.
10. Kellert, S.R.; Wilson, E.O. *The Biophilia Hypothesis*; Island Press: Avenue, NW, USA; Washington, DC, USA, 1993.
11. Kellert, S.R.; Heerwagen, J.; Mador, M. *Biophilic Design: The Theory, Science and Practice of Bringing Buildings to Life*; John Wiley and Sons: Hoboken, NJ, USA, 2011.
12. Ryan, C.O.; Browning, W.D.; Clancy, J.O.; Andrews, S.L.; Kallianpurkar, N.B. Biophilic design patterns: Emerging nature-based parameters for health and well-being in the built environment. *ArchNet-IJAR J. Archit. Plann. Res.* **2014**, *8*, 62. [CrossRef]
13. Kellert, S.R. *Nature by Design: The Practice of Biophilic Design*; Yale University Press: New Haven, CT, USA; London, UK, 2018.
14. Browning, W.; Kallianpurkar, N.; Ryan, C.; Labruto, L.; Watson, S.; Knop, T. *The Economics of Biophilia*; Terrapin Bright Green LLC.: New York, NY, USA, 2012.
15. Edge, S.; Hayles, C. Examining the economic, psychological and physiological benefits of retrofitting holistic sustainable and biophilic design strategies, for the indoor environment. In Proceedings of the AMPS Proceedings Series 9. Living and Sustainability: An Environmental Critique of Design and Building Practices, Locally and Globally, London, UK, 8–9 February 2017; AMPS: London, UK, 2017; pp. 515–525.
16. Beatley, T. *Handbook of Biophilic City Planning & Design*; Island Press: Washington, DC, USA, 2017.
17. Kuo, F.E.; Sullivan, W.C. Aggression and violence in the inner city: Effects of environment via mental fatigue. *Environ. Behav.* **2001**, *33*, 543–571. [CrossRef]
18. Schuetze, T.; Chelleri, L. Urban sustainability versus green-washing—Fallacy and reality of urban regeneration in downtown Seoul. *Sustainability* **2016**, *8*, 33. [CrossRef]
19. Kim, H.W.; Aaron McCarty, D.; Lee, J. Enhancing Sustainable Urban Regeneration through Smart Technologies: An Assessment of Local Urban Regeneration Strategic Plans in Korea. *Sustainability* **2020**, *12*, 6868. [CrossRef]
20. Zuo, J.; Dong, J.; Li, C. Environmental research on eco-complex network system construction in high-density areas based on urban regeneration. *Ekoloji* **2018**, *27*, 1479–1491.
21. Dargan, L. Participation and local urban regeneration: The case of the New Deal for Communities (NDC) in the UK. *Reg. Stud.* **2009**, *43*, 305–317. [CrossRef]
22. Curtis, S.; Cave, B.; Coutts, A. Is urban regeneration good for health? Perceptions and theories of the health impacts of urban change. *Environ. Plan. C Gov. Policy* **2002**, *20*, 517–534. [CrossRef]
23. Parry, J.; Laburn-Peart, K.; Orford, J.; Dalton, S. Mechanisms by which area-based regeneration programmes might impact on community health: A case study of the new deal for communities initiative. *Public Health* **2004**, *118*, 497–505. [CrossRef] [PubMed]
24. Miller, G.T. *Sustaining the Earth*; Thompson Learning Inc.: Novato, CA, USA, 2004.

25. AR5 Synthesis Report: Climate Change. 2014. Available online: https://www.ipcc.ch/report/ar5/syr/ (accessed on 27 January 2021).
26. Lynas, M. *Six Degrees: Our Future on a Hotter Planet*; National Geographic Books: London, UK, 2008.
27. Girgenti, G.; Prakash, V. *Winning the Green New Deal*; Simon & Schuster: New York, NY, USA, 2020.
28. Barbier, E. How is the global green new deal going? *Nature* **2010**, *464*, 832–833. [CrossRef]
29. Hockett, R.C.; Gunn-Wright, R. *The Green New Deal: Mobilizing for a Just, Prosperous, and Sustainable Economy*; Cornell Legal Studies Research Paper No.19-09; Elsevier: New York, NY, USA, 2019. [CrossRef]
30. Rifkin, J. *The Green New Deal: Why the Fossil Fuel Civilization Will Collapse by 2028, and the Bold Economic Plan to Save Life on Earth*; St. Martin's Press: New York, NY, USA, 2019.
31. Aronoff, K.; Battistoni, A.; Cohen, D.A.; Riofrancos, T. *A Planet to Win: Why We Need a Green New Deal*; Verso Books: London, UK, 2019.
32. Leiserowitz, A.A.; Maibach, E.; Roser-Renouf, C.; Feinberg, G.; Rosenthal, S. *Climate Change in the American Mind*; Yale University: New Haven, CT, USA, 2016.
33. Pachauri, R.K.; Allen, M.R.; Barros, V.R.; Broome, J.; Cramer, W.; Christ, R.; Church, J.A.; Clarke, L.; Dahe, Q.; Dasgupta, P. *Climate Change 2014: Synthesis Report. Contribution of Working Groups I, II and III to the Fifth Assessment Report of the Intergovernmental Panel on Climate Change*; IPCC: Geneva, Switzerland, 2014.
34. Richardson, K.; Steffen, W.; Liverman, D. *Climate Change: Global Risks, Challenges and Decisions*; Cambridge University Press: Cambridge, UK, 2011.
35. Lee, S.; Koh, M. *Climate Change and the Future of the Environment*; 21cbooks: Seoul, Korea, 2019.
36. Klein, R.J.; Schipper, E.L.F.; Dessai, S. Integrating mitigation and adaptation into climate and development policy: Three research questions. *Environ. Sci. Policy* **2005**, *8*, 579–588. [CrossRef]
37. Yohe, G.; Tol, R.S. Indicators for social and economic coping capacity—moving toward a working definition of adaptive capacity. *Glob. Environ. Chang.* **2002**, *12*, 25–40. [CrossRef]
38. The 8 Million Species We Don't Know. Available online: https://www.nytimes.com/2018/03/03/opinion/sunday/species-conservation-extinction.html (accessed on 8 August 2020).
39. Fromm, E. *The Heart of Man: Its Genius for Good and Evil*; Lantern Books: New York, NY, USA, 2011.
40. Holling, C.S. Resilience and stability of ecological systems. *Annu. Rev. Ecol. Evol. Syst.* **1973**, *4*, 1–23. [CrossRef]
41. Ulrich, R.S.; Simons, R.F.; Losito, B.D.; Fiorito, E.; Miles, M.A.; Zelson, M. Stress recovery during exposure to natural and urban environments. *J. Environ. Psychol.* **1991**, *11*, 201–230. [CrossRef]
42. Kaplan, R. *The Psychological Benefits of Nearby Nature*; Timber Press: Portland, OR, USA, 1992.
43. Arvay, C.G. *Biophilia in der Stadt*; Wilhelm Goldmann: München, Germany, 2018.
44. Lee, E.J.; Park, S.J. A Framework of Smart-Home Service for Elderly's Biophilic Experience. *Sustainability* **2020**, *12*, 8572. [CrossRef]
45. Butzer, K.W. Environment, Culture, and Human Evolution: Hominids first evolved in mosaic environments, but stone toolmaking accelerated the emergence of Homo, and both culture and environment subsequently served as catalysts for evolution. *Am. Sci.* **1977**, *65*, 572–584.
46. Orians, G.H. Habitat selection: General theory and applications to human behavior. In *The Evolution of Human Social Behavior*; Elsevier: Chicago, IL, USA, 1980.
47. Appleton, J. *The Experience of Landscape*; Wiley Chichester: New York, NY, USA, 1996.
48. Goldhagen, S.W. *Welcome to Your World*; HarperCollins: New York, NY, USA, 2017.
49. Beatley, T.; Newman, P. Biophilic cities are sustainable, resilient cities. *Sustainability* **2013**, *5*, 3328–3345. [CrossRef]
50. Mazuch, R. Salutogenic and biophilic design as therapeutic approaches to sustainable architecture. *Archit. Des.* **2017**, *87*, 42–47. [CrossRef]
51. Reeve, A.C.; Desha, C.; Hargreaves, D.; Hargroves, K. Biophilic urbanism: Contributions to holistic urban greening for urban renewal. *Smart Sustain. Built Environ.* **2015**, *4*, 215–233. [CrossRef]
52. Exploring the Nature Pyramid. Available online: https://www.thenatureofcities.com/2012/08/07/exploring-the-nature-pyramid/ (accessed on 21 July 2020).
53. Berman, M.G.; Jonides, J.; Kaplan, S. The cognitive benefits of interacting with nature. *Psychol. Sci.* **2008**, *19*, 1207–1212. [CrossRef] [PubMed]
54. Detweiler, M.B.; Murphy, P.F.; Kim, K.Y.; Myers, L.C.; Ashai, A. Scheduled medications and falls in dementia patients utilizing a wander garden. *Am. J. Alzheimer's Dis. Other Dement.* **2009**, *24*, 322–332. [CrossRef]
55. Ohtsuka, Y.; Yabunaka, N.; Takayama, S. Shinrin-yoku (forest-air bathing and walking) effectively decreases blood glucose levels in diabetic patients. *Int. J. Biometeorol.* **1998**, *41*, 125–127. [CrossRef]
56. Choi, D.Y.; Jung, S.-H.; Song, D.K.; An, E.J.; Park, D.; Kim, T.-O.; Jung, J.H.; Lee, H.M. Al-coated conductive fibrous filter with low pressure drop for efficient electrostatic capture of ultrafine particulate pollutants. *ACS Appl. Mater. Interfaces* **2017**, *9*, 16495–16504. [CrossRef]
57. Brown, D.K.; Barton, J.L.; Gladwell, V.F. Viewing nature scenes positively affects recovery of autonomic function following acute-mental stress. *Environ. Sci. Technol.* **2013**, *47*, 5562–5569. [CrossRef] [PubMed]
58. Tsunetsugu, Y.; Lee, J.; Park, B.-J.; Tyrväinen, L.; Kagawa, T.; Miyazaki, Y. Physiological and psychological effects of viewing urban forest landscapes assessed by multiple measurements. *Landsc. Urban Plan.* **2013**, *113*, 90–93. [CrossRef]

59. Van Den Berg, A.E.; Custers, M.H. Gardening promotes neuroendocrine and affective restoration from stress. *J. Health Psychol.* **2011**, *16*, 3–11. [CrossRef] [PubMed]
60. Figueiro, M.; Brons, J.; Plitnick, B.; Donlan, B.; Leslie, R.; Rea, M. Measuring circadian light and its impact on adolescents. *Light. Res. Technol.* **2011**, *43*, 201–215. [CrossRef]
61. Beckett, M.; Roden, L. Mechanisms by which circadian rhythm disruption may lead to cancer. *S. Afr. J. Sci.* **2009**, *105*, 415–420. [CrossRef]
62. Takano, T.; Nakamura, K.; Watanabe, M. Urban residential environments and senior citizens' longevity in megacity areas: The importance of walkable green spaces. *J. Epidemiol. Community Health* **2002**, *56*, 913–918. [CrossRef] [PubMed]
63. Chang, C.-Y.; Chen, P.-K. Human response to window views and indoor plants in the workplace. *HortScience* **2005**, *40*, 1354–1359. [CrossRef]
64. Kaplan, R. The role of nature in the context of the workplace. *Landsc. Urban Plan.* **1993**, *26*, 193–201. [CrossRef]
65. Biederman, I.; Vessel, E.A. Perceptual pleasure and the brain: A novel theory explains why the brain craves information and seeks it through the senses. *Am. Sci.* **2006**, *94*, 247–253. [CrossRef]
66. Taylor, A.F.; Kuo, F.E.; Sullivan, W.C. Coping with ADD: The surprising connection to green play settings. *Environ. Behav.* **2001**, *33*, 54–77. [CrossRef]
67. Mehta, R.; Zhu, R.; Cheema, A. Is noise always bad? Exploring the effects of ambient noise on creative cognition. *J. Consum. Res.* **2012**, *39*, 784–799. [CrossRef]
68. Franco, L.S.; Shanahan, D.F.; Fuller, R.A. A review of the benefits of nature experiences: More than meets the eye. *Int. J. Environ. Res. Public Health* **2017**, *14*, 864. [CrossRef] [PubMed]
69. Lichtenfeld, S.; Elliot, A.J.; Maier, M.A.; Pekrun, R. Fertile green: Green facilitates creative performance. *Psychol. Bull.* **2012**, *38*, 784–797. [CrossRef]
70. Ulrich, R.S. View through a window may influence recovery from surgery. *Science* **1984**, *224*, 420–421. [CrossRef] [PubMed]
71. Bergs, J. *Effect of Healthy Workplaces: Office Work, Well-Being, and Productivity*; Green Solar Architecture: Amersfoort, The Netherlands, 2002.
72. Elzeyadi, I. Daylighting-Bias and Biophilia: Quantifying the Impacts of daylight on Occupants Health. Available online: https://www.usgbc.org/sites/default/files/OR10_Daylighting%20Bias%20and%20Biophilia.pdf (accessed on 30 May 2020).
73. Wolfs, E.L. Biophilic Design and Bio-Collaboration: Applications and Implications in the Field of Industrial Design. *Arch. Des. Res.* **2015**, *28*, 71–89. [CrossRef]
74. Beatley, T. *Biophilic Cities: Integrating Nature into Urban Design and Planning*; Island Press: Washington, DC, USA, 2010.
75. Edwards, L.; Torcellini, P. *Literature Review of the Effects of Natural Light on Building Occupants*; National Renewable Energy Lab.: Golden, CO, USA, 2002.
76. Maas, J.; Van Dillen, S.M.; Verheij, R.A.; Groenewegen, P.P. Social contacts as a possible mechanism behind the relation between green space and health. *Health Place* **2009**, *15*, 586–595. [CrossRef] [PubMed]
77. Sullivan, S.; Ruffman, T. Emotion recognition deficits in the elderly. *Int. J. Neurosci.* **2004**, *114*, 403–432. [CrossRef] [PubMed]
78. Banks, M.R.; Willoughby, L.M.; Banks, W.A. Animal-assisted therapy and loneliness in nursing homes: Use of robotic versus living dogs. *J. Am. Med. Dir. Assoc.* **2008**, *9*, 173–177. [CrossRef]
79. Han, A.-R.; Park, S.-A.; Ahn, B.-E. Reduced stress and improved physical functional ability in elderly with mental health problems following a horticultural therapy program. *Complement. Ther. Med.* **2018**, *38*, 19–23. [CrossRef]
80. Troy, A.; Grove, J.M.; O'Neil-Dunne, J. The relationship between tree canopy and crime rates across an urban–rural gradient in the greater Baltimore region. *Landsc. Urban Plan.* **2012**, *106*, 262–270. [CrossRef]
81. Kim, S.-I. *Solution Green*; Medicimedia: Seoul, Korea, 2011.
82. Chen, Y. The Impact of Biophilic Design on Health and Wellbeing of Residents through Raising Environmental Awareness and Nature Connectedness. Ph.D. Thesis, University of Georgia, Athens, Georgia, 2017.
83. Mayrand, F.; Clergeau, P. Green roofs and green walls for biodiversity conservation: A contribution to urban connectivity? *Sustainability* **2018**, *10*, 985. [CrossRef]
84. Newman, P.; Hargroves, K.; Desha, C.; Reeve, A.; el-Baghdadi, O.; Bucknum, M.; Salter, R. *Can Biophilic Urbanism Deliver Strong Economic and Social Benefits in Cities*; The Sustainable Built Environment National Research Centre: Perth, Australia, 2012.
85. Depledge, M.H.; Stone, R.J.; Bird, W. Can natural and virtual environments be used to promote improved human health and wellbeing? *Environ. Sci. Technol.* **2011**, *45*, 4660–4665. [CrossRef]
86. Francis, R.A.; Lorimer, J. Urban reconciliation ecology: The potential of living roofs and walls. *J. Environ. Manag.* **2011**, *92*, 1429–1437. [CrossRef] [PubMed]
87. Parsaee, M.; Demers, C.M.; Hébert, M.; Lalonde, J.-F.; Potvin, A. Biophilic, photobiological and energy-efficient design framework of adaptive building façades for Northern Canada. *Indoor Built Environ.* **2020**, 1–27. [CrossRef]
88. Söderlund, J. *The Emergence of Biophilic Design*; Springer: Perth, Australia, 2019.
89. Xue, F.; Gou, Z.; Lau, S.S.-Y.; Lau, S.-K.; Chung, K.-H.; Zhang, J. From biophilic design to biophilic urbanism: Stakeholders' perspectives. *J. Clean. Prod.* **2019**, *211*, 1444–1452. [CrossRef]
90. Marshall, A.J.; Williams, N.S. Communicating Biophilic Design: Start With the Grasslands. *Front. Built Environ.* **2019**, *5*, 1. [CrossRef]
91. Kahn, P.H., Jr.; Kellert, S.R. *Children and Nature: Psychological, Sociocultural, and Evolutionary Investigations*; MIT Press: Cambridge, MA, USA, 2002.

92. Liu, J.; Kang, J.; Luo, T.; Behm, H. Landscape effects on soundscape experience in city parks. *Sci. Total Environ.* **2013**, *454*, 474–481. [CrossRef] [PubMed]
93. Diette, G.B.; Lechtzin, N.; Haponik, E.; Devrotes, A.; Rubin, H.R. Distraction therapy with nature sights and sounds reduces pain during flexible bronchoscopy: A complementary approach to routine analgesia. *Chest* **2003**, *123*, 941–948. [CrossRef]
94. Cheang, M. Urban Nature: Designing Apartment Unites with Nature Based on Biophilic Relationships. Ph.D. Thesis, University of Hawaii at Manoa, Honolulu, HI, USA, 2012.
95. White, M.; Smith, A.; Humphryes, K.; Pahl, S.; Snelling, D.; Depledge, M. Blue space: The importance of water for preference, affect, and restorativeness ratings of natural and built scenes. *J. Environ. Psychol.* **2010**, *30*, 482–493. [CrossRef]
96. Lee, E.J.; Park, S.J. Immersive experience model of the elderly welfare centers supporting successful aging. *Front. Psychol.* **2020**, *11*. [CrossRef]
97. Hedblom, M.; Heyman, E.; Antonsson, H.; Gunnarsson, B. Bird song diversity influences young people's appreciation of urban landscapes. *Urban For. Urban Green.* **2014**, *13*, 469–474. [CrossRef]
98. Yin, J. Bringing Nature Indoors With Virtual Reality: Human Reponses to Biophilic Design in Buildings. Ph.D. Thesis, Harvard University, Cambridge, MA, USA, 2019.
99. Benyus, J.M. *Biomimicry: Innovation Inspired by Nature*; William Morrow: New York, NY, USA, 1997.
100. Rivas-Sánchez, Y.A.; Moreno-Pérez, M.F.; Roldán-Cañas, J. Environment control with low-cost microcontrollers and microprocessors: Application for green walls. *Sustainability* **2019**, *11*, 782. [CrossRef]
101. Hardyanto, R.H.; Ciptadi, P.W.; Asmara, A. Smart Aquarium Based On Internet of Things. *Int. J. Bus. Inf. Syst.* **2019**, *1*, 48–53. [CrossRef]
102. Tapping into Nature. Available online: https://www.terrapinbrightgreen.com/tapping-into-nature/ (accessed on 16 October 2020).
103. Mazzoleni, I. *Architecture Follows Nature-Biomimetic Principles for Innovative Design*; NYCRC Press: New York, NY, USA, 2013; Volume 2.
104. Bejan, A.; Zane, J.P. *Design in Nature: How the Constructal Law Governs Evolution in Biology, Physics, Technology, and Social Organizations*; Doubleday: New York, NY, USA, 2012.
105. ASHRAE, A. *Standard 62.1-2013 Ventilation for Acceptable Indoor Air Quality*; American Society of Heating, Refrigerating and Air-Conditioning Engineers, Inc.: Atlanta, GA, USA, 2013; p. 40.

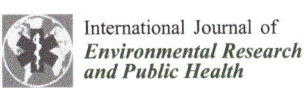

## Article

# Self-Administered Six-Minute Walk Test Using a Free Smartphone App in Asymptomatic Adults: Reliability and Reproducibility

Matheus Oliveira de Jesus [1], Thatiane Lopes Valentim Di Paschoale Ostolin [1], Neli Leite Proença [1], Rodrigo Pereira da Silva [1] and Victor Zuniga Dourado [1,2,*]

[1] Department of Human Movement Sciences, Federal University of São Paulo (UNIFESP), Santos 11015-020, SP, Brazil; matheus.oliveira93@hotmail.com.br (M.O.d.J.); thatiane.ostolin@unifesp.br (T.L.V.D.P.O.); nelieluana@gmail.com (N.L.P.); r.pereirads@hotmail.com (R.P.d.S.)
[2] Lown Scholars Program, Harvard T.H. Chan School of Public Health, Boston, MA 02115, USA
* Correspondence: victor.dourado@unifesp.br

**Abstract:** Background: The 6-min walk test (6MWT) is a simple, inexpensive, reliable, and reproducible test that provides a reasonable estimate of the cardiorespiratory fitness (CRF). We aimed to assess the reliability and reproducibility of a self-administered 6MWT in asymptomatic adults using a free smartphone app. Methods: In the 1st phase, 93 participants underwent a supervised 6MWT (6MWTsup) in a 30 m indoor corridor, using a triaxial accelerometer and their smartphones to compare the total step counts and to develop a 6-min walk distance (6MWD) prediction equation. In the 2nd phase, 25 participants performed the 6MWTsup and two self-administered 6MWTs outdoors (6MWTsa1 and 6MWTsa2, at least 48 h apart) using a free smartphone app. Results: The agreement between accelerometer- and app-based total step counts was limited (mean difference, −58.7 steps (−8.7%): 95% confidence interval, −326.5 (−46.8%) to 209.1 (29.3%)). The best algorithm for predicting the 6MWTsup$_m$ included: 795.456 + (0.815 height$_m$ app-steps) − (1.620 age$_{years}$) − (3.005 weight$_{kg}$) − (1.155 app-steps), $R^2$ = 0.609). The intraclass correlation coefficient between 6MWTsa2 and 6MWTsa1 was excellent (0.91: 0.81−0.96). The coefficient of variation was 6.4%. The agreement between the two self-administered tests was narrow (−1.9 (0.2%) meters: −57.4 (−9.5%) to 61.3 (9.9%)). Conclusions: The self-administered 6MWT has excellent reliability and reproducibility in asymptomatic adults, being a valuable tool for assessing CRF in community-based interventions.

**Keywords:** cardiorespiratory fitness; accelerometer; 6-minute walk test; physical activity level; health and public health; app; applications

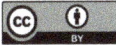

## 1. Introduction

Cardiorespiratory fitness (CRF) is one of the main domains of physical fitness. It refers to the cardiovascular, metabolic, and respiratory systems' ability to absorb, transport, and consume oxygen during the long-term physical effort of moderate-to-vigorous intensity [1]. High CRF is associated with lower cardiovascular and all-cause mortality [2,3]. In contrast, low CRF is considered one of the causes of diabetes mellitus, hypertension, coronary artery disease, and several types of cancer [4]. CRF alone holds predictive value for cardiovascular events, similar to the combination of classic cardiovascular risk factors [4]. CRF evaluation is essential to predict and assess the prognosis of several diseases [5] and the prescription of physical exercise and monitoring rehabilitation programs' results [4]. Accordingly, CRF has been considered a vital sign in cardiovascular health as a routine clinical practice strategy [4]. However, if the administration of the maximum exercise test is not possible, submaximal, and field tests—and even CRF estimation using prediction equations—must be performed in environments with few resources. Despite the evidence, the evaluation of CRF is yet to be incorporated as a routine strategy for screening cardiovascular risk.

The 6-min walk test (6MWT) is a simple, inexpensive, reliable, and reproducible test performed according to international standardization [6]. Initially, the 6MWT was developed to assess patients with cardiorespiratory diseases; however, it has already been validated in several diverse populations [7]. Furthermore, the 6MWT correlates consistently with the maximum oxygen consumption ($VO^2max$) both in patients with chronic diseases and in asymptomatic adults [8], and has several reference values [7]. The test is usually performed in a controlled environment [6] and has already been performed on thousands of patients with chronic diseases without any report of serious cardiovascular events [9,10], which suggests its safety. Therefore, the 6MWT provides a reasonable estimate of the CRF, especially in people with non-severe chronic diseases.

The six-minute walk test may be helpful in healthy asymptomatic subjects for cardiovascular risk screening in the clinical practice [4], due to its low cost, easy application, and performed in international standardization [6]. Furthermore, a walking distance below 96% of the predicted values can identify asymptomatic adults with low physical activity levels [11] and cardiorespiratory fitness [12]. Thus, it can be an excellent strategy to reduce the risk of cardiovascular disease.

The use of health applications (apps) has increased dramatically with the advent of mobile technology devices, such as smartphones and tablets. Their low cost and ease of use turned them into objects of epidemiological studies aiming at behavior changes through goal-setting, self-monitoring, and performance feedback [13]. Moreover, the efficiency of apps, combined with the ability to measure the distance covered by the Global Positioning System (GPS) and the number of steps using accelerometers built into the devices, opens up the possibility of using smartphone apps to self-administer the 6MWT. Thus, self-assessment of CRF would enable better cardiovascular risk screening and information for clinicians and primary care professionals. However, to the best of our knowledge, few studies have investigated the reliability and reproducibility of self-administration of the 6MWT [14–16], mainly involving patients in rehabilitation who undergo routine treatment with 6MWT and using paid apps. We are unaware of previous studies investigating the reliability and reproducibility of a self-administered 6MWT in the general population using a free smartphone app with a step-monitoring function.

Accordingly, this study aimed to assess the reliability and reproducibility of a self-administered 6MWT in asymptomatic adults using a free smartphone app for step counting.

## 2. Materials and Methods

### 2.1. Sample, Recruitment, and Design

The first phase of the study comprised 93 asymptomatic participants aged between 30 and 70 years old, with non-relevant cardiorespiratory, metabolic, or locomotor disorders that could preclude normal gait, as well as physical exercise. Participants should be engaged in technology, i.e., they use smartphone devices. We recruited participants through social networks, posters at regional universities, and local print media. Participants with abnormalities found during exercise testing, which could prevent the performance of unsupervised physical exercises, were excluded, such as an exam suggestive of myocardial ischemia, potentially lethal arrhythmias, and hyper-reactive blood pressure responses. We also excluded participants with spirometric abnormalities.

This phase's objective was to develop a 6MWT distance prediction equation using the number of steps performed and demographic and anthropometric attributes. The second phase consisted of 25 participants performing a supervised 6MWT (6MWTsup), and within the seven days after that, two more self-administered tests (6MWTsa) were performed, either indoors or outdoors, and in a safe environment, using a free smartphone app available at app stores. The study was submitted to, and approved by, the local Human Research Ethics Committee. All participants signed an informed consent form related to the study's objectives, methods, benefits, and possible risks.

The study participation was formalized by the signature of the free and informed consent form. The research was approved by the ethic in research committee of the Federal University of Sao Paulo, CEP/UNIFESP #1485/2017.

## 2.2. Application Choice

The researchers tested several free smartphone apps before starting the study; the most popular apps with a step count function that worked on the most popular operating systems (i.e., iOS and Android) were downloaded. In this list, we found applications such as Fitbit, Apple Health, Google fit, MyFitnessPal, MapMyWalk, Runtastic, and Runkeeper, among others. After a final meeting, we chose the app Pacer, mainly based on user ratings. Pacer has 4.9 rating stars in the app store and was reported by researchers as the most attractive. The researchers agreed with this choice due to some characteristics of the app mentioned above, which are as follows: (1) its proper functioning on the two most popular operating systems; (2) its accuracy in monitoring the number of daily steps; (3) the app's several gamification functions, such as goal setting, rewards, badges, progress bars, walking and running rankings, and forming groups with their social network. Although not necessary for the present study, these characteristics were decisive in stimulating technology to increase physical activity and fitness. Therefore, we investigated the agreement between the number of steps provided by the Pacer application and the triaxial accelerometer during the supervised six-minute walk test. We used the equation developed in the first phase to estimate the distance in the 6MWTsa performed with Pacer in the second phase.

## 2.3. Phase 1 Protocol

The phase 1 evaluation protocol was divided into two days, with a seven-day interval. On the first day of the evaluation, the participants underwent an initial health screening. After obtaining anthropometric measurements, we performed spirometry and cardiopulmonary exercise testing. On the second day, participants performed the 6MWTsup according to international recommendations [6].

## 2.4. Health Screening

We obtained from participants socio-demographic data (age, sex, schooling), health history, and classic cardiovascular risk factors for cardiovascular diseases, such as current smoking, obesity, high blood pressure, diabetes mellitus, dyslipidemia, and physical inactivity. Those who reported less than 150 min/week of moderate to intense physical activity or less than 75 min of intense physical activity per week were considered physically inactive [17]. We measured height (cm) and body mass (kg) using a digital scale with a stadiometer (Toledo™, Sao Paulo, Brazil) to calculate the body mass index (BMI) (kg/m$^2$). Obesity was considered when BMI $\geq$ 30 kg/m$^2$.

## 2.5. Supervised 6MWT

After seven days, participants performed the 6MWTsup in an indoor 30 m hallway under the supervision of two experienced examiners, following international recommendations [6]. The participants used a triaxial accelerometer (ActiGraph GTX3x+, MTI, Pensacola, FL, USA) to count the number of steps during the test. The participants simultaneously performed the 6MWTsup with their smartphones in their pocket to record the total number of steps obtained in the Pacer app. We recorded the distance covered in the 6MWT (6MWD) and the total accelerometer and app-based step counts.

## 2.6. Phase 2 Protocol

Phase two comprised 25 participants for the cross-validation sample, and participants performed a 6MWTsup in the same corridor adjacent to the laboratory, strictly equal to that performed in phase 1 for the first study sample.

*2.7. Self-Administered 6MWT*

The cross-validation sample ($n$ = 25) performed two tests at least 24 h apart. We instructed participants to measure baseline measurements of heart rate, perceived exertion, and blood pressure. Heart rate was measured by a validated smartphone app [18], and dyspnea and leg fatigue using the Borg scale [19]. We advised participants to use their own devices or visit a health facility (pharmacy, hospitals, or health centers) on the day of the test to measure their blood pressure.

For the test to be performed effectively, the participants were instructed to perform the tests on a straight course and, preferably, going back and forth over 20 m, in an open place with mild temperatures around 26 °C. The participants were also allowed to perform the tests indoors, as long as the course was long enough and straight. All were instructed to perform two 6MWTs in the same climatic conditions, time of day, and course.

The cardiopulmonary exercise test results, especially of the stress electrocardiogram, were discussed previously to ensure the participants' safety. Furthermore, four measurements of blood pressure at rest in the seven days of the protocol were performed, which allowed for rigorous screening of these participants with the cardiologist. All were advised not to perform the tests if the heart rate was above 120 bpm and/or blood pressure above 150/100 mmHg. The 6MWTsa distances were estimated based on the equation developed in phase 1 and then were compared to the 6MWTsup of phase 2.

*2.8. Statistical Analysis*

Statistical analysis was conducted using the statistical packages SPSS (IBM Corp., Armonk, NY, USA), version 23, and MedCalc (MedCalc Software Ltd., Ostend, Belgium), version 14. The data are presented as mean ± standard deviation for continuous variables, and counts/percentages for categorical variables.

2.8.1. Phase 1

The initial comparison was between the accelerometer- and app-based step counts obtained in the 6MWTsup in the initial sample ($n$ = 93). We compared means using Student's $t$-test. The reliability of the app was assessed by calculating the intraclass correlation coefficient (ICC) and its 95% confidence interval (95%CI), and the coefficient of variation (CV) of the mean difference to its standard deviation. We used the Bland plots method [20] to investigate the agreement between accelerometer- and app-based step counts by calculating the mean difference and its 95%CI against the average of the two approaches.

We fit stepwise multiple linear regressions to predict the 6MWTsup distance based on the total step counts and demographic (age and sex) and anthropometric (weight, height, and BMI) variables. A sensitivity analysis was used to identify the main predictors with linear models and a quadratic model, including age × age$^2$. The potential of the variable height × 0.41 and the interaction between height × number of steps was also investigated, as previously suggested [14]. We used the same sensitivity analysis to compare the step counts between the devices used (i.e., accelerometer vs. app). We found a stronger correlation of the distance walked with the app-based step counts, compared with that observed for the accelerometer-based counts. Because of the easier applicability of the app-based step counts in real life, the best equation was developed based on the app-based step counts. Considering an $R^2$ of this equation around 0.50 in previous studies [21], the statistical power of 80%, the alpha error of 0.05, and five predictors included in the analysis, 93 participants were needed to elaborate the equation in Phase 1 [22].

2.8.2. Phase 2

In a second cross-validation sample ($n$ = 25), the 6MWTsup was conducted under the same conditions to obtain the measured 6MWTsup distance. The Pacer app was used to evaluate the measurement properties of the 6MWTsa. The first and second 6MWTsa distances were estimated using the prediction equation developed in phase 1. We compared the distances using the paired Student's *t*-test. The reliability of the 6MWTsa was investigated by the ICC and 95%CI and by the CV. The reproducibility of the 6MWTsa was evaluated by the Bland and Altman plot [23] comparing the second 6MWTsa (6MWTsa2) and first 6MWTsa (6MWTsa1). We also investigated the agreement between 6MWTsa2 and 6MWTsup and 6MWTsa1 and 6MWTsup using the Bland and Altman method.

We considered the ICC values smaller than 0.5, between 0.5 and 0.75, between 0.75 and 0.9, and greater than 0.90 as indicative of weak, moderate, good, and excellent reliability, respectively [20]. For CV, the values considered acceptable were lower than 12%. We set the probability of alpha error for all tests at 5%.

## 3. Results

We evaluated 93 participants during phase 1 (39 men, 54 women). The participants were, on average, middle-aged and overweight. Except for a higher proportion of obese subjects and a slightly lower proportion of smokers, the other cardiovascular risk factors remained similar to the general population in Brazil [24] (Table 1). Phase 2's 25 participants were significantly younger, predominantly male, and represented a lower proportion of hypertensive and diabetic patients. However, they presented higher smoking and physical inactivity ratios (Table 2).

**Table 1.** General characteristics of sample enrolled in phase 1 to develop the prediction equation for six-minute walk distance (*n* = 93).

| Variables | Males (*n* = 39) | Females (*n* = 54) | Total Sample (*n* = 93) |
|---|---|---|---|
| Age (years) | 42 ± 6 | 46 ± 11 | 44 ± 10 |
| Weight (kg) | 81.0 ± 17.7 | 70.4 ± 11.8 | 74.8 ± 15.4 |
| Height (cm) | 173 ± 6 | 59 ± 6 | 165 ± 9 |
| BMI (kg/m$^2$) | 26.8 ± 4.4 | 27.6 ± 5.2 | 27.3 ± 4.9 |
| Cardiovascular risk factors, *n* (%) | | | |
| Arterial hypertension [a] | 6 (15.4) | 11 (20.4) | 17 (18.3) |
| Diabetes [a] | 2 (5.1) | 8 (14.8) | 10 (10.8) |
| Dyslipidemia [a] | 6 (15.4) | 11 (20.4) | 17 (18.3) |
| Obesity | 8 (20.5) | 16 (29.6) | 24 (25.8) |
| Current smoking [a] | 3 (7.7) | 7 (13) | 10 (10.8) |
| Physical inactivity | 4 (10.3) | 3 (5.6) | 7 (7.5) |
| Six-minute walk distance (m) | 670 ± 65 | 602 ± 81 | 633 ± 81 |
| Step counts (accelerometer) | 767 ± 84 | 758 ± 76 | 762 ± 79 |
| Step counts (application) | 721 ± 112 | 686 ± 111 | 704 ± 112 |

Data were expressed as mean ± standard deviation of frequency (%). BMI: Body Mass Index. [a]: cardiovascular risk factor self-reported.

The distance covered in the 6MWTsup was significantly correlated with age, height, BMI, accelerometer-based step counts, and app-based step counts. Although it did not reach statistical significance, weight presented a weak correlation with 6MWTsup (Table 3). After stepwise multiple regression analysis, the interaction between height and app-based step counts, age, weight, and app-based step counts was the main predictor of 6MWDsup, explaining almost 61% of outcome variability (Table 4).

The mean difference between measured and estimated 6MWD calculated using the equation developed in phase 1 was only −2.1 m (0.6%) with a 95% confidence interval (95%CI) from −110.4 (−17.4%) to 106.2 (16.1%) (Figure 1a,b). The correlation between values was strong (r = 0.77; *p* < 0.001; R$^2$ = 0.59). The ICC was good (0.855: 0.671–0.936), as was the CV (6.1%). Although it did not reach statistical significance, the mean values of 6MWD tended to be positively correlated with the mean difference (*p* = 0.07).

The agreement between accelerometer- and app-based total step counts during the 6MWTsup was limited (mean difference, −58.7 steps (−8.7%): 95% confidence interval, −326.5 (−46.8%) to 209.1 (29.3%)) (Figure 2a,b). The correlation between the two measurements was non-significant (r = 0.13; *p* = 0.832) and the CV was higher than 12% (16.4%).

Table 2. General characteristics of the sample used for cross-sectional validation (n = 25).

| Variables | Males (n = 16) | Females (n = 9) | Total Sample (n = 25) |
|---|---|---|---|
| Age (years) | 38 ± 8 | 41 ± 10 | 36 ± 9 |
| Weight (kg) | 88.6 ± 18.4 | 70.2 ± 13.5 | 82.0 ± 18.8 |
| Height (cm) | 176 ± 6 | 162 ± 5 | 171 ± 9 |
| BMI (kg/m$^2$) | 28.4 ± 5.0 | 26.6 ± 5.0 | 27.8 ± 5.0 |
| Cardiovascular risk factors, n (%) | | | |
| Arterial hypertension [a] | 2 (12) | 0 (0) | 2 (8) |
| Diabetes [a] | 0 (0) | 0 (0) | 0 (0) |
| Dyslipidemia [a] | 3 (18) | 3 (33) | 6 (24) |
| Obesity | 3 (18) | 2 (22) | 5 (20) |
| Current smoking [a] | 3 (18) | 1 (11) | 4 (16) |
| Physical inactivity | 4 (25) | 5 (55) | 9 (36) |
| Six-minute walk distance (m) | 663 ± 79 | 640 ± 69 | 648 ± 84 |
| Step counts (accelerometer) | 754 ± 105 | 761 ± 93 | 754 ± 98 |
| Step counts (application) | 707 ± 112 | 644 ± 138 | 680 ± 123 |

Data were expressed as mean ± standard deviation of frequency (%). BMI: Body Mass Index. [a]: cardiovascular risk factor self-reported.

Table 3. Correlation matrix between the distance covered in the supervised 6MWT (6MWD), demographic, anthropometric attributes and the total number of steps performed in the test (n = 93).

| Variables | | 6MWD (m) | Age (years) | Height (cm) | Weight (kg) | BMI (kg/m$^2$) | Accelerometer-Based Step Counts | App-Based Step Counts |
|---|---|---|---|---|---|---|---|---|
| 6MWD (m) | r | 1 | −0.499 ** | 0.459 ** | −0.166 | −0.512 ** | 0.350 ** | 0.351 ** |
| | p | | 0.000 | 0.000 | 0.073 | 0.000 | 0.000 | 0.003 |
| Age (years) | r | −0.499 ** | 1 | −0.427 ** | −0.124 | 0.155 | −0.215 * | −0.021 |
| | p | 0.000 | | 0.000 | 0,180 | 0.094 | 0.020 | 0.864 |
| Height (cm) | r | 0.459 ** | −0.427 ** | 1 | 0.505 ** | −0.091 | −0.130 | 0.061 |
| | p | 0.000 | 0.000 | | 0.000 | 0.327 | 0.162 | 0.611 |
| Weight (kg) | r | −0.166 | −0.124 | 0.505 ** | 1 | 0.805 ** | −0.378 ** | 0.016 |
| | p | 0.073 | 0.180 | 0.000 | | 0.000 | 0.000 | 0.894 |
| BMI (kg/m$^2$) | r | −0.512 ** | 0.155 | −0.091 | 0.805 ** | 1 | −0.347 ** | −0.032 |
| | p | 0.000 | 0.094 | 0.327 | 0.000 | | 0.000 | 0.792 |
| Accelerometer-based step counts | r | 0.350 ** | −0.215 * | −0.130 | −0.378 ** | −0.347 ** | 1 | 0.025 |
| | p | 0.000 | 0.020 | 0.162 | 0.000 | 0.000 | | 0.834 |
| App-based step counts | r | 0.351 ** | −0.021 | 0.061 | 0.016 | −0.032 | 0.025 | 1 |
| | p | 0.003 | 0.864 | 0.611 | 0.894 | 0.792 | 0.834 | |

* $p < 0.05$; ** $p < 0.01$; BMI: Body Mass Index.

Table 4. Predictive model for six-minute walk distance.

| Variables | Unstandardized Coefficients | | Standardized Coefficients | | | | 95% Confidence Interval of B | |
|---|---|---|---|---|---|---|---|---|
| | B | Standard Error | Beta | Partial R$^2$ | ΔR$^2$ | p | Lower Limit | Upper LIMIT |
| Constant | 795.456 | 593.820 | | | | 0.000 | 676.021 | 914.891 |
| Height$_m$ × app-based step counts | 0.815 | 0.121 | 2.114 | 0.230 | 0.230 | 0.000 | 0.574 | 1.056 |
| Age (years) | −1.620 | 0.754 | −0.185 | 0.348 | 0.119 | 0.035 | −3.125 | −0.115 |
| Weight (kg) | −3.005 | 0.482 | −0.597 | 0.437 | 0.088 | 0.000 | −3.967 | −2.042 |
| App-based step counts | −1.155 | 0.214 | −1.634 | 0.609 | 0.172 | 0.000 | −1.583 | −0.727 |

Model R$^2$ = 0.609; Standard error of estimate = 51.3 m. App-based step counts: total number of steps obtained through smartphone app at the end of six-minute walk test.

In phase 2 of the study, the self-administered 6MWD showed excellent reproducibility. The 6MWTsa2 was less than two meters different from the 6MWTsa1 (mean difference, 1.94 ± 30.27 m; p 0.761), and the difference was normally distributed. Confidence limits were shallow in 22 of 25 participants and were less than 10% (Figure 3a,b). The correlation between the mean difference and the mean values was not significant. Reliability between measurements was also excellent (ICC, 0.91: 95%CI, 0.81–0.96; CV = 6.4%).

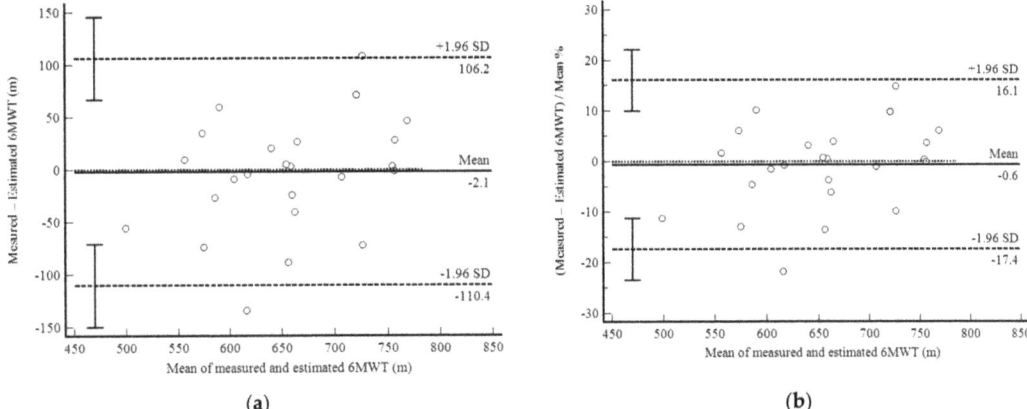

**Figure 1.** Bland and Altman graphic method with limits of agreement and 95% confidence interval (95%CI) between the measured and estimated six-minute walk test (6MWT) using the equation developed in the present study (Phase 1). (**a**) absolute values; (**b**) percentage values.

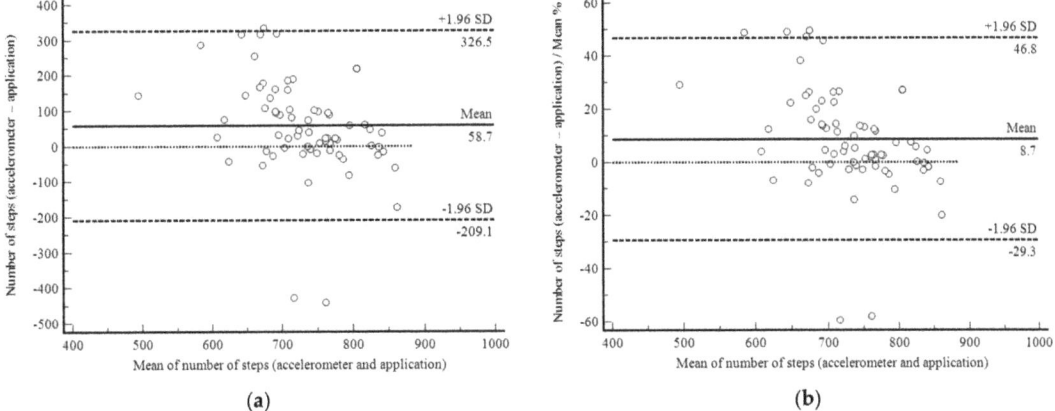

**Figure 2.** Bland and Altman graphic method with limits of agreement and 95% confidence interval (95%CI) between the accelerometer- and app-based number of steps during the supervised six-minute walk test in 93 subjects enrolled in Phase 1 of the present study. (**a**) absolute values; (**b**) percentage values.

The 6MWTsa1 was not significantly different from the 6MWTsup (mean difference, 1.68 ± 61.00 m; $p = 0.894$). The reliability of this evaluation was moderate (ICC, 0.75: 95%CI, 0.42–0.89; CV = 27.5%). The confidence limits were acceptable around 19%, but with a significant negative correlation between the mean difference and the mean values, i.e., the 6MWDsa1 overestimated the results of the subjects who took fewer steps and underestimated the ones who took more steps (Figure 4a,b).

We observed similar results for 6MWDsa2 as above mentioned. Although the mean difference was not statistically significant (3.64 ± 60.57 m; $p$ = 0.776), reliability was considered good (ICC, 0.79: 95%CI, 0.50–0.91; CV = 6.0%). Confidence limits of agreement were acceptable, lower than 19%, but with a significant negative correlation similar to that described for the 6MWTsa1 (Figure 5a,b).

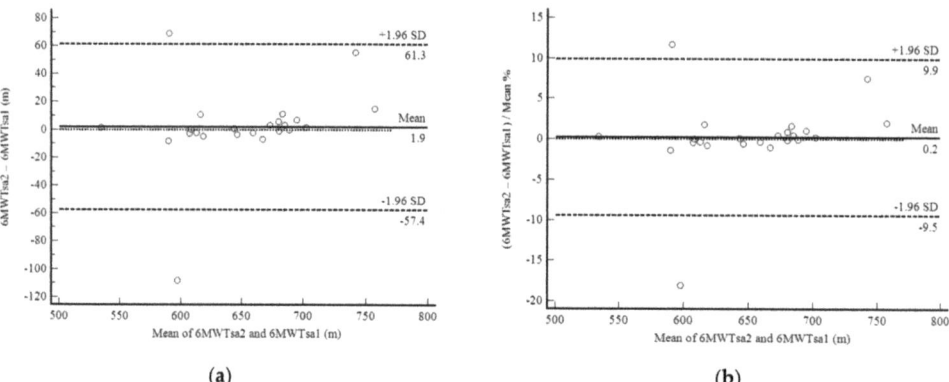

**Figure 3.** Bland and Altman graphic method with limits of agreement and 95% confidence interval (95%CI) between the distance walked estimated by the number of steps and demographic and anthropometric attributes in the second self-administered six-minute walk test (6MWTsa2) and first (6MWTsa1). (**a**) absolute values; (**b**) percentage values.

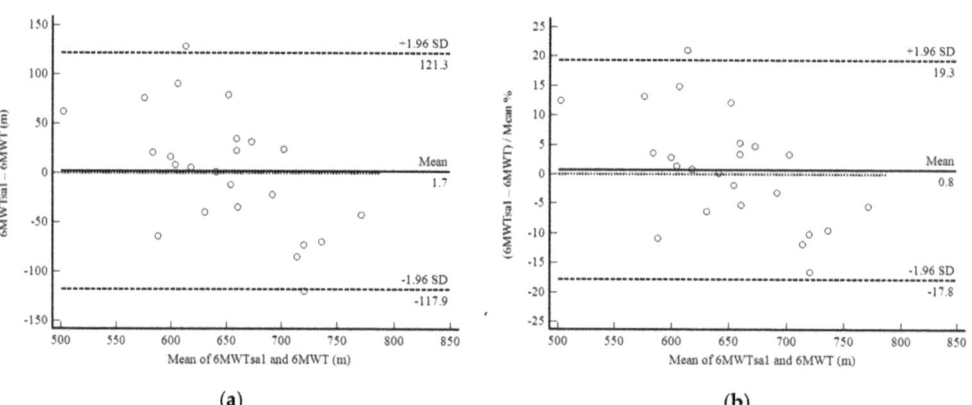

**Figure 4.** Bland and Altman graphic method with limits of agreement and 95% confidence interval (95%CI) between the distance walked estimated by the number of steps and demographic and anthropometric attributes in the first self-administered six-minute walk test (6MWTsa1) and the supervised six-minute walk test distance (6MWT). (**a**) absolute values; (**b**) percentage values.

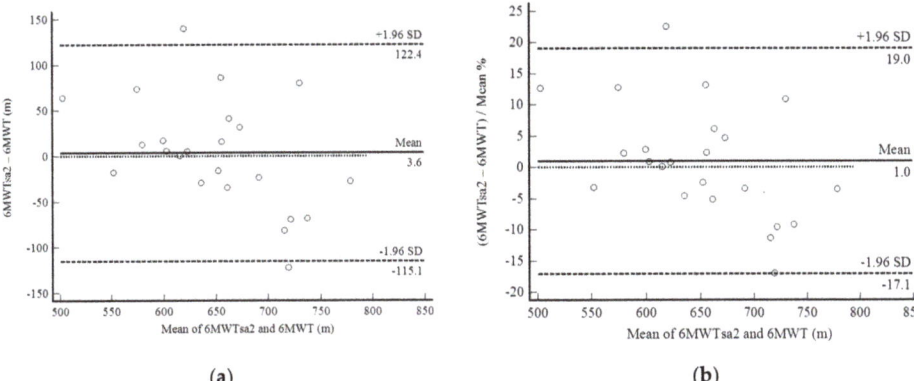

**Figure 5.** Bland and Altman graphic method with limits of agreement and 95% confidence interval (95%CI) between the distance walked estimated by the number of steps and demographic and anthropometric attributes in the second self-administered six-minute walk test (6MWTsa2) and the supervised six-minute walk test distance (6MWT). (**a**) absolute values; (**b**) percentage values.

## 4. Discussion

This study showed the excellent reliability and reproducibility of the self-administered 6MWT in asymptomatic adults using a free-of-charge smartphone app. Although the results were less consistent, the self-administered tests also managed to estimate the accurate distance covered in the 6MWT in a wide range of physical fitness without significant differences. These results were observed despite the low accuracy of the number of steps quantified by the smartphone concerning the direct reference method, i.e., triaxial accelerometer. Nevertheless, demographic, anthropometric attributes, and the interaction between height and app-based step counts ensured greater validity of the proposed estimates.

The main finding was the excellent reliability and reproducibility of 6MWDsa2 with 6MWDsa1. Reliability measures (ICC = 0.91: 0.81–0.96; CV = 6.4%) were excellent and the confidence limits were narrow, below 10% bias. Our results for asymptomatic adults are even more consistent than those previously described for heart failure patients [14] and cancer [15]. Brooks et al. [14] evaluated patients with heart failure in a very similar design to our study. The reliability of the measurements was also high (ICC = 0.88, 95% = 0.77–0.98, IC = 4.7%) after performing the self-administered 6MWT per week (3.2 ± 1.0). The mean difference between the distances was only 7.6 ± 26 m and was less than 15% in 100% of the patients evaluated in Brooks et al. [14]. Through a similar equation and involving the interaction between height and app-based step counts, we observed a mean difference of only 1.94 ± 30.27 m, less than 10% in 96% of cases. These results are encouraging. Our study also presents the advantage of a free app available in the two largest app stores, with good functionality in both iOS and Android systems. We were unable to find the app SA-6MWT to be downloaded, which is the one used in the study by Brooks et al. [14]. Douma et al. [15] used an app also available free of charge (Walkmeter) for self-administration of 6WMT. Reliability values were adequate (ICC = 0.88: 0.74–0.94), unlike the limits of agreement that were limited; lower agreement can be attributed to the fact that the distance traveled in the self-administered tests was quantified with GPS signal since the used app does not have measurements of the number of steps. The results indicate that the self-administration of the 6MWT is promising in patients and asymptomatic adults and that the number of steps, combined with demographic and anthropometric attributes, can improve the effectiveness of this strategy [25].

Regarding the reliability and agreement of 6MWDsa with 6MWDsup, our results were less consistent than those mentioned above. However, the equation developed in our study was able to estimate the 6MWDsa without statistically significant differences for 6MWDsup. The 6MWDsa1 was only 1.68 ± 61.00 m higher than 6MWDsup, while the 6MWDsa1 was 3.64 ± 60.57 m higher. The reliability of the 6MWDsa2 was also good (ICC, 0.79: 95%CI, 0.50–0.91; CV = 6.0%). The limits of agreement were lower than 20%. The results of Brooks et al. [14] were similar to 91% of patients showing differences of less than 15%. These limits of reliability are within what is considered acceptable. Again, the use of GPS in the study by Douma et al. [15] in cancer patients showed limitations to the actual estimation of 6MWD in supervised testing. However, both in our study and Brooks et al. [14], there was a correlation between the mean difference and the mean values of the 6MWD, indicating bias in physical fitness extremes. Our results indicate that the equation developed underestimates the real 6MWD, especially in those with a higher CRF level who took more steps during the 6MWT. Similar results were described for another physical activity monitor, with overestimation at lower walking speeds and underestimation at higher speeds [26]. Our equation should thus be used with caution in fitter individuals.

Our results suggest that the 6MWDsa assessed in this study is very precise, considering its excellent reproducibility; however, its accuracy is limited, especially in individuals with more significant physical fitness. However, we can suggest the great practical applicability of our results. High CRF is a vital health index [2,3], and the VO2max measurement is the only index capable of increasing the predictive power of cardiovascular risk scores containing classic risk factors [4]. Adding CRF to traditional risk factors means reclassifying the risk of poor health outcomes. Even globally used and recognized cardiovascular risk scores such as Framingham's can be improved with CRF in the prediction model [27]. The justification for the non-inclusion of CRF in cardiovascular event prediction models lies in its need for sophisticated equipment and highly trained human resources make it challenging to use on a large scale. However, clinical field tests such as the 6MWT can make this assessment more feasible in the clinical and public health environment. The literature, although still controversial, shows that VO2max can be estimated through 6MWD, both in patients with chronic diseases and in asymptomatic individuals [5,8]. Although the accuracy of the 6MWD estimate of the present study may be questioned, we still suggest that the proposed strategy is valid. If we are unable to measure VO2max, it is recommended to use submaximal tests, field tests, and even estimates without exercise [4]. The latter presents an error in the VO2max estimate around 2.98 to 6.90 mL/min/kg, similar to the error described for submaxims [28]. Regardless of the questionable accuracy of these CRF prediction equations, two of them—by Jurca et al. [29] and Nes et al. [30]—showed a reduction in the risk of long-term mortality [31,32], as well as reduction of cardiovascular risk compatible with the reduction described for the direct CRF measurement [33]. Thus, our strategy can be useful for the periodic evaluation of CRF and places it as a vital sign in the clinical environment and public health [4].

Our results indicated the app's tendency to underestimate the actual number of steps performed (8.7%; 58.7 steps). Our results are following the previously described. Green et al. [21] compared the number of steps quantified by smartphone apps, both iOS and Android, with the direct visual measurement evaluated by video at three treadmill walking speeds (2.5, 5, and 7.7 km/h). The biases described were 9%, 5.5%, and 12.8%, respectively. There were no significant differences between the various smartphone brands. Considering that the 6MWD of asymptomatic adults varies between 450 and 790 m, which corresponds to speeds between 4.5 and 7.9 km/h, our results were very similar to those described by Green et al. [21]. The literature shows that the different apps' algorithms influence the measurements more than the smartphone brand.

Some limitations of our study must be addressed. Our cross-validation sample presented some distinct characteristics of the sample used to elaborate the 6WMD prediction equation, due to our convenience sample. Also, we used the available sample at our convenience for the cross-validation phase. Even though we did not calculate a sample size a priori, we used the MedCalc software version 14 to calculate the mean difference and its standard deviation, and the maximum allowed difference for a sample size of 25 as in the present study. Considering the best scenario of a mean difference of zero and a standard deviation of the mean difference of 53 m in our previous experience in asymptomatic subjects [12], we found the maximum allowed difference of 170 m. This distance traveled is much larger than found in our 6MWDsa2 vs. 6MWDsa1 Bland and Altman plot (61.3 m), and even more extensive than our worse result of 122.4 m. Thus, we are confident that our limits of agreement support our conclusions. Nevertheless, our results were valid, and we believe them to be helpful in both cases. Regarding measurement properties, the responsiveness of the 6MWTsa was not evaluated in this study, as well as in previous studies. Therefore, this property, both in apparently healthy people and in patients with chronic diseases, remains unknown. Nonetheless, given the excellent responsiveness of the supervised 6MWT, including the minimum clinically relevant distance available, we can expect the 6MWT to have good responsiveness. We also performed the 6MWTsup in the 25 participants in the cross-validation section. Thus, they could have learned how to do the 6MWT correctly. However, whether our results can be applied to an utterly naïve app user remains unknown. Finally, considering the increase in cardiovascular health problems in people under 40 years of age, we decided to include younger adults between 30 and 39 years of age who presented lower cardiovascular risk and higher CRF, which may have contributed to underestimating 6MWT by the equation developed.

This study presents considerable potential. To the best of our knowledge, this is the first study to evaluate the measurement properties of the self-administered 6MWT in a sample of asymptomatic adults, which allows us to suggest the use of this strategy in primary care in CRF monitoring and health promotion programs. We also developed the equation of predicting 6MWD in a sufficient sample of individuals, which increases the internal validity of our results. Additionally, our study used a free app with optimal functionality on the two most popular smartphone operating systems, unlike the unavailable app developed by Brooks et al. [14] and the free app lacking step count monitoring as investigated by Douma et al. [15].

Our results present great practical applicability. The incremental and symptom-limited CPET requires sophisticated, expensive equipment and requires highly skilled staff. Although the incremental walk test is a field test, it has the characteristic of controlled speed, which allows exercise at high and even maximum intensity in the asymptomatic population [7]. The 6MWT, in turn, presents extensive validity, reliability, reproducibility, and responsiveness determined in the literature [6,34]. The test has been widely used to monitor the progression of functional exercise capacity and the results of several interventions [4]. Thus, the self-administration of this test would allow the self-monitoring of several morbidities and chronic diseases. Because it is a submaximal test, it has already been applied to thousands of patients with severe diseases without reports of adverse effects and non-fatal or fatal events [4]. Probably because of this, the 6MWT is less intimidating in more severe health conditions [35]. Therefore, the self-administered 6MWT is promising in achieving the AHA (American Heart Association) objectives to include periodic evaluation of CRF definitively as a vital sign in the clinical environment.

## 5. Conclusions

We can conclude that the self-administration of the 6MWT in asymptomatic adults using a smartphone app is valid and presents excellent reliability and reproducibility. This strategy may be useful for the periodic evaluation of CRF in the clinical environment and in primary care. However, our results suggest that the 6MWT should be used with caution in people with higher CRF.

**Author Contributions:** Conceptualization, M.O.d.J. and V.Z.D.; methodology, M.O.d.J., T.L.V.D.P.O. and V.Z.D.; software, V.Z.D.; validation, M.O.d.J., T.L.V.D.P.O. and V.Z.D.; formal analysis, V.Z.D.; investigation, M.O.d.J., T.L.V.D.P.O., N.L.P., R.P.d.S. and V.Z.D.; resources, V.Z.D.; data curation, M.O.d.J., T.L.V.D.P.O. and V.Z.D.; writing—original draft preparation, M.O.d.J., T.L.V.D.P.O., N.L.P., R.P.d.S. and V.Z.D.; writing—review and editing, M.O.d.J., T.L.V.D.P.O., N.L.P., R.P.d.S. and V.Z.D.; visualization, M.O.d.J., T.L.V.D.P.O. and V.Z.D.; supervision, V.Z.D.; project administration, V.Z.D.; funding acquisition, V.Z.D. All authors have read and agreed to the published version of the manuscript.

**Funding:** This research was funded by São Paulo Research Foundation (FAPESP), grant number #2016/50249-3 and #2011/07282-6.

**Institutional Review Board Statement:** The study was conducted according to the guidelines of the Declaration of Helsinki and approved by the Research Ethics Committee of Federal University of São Paulo (#186.796/2013 and #1485/2017).

**Informed Consent Statement:** Informed consent was obtained from all subjects involved in the study.

**Data Availability Statement:** The datasets used and/or analyzed during the current study are available from the corresponding author on reasonable request and with permission of Victor Dourado.

**Acknowledgments:** The authors are grateful to the Lown Scholars Program for their support and the payment of the manuscript fee. We also would like to thank all the other researchers who are part of the EPIMOV Study team.

**Conflicts of Interest:** The authors declare no conflict of interest. The funders had no role in the design of the study, in the collection, analyses, or interpretation of data; in the writing of the manuscript, or in the decision to publish the results.

## References

1. Herdy, A.H.; Uhlendorf, D. Reference values for cardiopulmonary exercise testing for sedentary and active men and women. *Arq. Bras. Cardiol.* **2011**, *96*, 54–59. [CrossRef] [PubMed]
2. Hung, T.H.; Liao, P.A.; Chang, H.H.; Wang, J.H.; Wu, M.C. Examining the relationship between cardiorespiratory fitness and body weight status: Empirical evidence from a population-based survey of adults in Taiwan. *Sci. World J.* **2014**, *2014*, 463736. [CrossRef] [PubMed]
3. Myers, J.; Kaminsky, L.A.; Lima, R.; Christle, J.W.; Ashley, E.; Arena, R. A reference equation for normal standards for $VO_2$ max: Analysis from the fitness registry and the importance of exercise national database (FRIEND Registry). *Prog. Cardiovasc. Dis.* **2017**, *60*, 21–29. [CrossRef] [PubMed]
4. Ross, R.; Blair, S.N.; Arena, R.; Church, T.S.; Despres, J.P.; Franklin, B.A.; Haskell, W.L.; Kaminsky, L.A.; Levine, B.D.; Lavie, C.J.; et al. Importance of assessing cardiorespiratory fitness in clinical practice: A case for fitness as a clinical vital sign: A scientific statement from the American Heart Association. *Circulation* **2016**, *134*, e653–e699. [CrossRef]
5. Belli, K.C.; Callegaro, C.C.; Richter, C.M.; Klafke, J.Z.; Stein, R.; Viecili, P.R. Cardiorespiratory fitness of a Brazilian regional sample distributed in different tables. *Arq. Bras. Cardiol.* **2012**, *99*, 811–817. [CrossRef]
6. Holland, A.E.; Spruit, M.A.; Troosters, T.; Puhan, M.A.; Pepin, V.; Saey, D.; McCormack, M.C.; Carlin, B.W.; Sciurba, F.C.; Pitta, F.; et al. An official European Respiratory Society/American Thoracic Society technical standard: Field walking tests in chronic respiratory disease. *Eur. Respir. J.* **2014**, *44*, 1428–1446. [CrossRef]
7. Dourado, V.Z. Reference equations for the 6-minute walk test in healthy individuals. *Arq. Bras. Cardiol.* **2011**, *96*, e128–e138. [CrossRef]
8. Sperandio, E.F.; Arantes, R.L.; Matheus, A.C.; Silva, R.P.; Lauria, V.T.; Romiti, M.; Gagliardi, A.R.T.; Dourado, V.Z. Intensity and physiological responses to the 6-minute walk test in middle-aged and older adults: A comparison with cardiopulmonary exercise testing. *Braz. J. Med. Biol. Res.* **2015**, *48*, 349–353. [CrossRef]
9. Bittner, V.; Weiner, D.H.; Yusuf, S.; Rogers, W.J.; McIntyre, K.M.; Bangdiwala, S.I.; Kronenberg, M.V.; Kostis, J.B.; Kohn, R.M.; Woods, P.A.; et al. Prediction of mortality and morbidity with a 6-minute walk test in patients with left ventricular dysfunction. SOLVD Investigators. *JAMA* **1993**, *270*, 1702–1707. [CrossRef]
10. Diniz, L.S.; Neves, V.R.; Starke, A.C.; Barbosa, M.P.T.; Britto, R.R.; Ribeiro, A.L.P. Safety of early performance of the six-minute walk test following acute myocardial infarction: A cross-sectional study. *Braz. J. Phys. Ther.* **2017**, *21*, 167–174. [CrossRef]
11. Sperandio, E.F.; Arantes, R.L.; Silva, R.P.; Matheus, A.C.; Lauria, V.T.; Bianchim, M.S.; Romiti, M.; Gagliardi, A.R.T.; Dourado, V.Z. Screening for physical inactivity among adults: The value of distance walked in the six-minute walk test. A cross-sectional diagnostic study. *Sao Paulo Med. J.* **2016**, *134*, 56–62. [CrossRef]
12. Dourado, V.Z.; Kan, R.; Simões, M.S.M.P.; Lauria, V.T.; Tanni, S.E.; Godoy, I.; Gagliardi, A.R.T.; Romiti, M.; Arante, R.L. Classification of cardiorespiratory fitness using the six-minute walk test in adults: Comparison with cardiopulmonary exercise testing. *Pulmonology* **2021**, *27*, 500–508. [CrossRef]
13. Direito, A.; Dale, L.P.; Shields, E.; Dobson, R.; Whittaker, R.; Maddison, R. Do physical activity and dietary smartphone applications incorporate evidence-based behaviour change techniques? *BMC Public Health* **2014**, *14*, 3. [CrossRef]
14. Brooks, G.C.; Vittinghoff, E.; Iyer, S.; Tandon, D.; Kuhar, P.; Madsen, K.A.; Marcus, G.M.; Pletcher, M.J.; Olgin, J.E. Accuracy and usability of a self-administered 6-minute walk test smartphone application. *Circ. Heart Fail.* **2015**, *8*, 905–913. [CrossRef]
15. Douma, J.A.J.; Verheul, H.M.W.; Buffart, L.M. Feasibility, validity and reliability of objective smartphone measurements of physical activity and fitness in patients with cancer. *BMC Cancer* **2018**, *18*, 3. [CrossRef]

16. Salvi, D.; Poffley, E.; Orchard, E.; Tarassenko, L. The mobile-based 6-minute walk test: Usability study and algorithm development and validation. *JMIR mHealth uHealth* **2020**, *8*, e13756. [CrossRef]
17. World Health Organization. Guidelines on Physical Activity and Sedentary Behavior. Available online: https://www.who.int/publications/i/item/9789240015128 (accessed on 18 August 2021).
18. Poh, M.Z.; Poh, Y.C. Validation of a standalone smartphone application for measuring heart rate using imaging photoplethysmography. *Telemed. e-Health* **2017**, *23*, 678–683. [CrossRef]
19. Borg, G.A. Psychophysical bases of perceived exertion. *Med. Sci. Sports Exerc.* **1982**, *14*, 377–381. [CrossRef]
20. Koo, T.K.; Li, M.Y. A guideline of selecting and reporting intraclass correlation coefficients for reliability research. *J. Chiropr. Med.* **2016**, *15*, 155–163. [CrossRef]
21. Green, A.; Coopoo, Y.; Borman, A. Physical activity tracking using mobile devices: Can a heterogeneous sample of smart phones accurately quantify steps? *Afr. J. Phys. Act. Health Sci.* **2018**, *24*, 514–524.
22. Field, A. *Discovering Statistics Using IBM SPSS Statistics*, 4th ed.; Sage Publications: London, UK, 2013.
23. Bland, J.M.; Altman, D.G. Statistical methods for assessing agreement between two methods of clinical measurement. *Lancet* **1986**, *327*, 307–310. [CrossRef]
24. Ministério da Saúde. Secretaria de Vigilância em Saúde. Departamento de Vigilância de Doenças e Agravos não Transmissíveis e Promoção de Saúde. Vigitel Brasil 2019: Vigilância de Fatores de Risco e Proteção para Doenças crônicas por Inquérito Telefônico. Available online: https://bvsms.saude.gov.br/bvs/publicacoes/vigitel_brasil_2019_vigilancia_fatores_risco.pdf (accessed on 13 December 2021).
25. Du, H.; Newton, P.J.; Salamonson, Y.; Carrieri-Kohlman, V.L.; Davidson, P.M. A review of the six-minute walk test: Its implication as a self-administered assessment tool. *Eur. J. Cardiovasc. Nurs.* **2009**, *8*, 2–8. [CrossRef]
26. Takacs, J.; Pollock, C.L.; Guenther, J.R.; Bahar, M.; Napier, C.; Hunt, M.A. Validation of the Fitbit One activity monitor device during treadmill walking. *J. Sci. Med. Sport* **2014**, *17*, 496–500. [CrossRef]
27. Arena, R.; McNeil, A. Let's talk about moving: The impact of cardiorespiratory fitness, exercise, steps and sitting on cardiovascular risk. *Braz. J. Cardiovasc. Surg.* **2017**, *32*, 3–5. [CrossRef] [PubMed]
28. Maranhao Neto, G.A.A.; Lourenco, P.M.C.; Farinatti, P.d.T.V. Prediction of aerobic fitness without stress testing and applicability to epidemiological studies: A systematic review. *Cad. Saude Publica* **2004**, *20*, 48–56. [CrossRef]
29. Jurca, R.; Jackson, A.S.; LaMonte, M.J.; Morrow, J.R., Jr.; Blair, S.N.; Wareham, N.J.; Haskell, W.L.; Van Mechelen, W.; Churc, T.S.; Jakicic, J.M.; et al. Assessing cardiorespiratory fitness without performing exercise testing. *Am. J. Prev. Med.* **2005**, *29*, 185–193. [CrossRef] [PubMed]
30. Nes, B.M.; Janszky, I.; Wisloff, U.; Stoylen, A.; Karlsen, T. Age-predicted maximal heart rate in healthy subjects: The HUNT fitness study. *Scand. J. Med. Sci. Sports* **2013**, *23*, 697–704. [CrossRef] [PubMed]
31. Kokkinos, P.; Manolis, A.; Pittaras, A.; Doumas, M.; Giannelou, A.; Panagiotakos, D.B.; Faselis, C.; Narayan, P.; Singh, S.; Myers, J. Exercise capacity and mortality in hypertensive men with and without additional risk factors. *Hypertension* **2009**, *53*, 494–499. [CrossRef]
32. Stamatakis, E.; Hamer, M.; O'Donovan, G.; Batty, G.D.; Kivimaki, M. A non-exercise testing method for estimating cardiorespiratory fitness: Associations with all-cause and cardiovascular mortality in a pooled analysis of eight population-based cohorts. *Eur. Heart J.* **2013**, *34*, 750–758. [CrossRef]
33. Kodama, S.; Saito, K.; Tanaka, S.; Maki, M.; Yachi, Y.; Asumi, M.; Sugawara, A.; Totsuka, K.; Shimano, H.; Ohashi, Y.; et al. Cardiorespiratory fitness as a quantitative predictor of all-cause mortality and cardiovascular events in healthy men and women: A meta-analysis. *JAMA* **2009**, *301*, 2024–2035. [CrossRef]
34. Morakami, F.K.; Morita, A.A.; Bisca, G.W.; Felcar, J.M.; Ribeiro, M.; Furlanetto, K.C.; Hernandes, N.A.; Pitta, F. Can the six-minute walk distance predict the occurrence of acute exacerbations of COPD in patients in Brazil? *J. Bras. Pneumol.* **2017**, *43*, 280–284. [CrossRef]
35. Gary, R.A.; Sueta, C.A.; Rosenberg, B.; Cheek, D. Use of the 6-minute walk test for women with diastolic heart failure. *J. Cardiopulm. Rehabil.* **2004**, *24*, 264–268. [CrossRef]

MDPI
St. Alban-Anlage 66
4052 Basel
Switzerland
Tel. +41 61 683 77 34
Fax +41 61 302 89 18
www.mdpi.com

*International Journal of Environmental Research and Public Health* Editorial Office
E-mail: ijerph@mdpi.com
www.mdpi.com/journal/ijerph

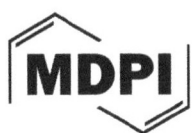

www.ingramcontent.com/pod-product-compliance
Lightning Source LLC
LaVergne TN
LVHW070358100526
838202LV00014B/1343